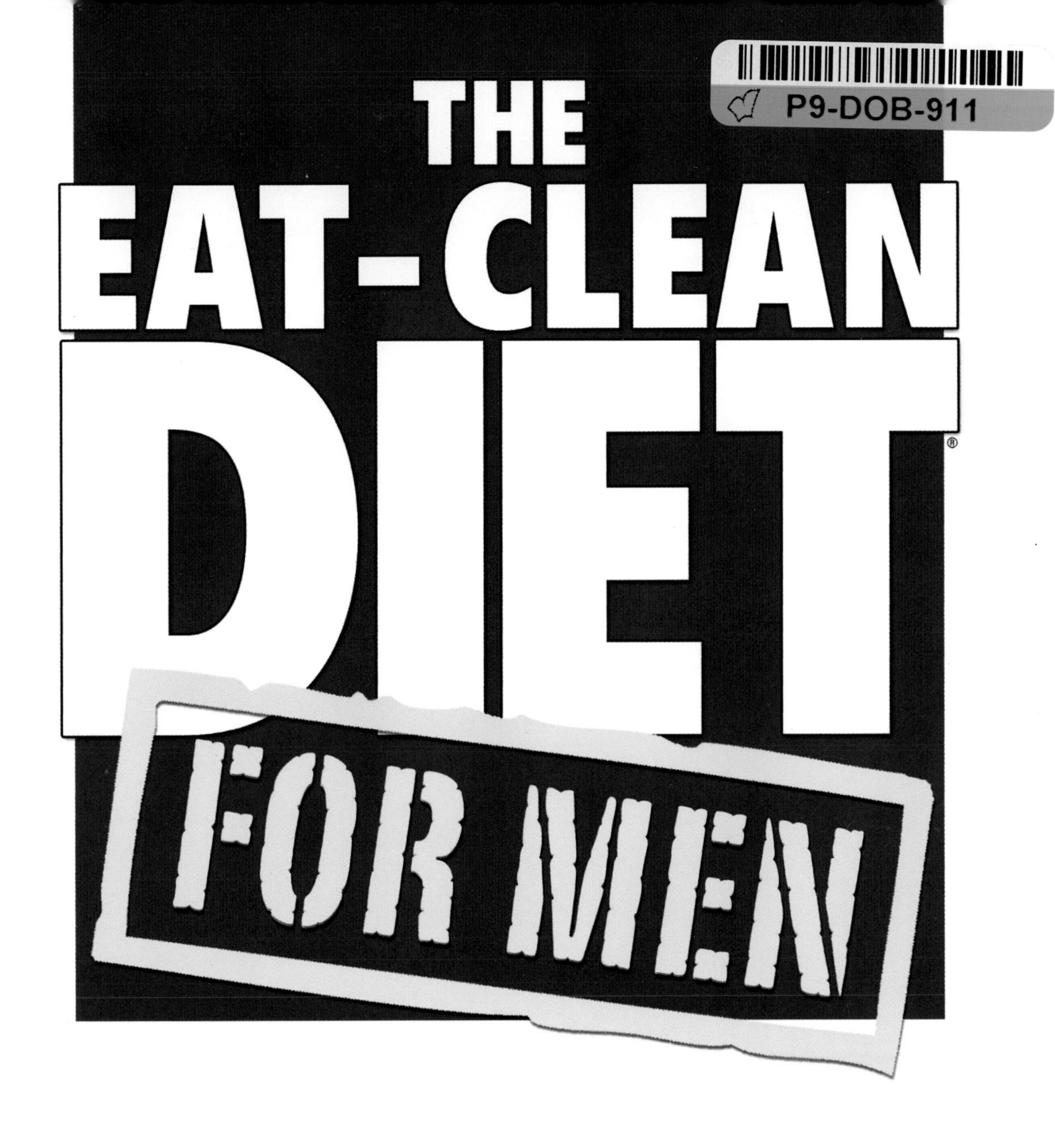
THE
EAT-CLEAN
DIET®
FOR MEN

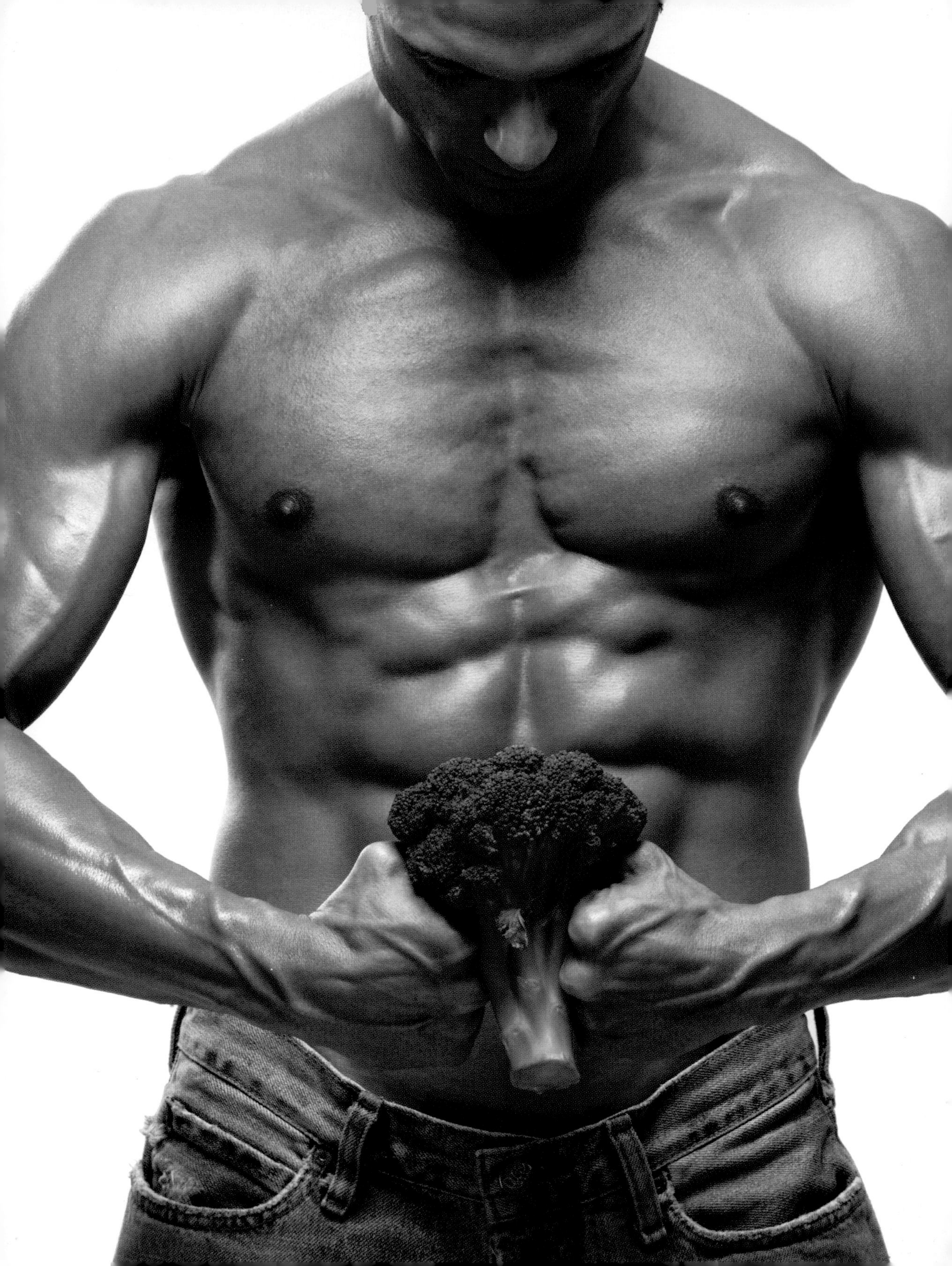

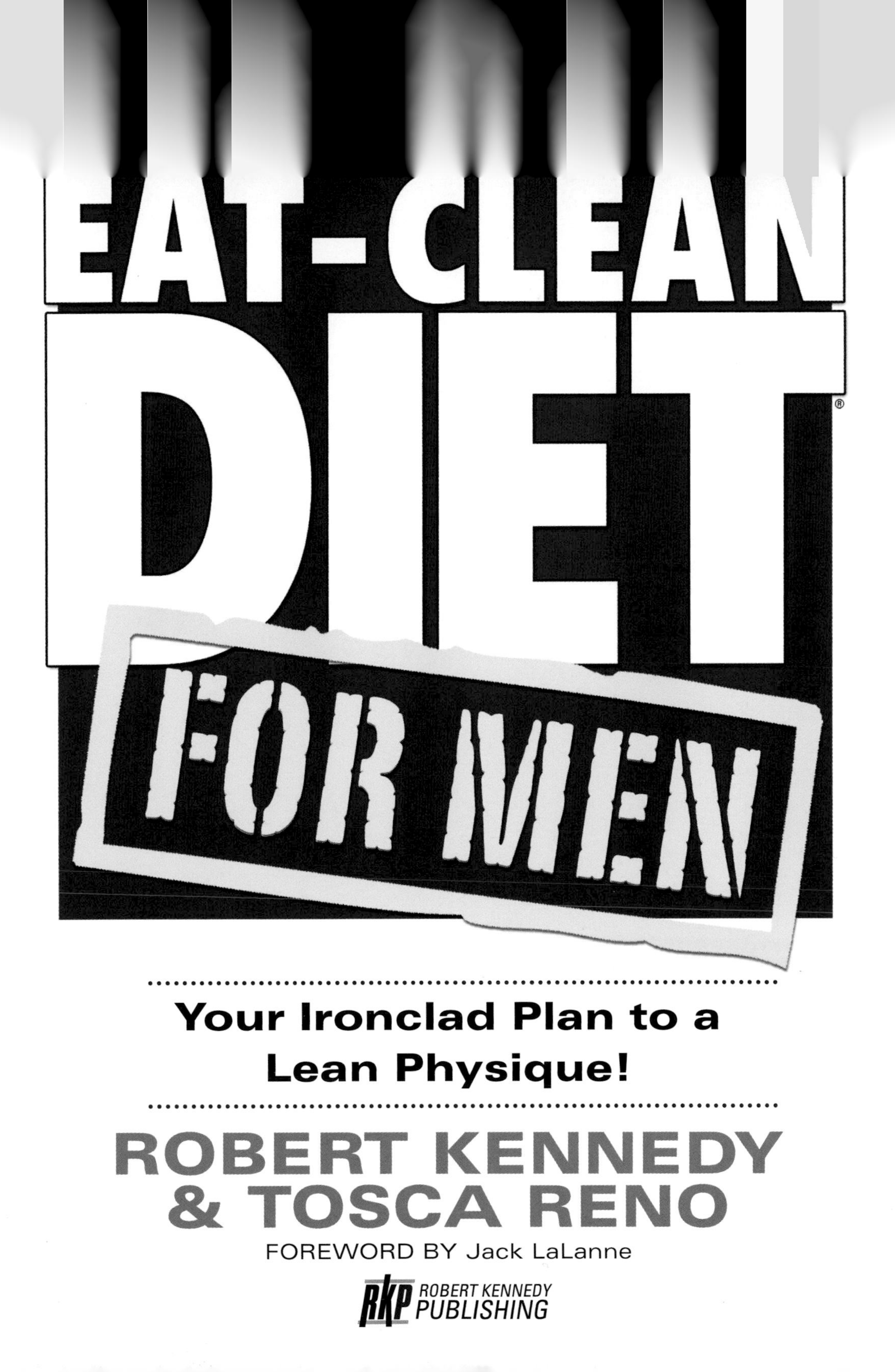
EAT-CLEAN
DIET®
FOR MEN
Your Ironclad Plan to a
Lean Physique!
ROBERT KENNEDY
& TOSCA RENO
FOREWORD BY Jack LaLanne
RKP ROBERT KENNEDY
PUBLISHING

Published by Robert Kennedy Publishing
400 Matheson Blvd. West
Mississauga, ON
L5R 3M1 Canada
Visit us at **www.eatcleandiet.com** and
**www.toscareno.com**

**Senior Production Editor:** Wendy Morley
**Online and Associate Editor:** Vinita Persaud
**Editorial Assistant:** Antonia McGuire
**Proofreader:** Kimberly Dunlop
**Art Director:** Gabriella Caruso Marques
**Editorial Designers:** Jessica Pensabene, Brian Ross

Library and Archives Canada Cataloguing in Publication

Kennedy, Robert, 1938-
The Eat-Clean Diet for Men : Your Ironclad Plan to a Lean Physique / Robert Kennedy, Tosca Reno.

Includes index.
ISBN 978-1-55210-056-1.--ISBN 1-55210-056-1

1. Men--Nutrition. 2. Men--Health and hygiene.
I. Reno, Tosca, 1959- II. Title.

RA777.8.K46 2009 613'.04234 C2008-907804-7

10 9 8 7 6 5 4 3 2 1

Distributed in Canada by
NBN (National Book Network)
67 Mowat Avenue, Suite 241
Toronto, ON
M6K 3E3

Distributed in USA by
NBN (National Book Network)
15200 NBN Way
Blue Ridge Summit, PA
17214

Printed in Canada

## IMPORTANT

The information in this book reflects the authors' experiences and opinions and is not intended to replace medical advice.

Before beginning this or any nutritional or exercise regimen, consult your physician to be sure it is appropriate for you. Ask for a physical stress test.

For all the men who thought Eating Clean was only for women. You are going to love the results!

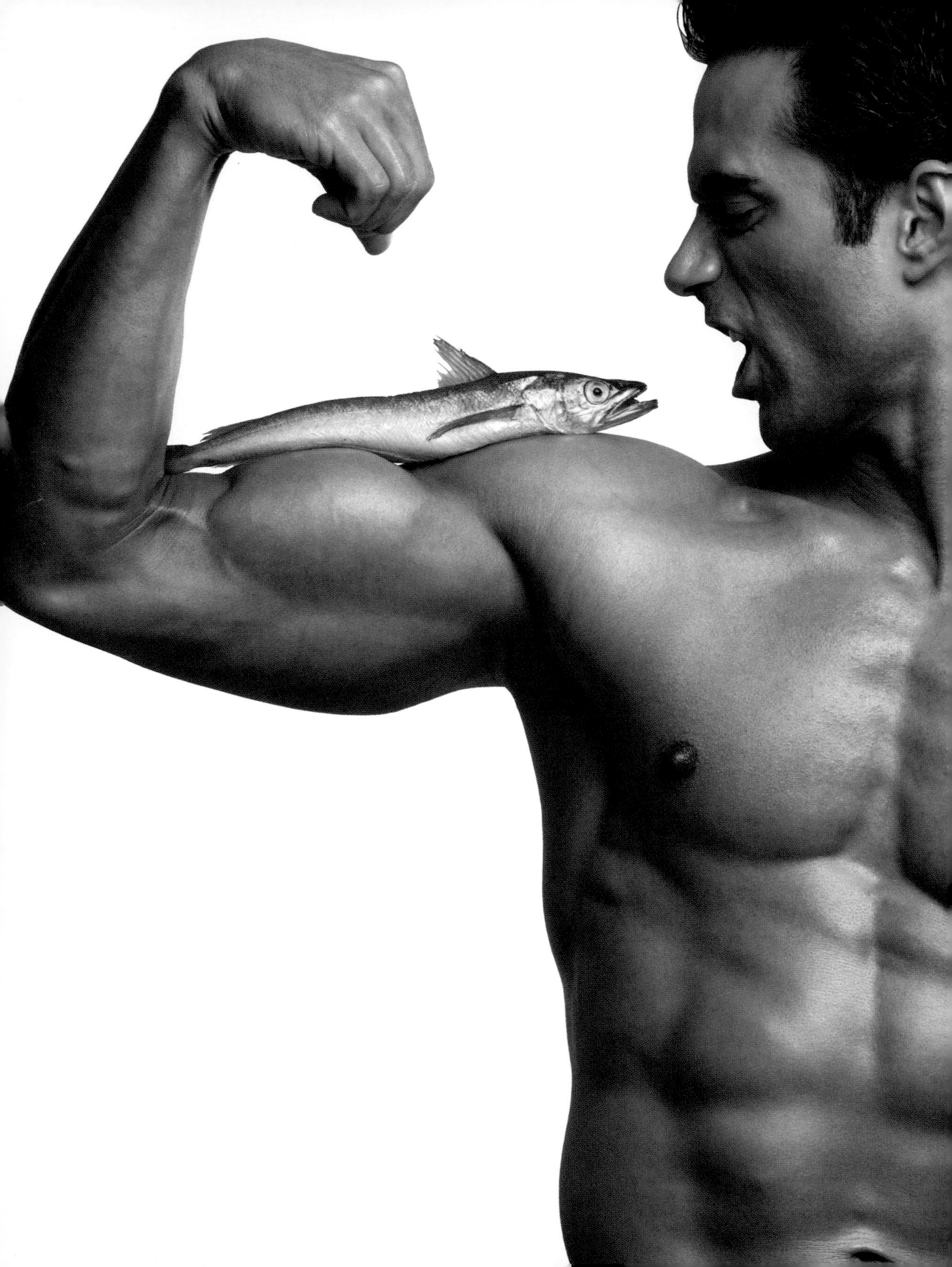

# [CONTENTS]

# [FOREWORD]

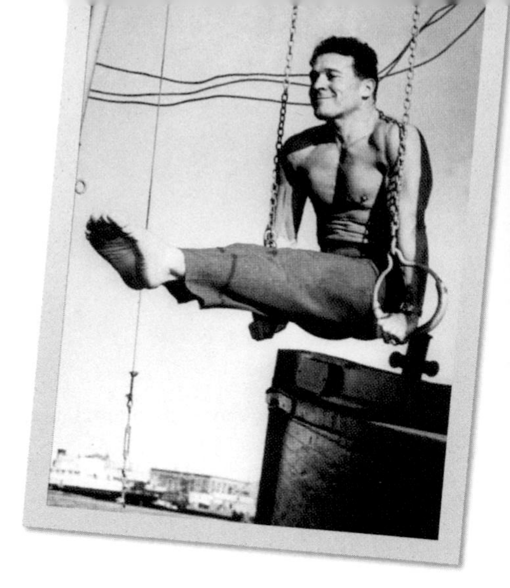

I often tell the guys and gals who attend my seminars to get out their calendars or diaries and put a circle around the date, because this is the first day of the rest of their lives. How true it is!

As I write this I am nearly 95 years young and rarin' to go. But this wasn't always the case. As a youngster brought up on a farm, I had access to an abundance of nature's healthy produce, yet I would frequently fill up on ice cream and cookies. I was a sugarholic. I wore glasses and arch supports, and my face was full of pimples, boils and acne. I constantly had headaches. Worst of all I developed a bad attitude and a nasty temper. I was weak and sick and troubled, so much so in fact that I had to drop out of school for six months.

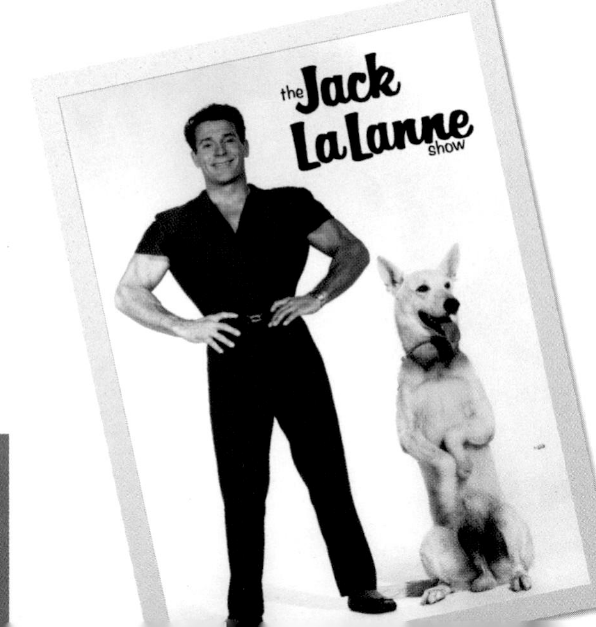


Then I attended a chance seminar with my mother and it changed my life completely. The health lecturer Paul Bragg said I could be born again. His advice went straight to my heart. I had always wanted to have a healthy body, play sports and be popular with girls. I got myself a copy of *Gray's Anatomy* and learned almost every line by heart. I wanted to be outstandingly fit and healthy. I yearned for a "Mr. America-type" body. As I exercised and improved my nutrition, I first became the captain of our high-school football team, then an AAU (Amateur Athletic Union) state wrestling champion. I never looked back. Every day of my life since Paul Bragg's message registered in my head has been a joy, my waking moments filled with strength, energy and personal fulfillment. As time went on I opened a gym, had my own TV fitness show for 34 years – the longest-running fitness show on TV – lectured to literally hundreds of thousands, and performed many feats of strength and stamina, the records of which still stand today.

In the United States almost one billion workdays a year are lost because of disability or chronic disease. The vast majority of these illnesses are the result of inactivity and poor eating choices, and can be avoided with good eating practices. Now Robert Kennedy and his wife Tosca Reno have put together *The Eat-Clean Diet for Men*, and the concept of eating clean is exactly the way I have eaten for almost 80 years, so I know it works!

Diets have long been the domain of women. Here we have a diet for men. But in truth, it is more than a diet. It is a lifestyle of eating only the most nourishing and healthy foods. You are not going to feel hungry. How could you when you eat rice, chicken, sweet potatoes, whole grains, fish, lean beef, nuts, fruits and vegetables of all kinds?

Robert Kennedy and Tosca Reno have produced a book that will not only help you feel more energetic and alive, but will in all likelihood reduce your risk of heart attack or stroke. *The Eat-Clean Diet for Men* fuels your body naturally. There is no place for skyrocketing your cholesterol level. No place to eat junk food that leads to life-shortening obesity. And no place to be anything but fit and healthy for the rest of your days. Enjoy and benefit from this book. It recommends everything I believe in and have followed over the last 80 years, and if you need an example of a vital, active, long life you need look no further than me!

I have no way of knowing how tall or short, fat or thin, young or not so young you happen to be. Maybe you've exercised and eaten well all your life. Or perhaps the opposite is true. You've let yourself go. Whatever the case, check with your healthcare provider and make sure you are suited to both exercise and changing your eating habits as described in this book. When you get the green light to go ahead you'll be energized to train regularly and eat correctly. And what a joy your life will become! Remember, when things seem difficult or even impossible, that is the time to cement your commitment. There is no substitute for perseverance. You will succeed in gaining back your health, your lean physique and your fitness level of days gone by – or maybe even achieve a level of health and fitness you've never seen before. My thoughts are with you. I envy you your chances.

Jack LaLanne

Jack LaLanne

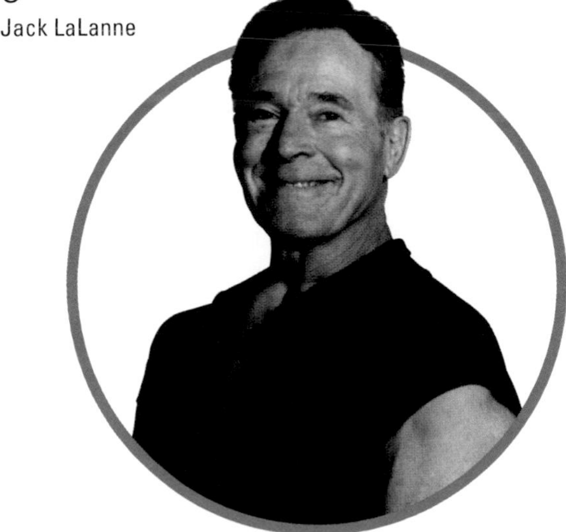

# [INTRODUCTION]

We wrote and published *The Eat-Clean Diet* to share Tosca's weight-loss success story with others, never foreseeing how incredibly well it would be received. The demand for a cookbook to follow it up necessitated spending the next summer cooking, tasting, and testing hundreds of recipes to satisfy the appetites of happy Clean Eaters. Both of these books have been on the best-seller list in their categories since they were published, a testament to their simple but powerful message – to Eat Clean is to Live Well.

Parents clamored for a Clean-Eating guidebook to use as a tool to help ward off the growing obesity and health crisis seen in our young. *The Eat-Clean Diet for Family and Kids* was the result, and it too is doing well internationally.

Now it is time for the men to be addressed. We did not want to omit an entire segment of the population, especially since some of the most powerful weight-loss and health-improvement stories we've received are from men. So men, stop worrying! This book is devoted solely to you and your attitudes to nutrition, training and

**[ So men, stop worrying! This book is devoted solely to you and your attitudes to nutrition, training and health. ]**

health. Through email after email, you men persuaded us that this book was necessary. Your words gave us our voice. Your questions are insightful and thought provoking, and they need to be answered. Basically you asked, "What about me?" We heard you and this book is our response.

Women may be the stereotype, but men love to talk too – especially about their own situations and experiences, and even more about their bodies! Who knew? There is plenty of room in the henhouse for you, Clean-Eating man. Welcome aboard.

The humor and sadness we encountered while working on this book sustained our spirit and fueled our passion to write not just a book of advice and words strung together with punctuation and chapter headings, but a story. A man we heard from named Larry put it well: "I rarely take any book to read in bed, let alone a diet book. But yours is a story. I love a story. It doesn't feel like work. It feels like you are talking to me."

This is our story for you.
Remember, we are always listening.

Robert Kennedy
Tosca Reno

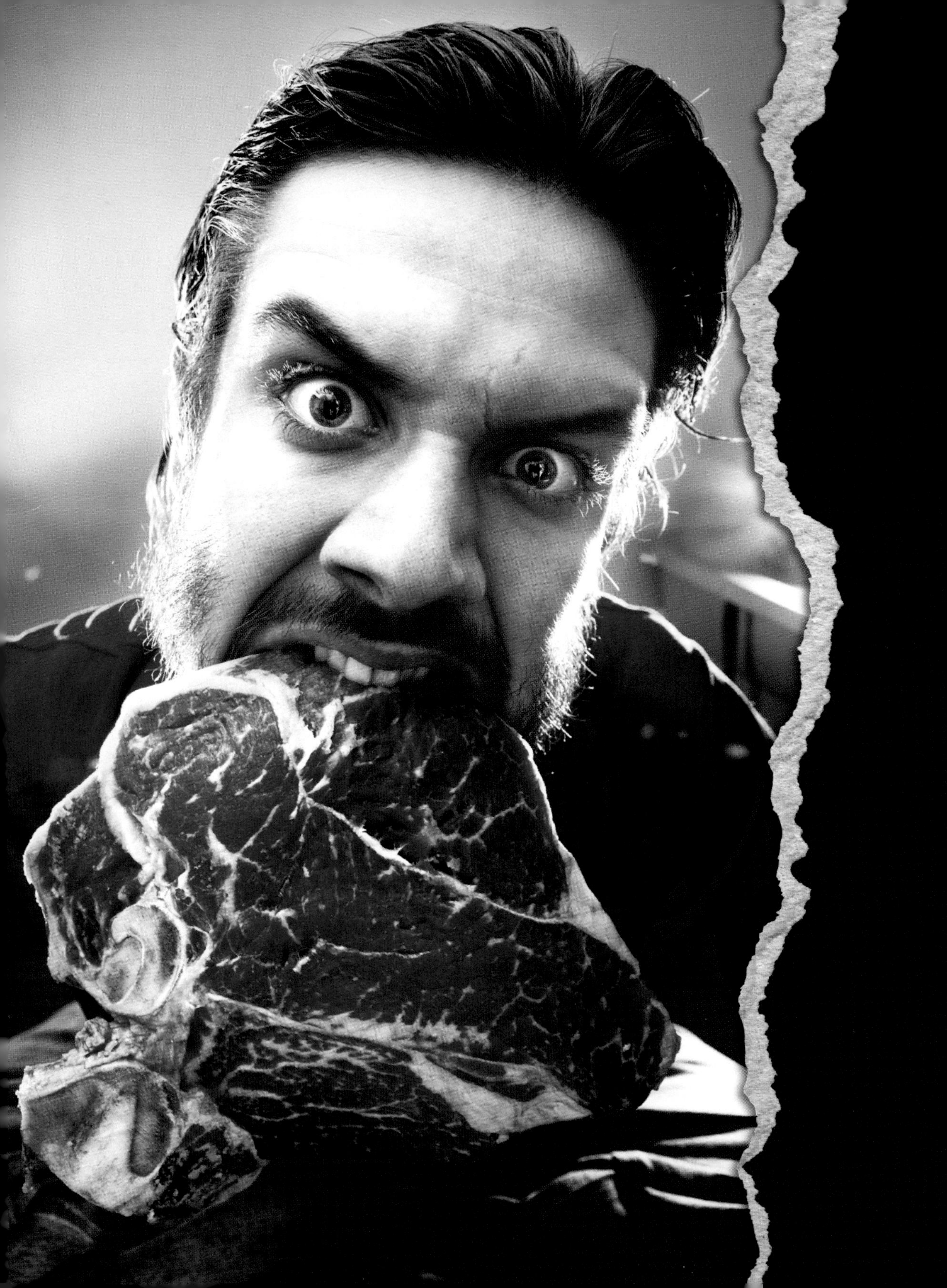

# [CHAPTER ONE]

# TODAY'S ANSWER TO "WHAT CAN I EAT?"

## WHY SHOULD MEN EAT CLEAN?

All around are men who charge through their day full steam ahead, rarely taking the time to look in the rearview mirror to see what's behind them. Careers, mortgages, wives, families, passions and more distractions make good health disappear in a blur miles behind them as they speed forward. This is concerning. So many men have health problems that seriously impact on their lives and the lives of their loved ones. This health problem might be diabetes, for which blood sugar must constantly be measured and insulin injected, or it might be a heart attack. Sooner or later this health problem will likely result in death.

Earlier today we were sitting in an airport lounge surrounded by men pushing tiny BlackBerry buttons, pounding out messages on computer keyboards, talking about IT concepts, programs and deals that must be made. Every single one of these men happened to be overweight in varying degrees. They were tired and grumpy looking. Airports can do that to you, but so can carrying too much weight. The average man will gain half a pound each year in his adult life – more if eating is unchecked. This is worrisome. As has been predicted by many in the health industry, including James Hill, dean of American obesity studies at the University of Colorado: "If the fat epidemic goes unchecked, most Americans will be overweight within a few generations."[1]

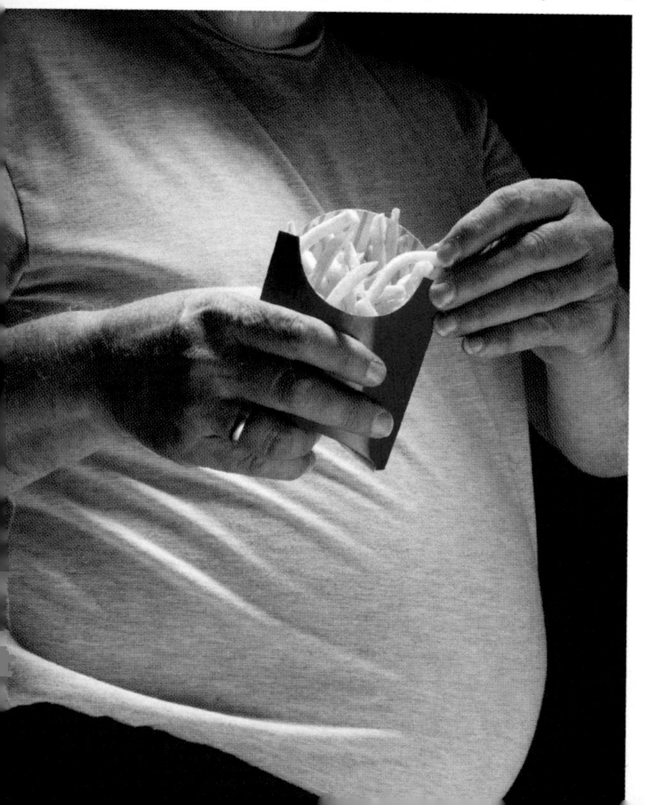

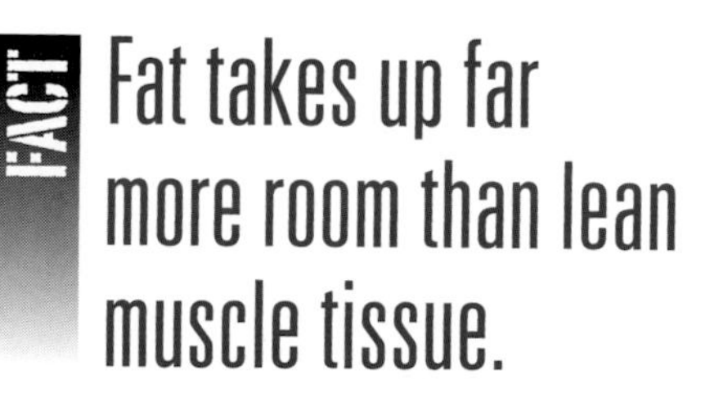
FACT
Fat takes up far more room than lean muscle tissue.

The reasons for considering a new way of eating, that is Eating Clean, are many. If you need an obvious one, then being overweight is it. Since there are currently millions of North American men and women who are either overweight or obese – as much as 67 percent of the population earns this dubious distinction – it is all too likely you may fall into this category. However, being overweight is not the only reason to consider a new way of eating. Perhaps the most significant reason is that the current way is not working. It is easy to grow complacent with good health when you have it. When you are young and all systems appear to be running in good order, you don't even think about health much – good, bad or otherwise. You feel invincible, vibrant and infallible. What could possibly go amiss?

The trouble sets in when the pounds accumulate. With as little as five pounds of weight gain, the body must begin to make changes to accommodate the load. Five pounds isn't much, but have you ever looked at five pounds of fat? It's heavy, revolting and takes up a lot of space. Fat takes up far more room than lean muscle tissue does. Granted we do need some fat, especially deep brown fat for fuel and warmth, but yellow, subcutaneous fat is not ideal. With weight gain the body rearranges itself physically and chemically to support the excess – joints, muscles, organs, blood vessels, sweat glands – every tiny detail inside you is affected by weight gain. Try walking around with a 15-pound weight belt strapped to your waist. It hurts your hips and knees, challenges your lungs and heart and makes you tired.

## IS IT TRUE? I CAN EAT MORE BUT WEIGH LESS?

Eating Clean is a way to eat that supports a healthier lifestyle. Through it you will eat more, but make improved food choices, eat more regularly and exchange a sluggish, sloppy body for a tight, lean,

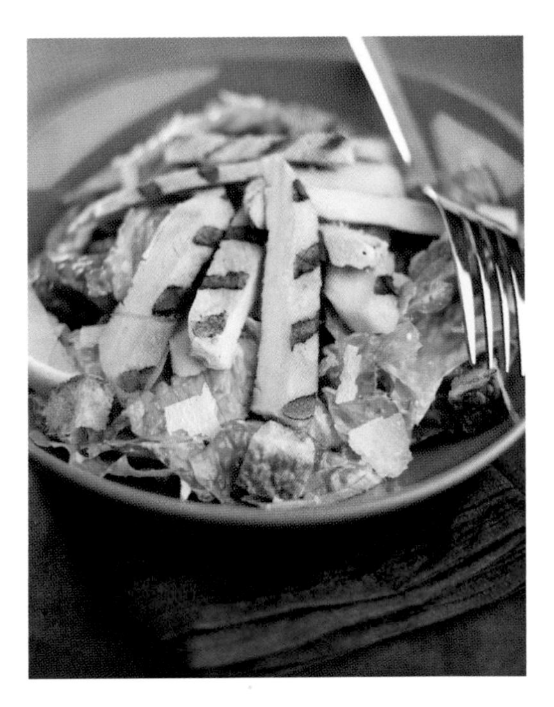

energy-filled physique – all through excellent nutrition with Clean food. Fueling up on superior foods does not just mean you are just chasing fat from your body to achieve a leaner, tighter physique. It means you are also voting with your hard-earned dollars to choose Clean, nutritious fuel to charge your engine, whether that engine is a Mercedes, a yacht, a Hummer, a bicycle, a Russian MIG or your very own body.

With an appropriately fueled engine, you will undoubtedly be amazed at how much better you will look and feel. Think of your own vehicle. No matter how old a car is or what make it may be, the better the fuel you pump into it and the more

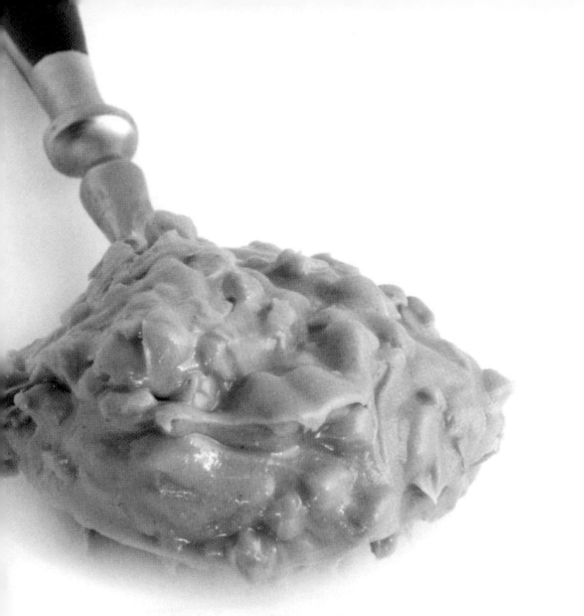

**Nut butter is an excellent Clean-Eating choice.**

conscientiously you maintain it, the better it looks and performs. Do you notice how much better your car drives after a tune-up and oil change? Your body is just like that. Conversely, if you pump your body (or car) full of energy-poor fuel it will begin to show signs of wear and tear. Imagine using saturated kitchen grease in your car. Your Jaguar would become a jalopy. No one wants to live in a body that shows signs of disrepair. The fun of eating junk food wanes quickly with repeated trips to doctors, hospitals and clinics.

Eating Clean is a simple, easily learned way of nourishing the body for optimum health and performance. It will keep you full, lean, active and living the best life ever. It's the answer for this nation of folks who are searching for the magic fat-burning pill that is nowhere to be found but inside you! The best part about Eating Clean is that you are able to eat more, not less. We are not suggesting that you eat more Dirty foods – chips, pizzas, greasy burgers and fries – no, not those! The idea is to eat more of the good foods that will fuel you properly.

## WHAT ARE THE CLEANEST FOODS?

Reaching for nutritious, Clean foods is going to build you the best physique ever. What will you be eating? That is an excellent question. These foods will be the most natural, wholesome and nutrient-packed foods available. Coincidentally, Clean foods do not require environmentally unfriendly packaging! These foods are readily available if you know what to look for. We encourage you to think of food differently when you next step into the supermarket. Not all food is good food. Not all food is Clean-Eating food.

Ideal Clean foods include lean protein, complex carbohydrates and healthy fats. If you are a vegetarian don't worry, Clean Eating is still for you since lean protein comes in the form of excellent vegan sources such as tofu and other soy products, hemp, whole grains such as quinoa, nuts and nut butters, and dairy if you allow it. More on the subject of protein in Chapter 4.

Dietary protein kick-starts your metabolism because it has a direct stimulating effect on the fat-busting hormone glucagon, and on metabolically

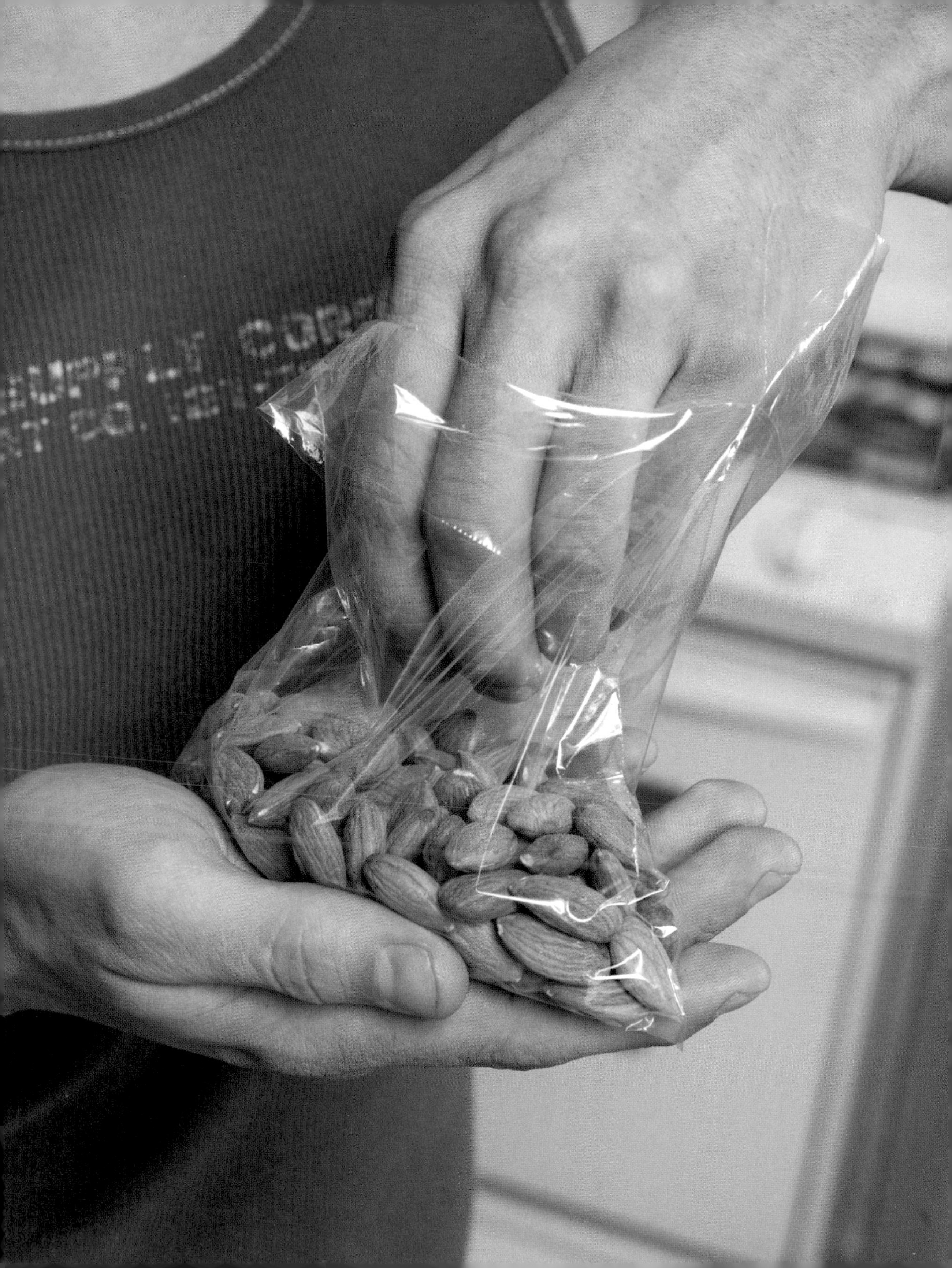

active muscle. When the body processes protein, it initiates a response called thermogenesis – which means the production of heat. When your body is packed with lean muscle tissue, extra heat is created through thermogenesis and this causes body fat to be burned away.

The best sources of lean protein include not only the vegetarian options suggested above, but also game meats such as bison, venison, elk and grass-fed beef as well as free-range poultry, game birds, wild fish, egg whites, pork tenderloin, cottage cheese, plain yogurt and some seafood. The list is long and specific. From here on in, no more fatty cuts of meat!

It is not enough to consume just lean protein. This muscle-building nutrient is best absorbed by the body when consumed with complex carbohydrates. Every meal should include complex carbohydrates from either fresh fruit or vegetables, and sometimes from whole grains. The more processed the carbohydrate the more detrimental to health. Refined carbohydrates flood the body with a flash of instant energy in the form of sugar. Too much of it shoots blood-sugar levels through the roof, a decidedly unhealthy side effect. By consuming unrefined carbs, you will avoid these erratic highs and lows in blood-sugar levels. A slow-burning carb lengthens the digestion and absorption processes, helping to keep your blood sugar on an even keel.

## FATS – THE FOUR-LETTER WORD YOU NEED TO KNOW

Most of us are freaked out about fats. The word conjures up images of jiggly thighs, a beer belly hanging over pants and globs of grease clogging up

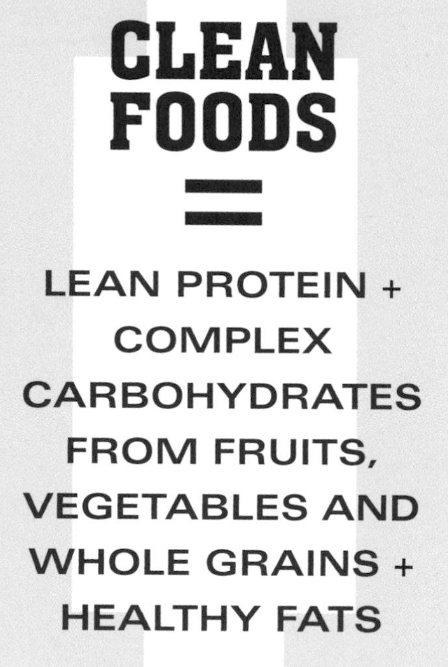

CLEAN
FOODS
=
LEAN PROTEIN +
COMPLEX
CARBOHYDRATES
FROM FRUITS,
VEGETABLES AND
WHOLE GRAINS +
HEALTHY FATS

the drain. But fats have a Jekyll-and-Hyde nature. Unhealthy fats, including saturated and trans fats, have no place in a Clean diet. You will find these in processed, factory-made foods. However, healthy fats are necessary for good health and, ironically, for successful weight loss. Include enough nuts, nut butter, seeds, unsaturated oils and deep-sea fish so about 15 percent of your diet comes from EFAs, or essential fatty acids.

## WHAT ARE THE DIRTIEST FOODS?

If lean protein, complex carbohydrates and healthy fats are the good guys then who are the villains? If you consider the Standard North American Diet for a moment it won't take long to figure out who they are. The Standard North American Diet includes predominantly these ingredients: toxins, chemicals, preservatives, food coloring, saturated and trans fats, empty calories, insufficient fiber, too many refined simple carbohydrates including sugar, and a host of unknowns that have been embedded into each and every cell in our body since birth. It might be safe to say much of what we eat is manufactured food that has little to do with the original source of whatever that food might be. Think about it! What exactly is a Twinkie? Or a Cheezie?

## TOSCA'S LIST –

# TEN OF THE UGLIEST FOODS YOU NEVER WANT TO EAT!

### DONUTS

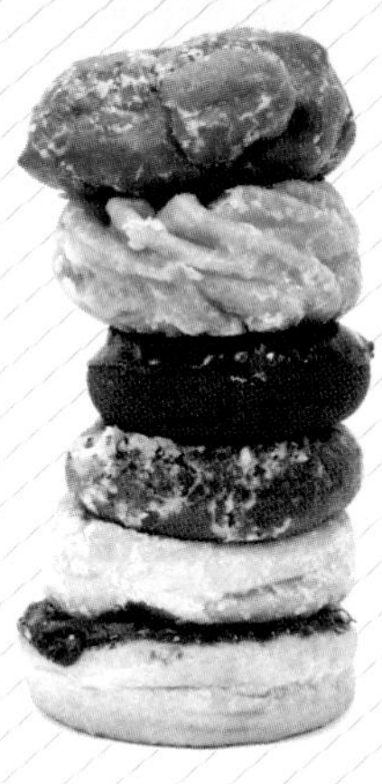

There are many ways to start your day but a donut should not be one of them. An ordinary donut can contain as many as 490 calories, most of them empty, and at least 30 grams of fat. If your donut is dressed with jelly, sugar, whipped cream or other such notions, you can count on much bigger, uglier numbers, none of them good for your waistline. The refined flours and sugars in the donut will send your blood-glucose levels through the roof and put the brakes on your metabolism.

### MARSHMALLOW FLUFF

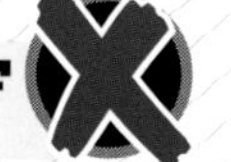

Here is some stuff that is all fluff. In my books Marshmallow Fluff and marshmallows are equally ridiculous foods, neither of which contributes to good health. One teaspoon of Fluff contains 60 calories but again it is the sugar that is most detrimental to you, making blood-sugar levels skyrocket. The other ingredients include gelatin and corn syrup – the latter is just another word for more sugar. We've nicknamed this stuff chemical puff!

### COLAS, SODAS AND CARBONATED BEVERAGES

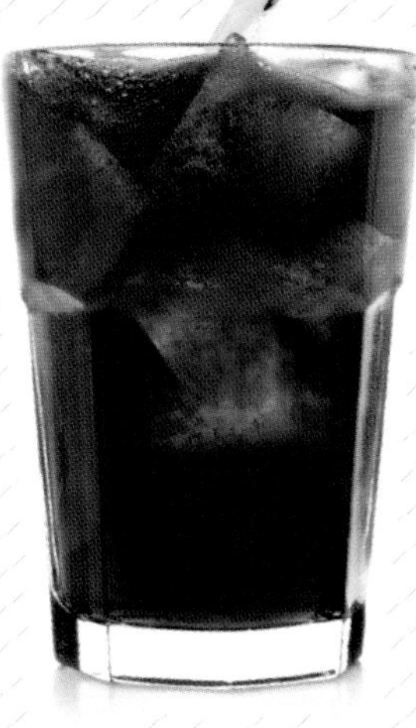

I have witnessed a disturbing sight – that of a father pouring Coca-Cola into an infant baby bottle and feeding it to the child! I am still shocked years later, but such is the addiction to these bubbly beverages. The average can of carbonated beverage contains nine teaspoons of sugar. Nine! That is about the same amount consumed in a Thanksgiving meal. Who could possibly process that much sugar in one go and still be healthy? Imagine the effect on a baby! Even those beverages claiming to be sugar free are dangerous, because fake sugars are equally unhealthy. Gentlemen, try to curb your consumption of such drinks as much as possible, and entirely for your best health.

### BACON, DELI MEATS & PROCESSED MEATS

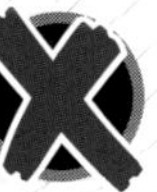

These items are hotbeds of preservatives and chemicals. They say there are two things you never want to see being made, and one of them is a hot dog. A hot dog is nothing more than a receptacle for the unwanted bits and pieces from slaughtered animals. Hot dogs, breakfast sausages and bologna contain high amounts of unhealthy fats. They also contain sugar and preservative chemicals including nitrates, sodium and nitrites. Many of these are implicated in such diseases as cancer.

## SUGARY BREAKFAST CEREALS

If ever an aisle at the supermarket were booby-trapped, the cereal aisle would be it. There is so much trickery going on here that you, the customer, must be ever on the alert for hidden empty calories. Many cereals boast high nutrition to convince you to pull your money out of your pocket to buy the stuff, but in reality they offer high quantities of nothing but added sugar. The obviously unhealthy Froot Loops contains 15 grams of sugar in a suggested serving of one cup of cereal. Fifteen grams! That is a huge dose of sugar, as much, in fact, as a Kit Kat bar. But the healthy-sounding Crunchy Almond Oatmeal Crisp has *16 grams* of sugar per one-cup serving! Better think again when standing in front of the cereal boxes! Rolled oats made into a bowl of steaming oatmeal is an excellent alternative.

## FRUIT JUICES AND FAKES

Fake fruit drinks do not generally brag about how healthy they are for you; they tell you instead about how much energy they will give you – that is called a sugar rush – and how good they taste – thanks to sugar. All that added sugar adds up to a big problem when your body starts metabolizing the stuff. Your poor body gets tired of producing insulin and sometimes wears out, causing a diabetic situation. Fruit juices can be equally deceptive. They are made from fruit, it is true, but not always pure fruit juice. When they *are* made with 100% fruit juice we think we can drink a huge glass and that it's good for us. But it's not. A 12-ounce glass of fresh-squeezed orange juice contains 36 grams of sugar. Yes it is natural sugar, but the body still has to mop up 36 grams of the stuff. This is far too much. Like most fruits, the orange was packaged perfectly for one serving and that is what the body can handle, about 9 grams of natural sugar, with fiber. If you really must drink juice, then either drink an actual serving of four ounces along with some protein, or dilute the juice one part juice to two parts water.

## JUNK FOOD

It hardly needs to be said that junk food is not good for you. I know plenty of men who can lie down on the couch and munch down an entire family-sized bag of chips. Then they wonder why they have a gut. Okay, junk food is crunchy, salty and sometimes just plain fun to eat, but it should be done in moderation on occasion, not as a regular part of your life. Most junk food contains an unwelcome mix of empty calories, trans and saturated fats and sodium. They definitely contribute to an expanding waistline and progressively poor health. Stay away from these or measure a small amount of an unoffending snack like unsalted nuts into a bowl.

## CANDY

Candy is not exactly a food group but boy does it have universal appeal! Candy should be considered an occasional treat, not a full-time job. This much-consumed item is always calorie dense and loaded with sugar, artificial food colorings, and often a lot of other ingredients that help push out your waistline. Candy overconsumption has been implicated in many health disorders, from ADD to autism. Cotton candy is lumped into the candy group too – it is made from spun sugar and food coloring.

## FRENCH FRIES

The traditional French fry has become North America's most consumed "vegetable." This is a dubious honor, since fries are far from being healthy fare. They are normally cooked in enormous vats of hydrogenated oil that has been heated and reheated many times over. As if the trans fat weren't bad enough already, this reheating of oil causes free radicals to form in the oil, and these free radicals transfer into the fries, which are then consumed by you. Free radicals are often the precursors to disease, especially cancer. The oil also contributes a significant unhealthy element since it is a kind of fat that causes an increase in LDL, or "bad" cholesterol, and a decrease in HDL, or "good" cholesterol. This leads to atherosclerosis, or hardening of the arteries, among other health concerns. Fries should be eaten in moderation if at all. Have some healthy oven fries made with olive oil instead of these killers.

## TWINKLE, TWINKIE!

You and yours have probably eaten many a Twinkie. The book *Deconstructing a Twinkie* sheds light on the numerous ingredients that go into the making of this little pastry. As benign as it looks, beware! Twinkies have been engineered to last. During the 1960s when the fear of being bombed was prevalent, Twinkies were stockpiled more than any other food in bomb shelters. They do not decay for an unreasonably long time. They are full of sugars, refined flours, trans fats, preservatives and other manufactured ingredients that have no business going into your body!

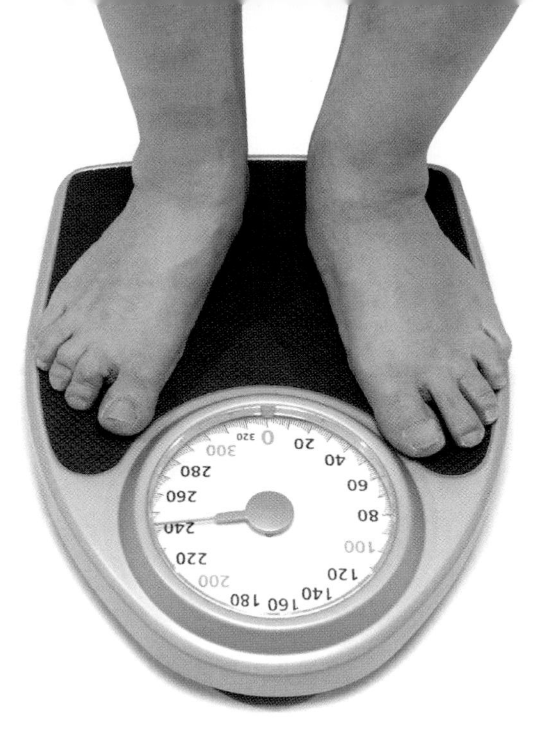

# WHAT CAN CLEAN EATING DO FOR YOU?

Food is the life force that sustains us. The quality of that food matters more than you may previously have realized. So much does it factor into health and fitness that it's worth the effort to procure the highest-quality food you can. Food helps to minimize the negative effects of life – the very life you are living right now.

Our planet does not score as well as it used to on its own health report card. The haze clinging to the city skyline in many parts of the country is a certain indication of that. Waters blanketing the earth have become cesspools in many areas. This less-than-pure environment is where our food is grown and manufactured. Whatever has found its way into our soil, air and water, good or bad, will also find its way into our food, and thus our bodies.

Eating Clean is a way to simplify eating. It is a way to overhaul your current eating habits and embrace whole, natural foods – particularly those that have not been refined. The refining process generally means most of the goodness has been stripped away. Foods containing healthful nutrients including vitamins, minerals, fats, protein, enzymes and phytochemicals factor heavily in a Clean-Eating diet. When you begin to consume Clean foods the body responds in often astounding ways because it is finally receiving the most essential and valuable ingredients with which to repair and rebuild itself in an efficient manner.

Where once you may have felt sluggish and fatigued during the day, you will be able to fly through the hours with abundant energy. If you carry those few extra pounds, through Eating Clean you will be able to shed them at an average rate of three pounds per week. If you carry even more excess weight, then your rate of weight loss could be greater. But weight loss will happen safely, because you are not depriving your body of essential nutrients. Once you have reached your ideal weight, maintenance becomes simple because you will rely on the same healthy foods to keep you at your goal weight as you depended on to lose weight. A fad diet can never promise long-term results, because the measures you take to lose weight are often drastic and unsustainable in the long run. If you replace empty foods with hard-working protein and complex carbohydrates, these will become the backbone of your diet in the truest sense of the word. The word "diet" describes the food you eat every day over long periods of time. Eating Clean is not so much a die-t as a live-it!

Once you discover what nutritious foods can do, you will experience a sense of liberation. Finally you will be free from the grip of food and the often-negative power it has on you. Knowing what to eat, how often to eat and how much to eat gives you a wonderful feeling of being able to navigate the world of food in a positive way. Consuming lean proteins such as chicken, turkey, fish, beef, bison, egg whites and so on will reward you by building lean muscle tissue. Complex carbohydrates from whole grains and fresh fruit and vegetables fortify the body when partnered with lean protein, and provide you with abundant energy as well as a host of other healthful qualities. Once you learn how Clean foods can transform your body you will rarely debate whether or not to eat that gigantic greasy burger and plate of fries.

Eating Clean will help you create a strong and healthy immune system as well as a muscled, powerful body. Simply exchanging fatty tissue for muscle tissue positively alters the blood and body chemistry. Many people find they are rarely ill once they embark on Eating Clean. They notice improved energy, heightened mental clarity, renewed libido, brighter skin, lustrous hair, fewer cravings, reduced headaches and much more. Some of the most exciting letters we receive from readers are those that say a loved one was able to reduce or go off insulin, blood-pressure or heart medications altogether thanks to Eating Clean. Neither of us are doctors so we will never tell you that Clean Eating is the answer to all your medical problems, but it is a fact that higher-quality nutrition will deliver improved health.

## SIGNS OF TOXICITY

You may be wondering if your current grade of fuel/food is making you toxic. Your body is always talking to you, so chances are you probably already know whether you are toxic. Toxicity in the body is an accumulation of unwanted, unhealthy chemicals that pile up inside us, thanks to the consumption of low-grade foods and thanks to living on this polluted planet. Hundreds of billions of pounds of chemicals are manufactured every year and they end up in what we eat and in us. Many chemicals seep inside through the skin and via our lungs. It is virtually impossible to escape from the toxic environment we have created, but we can certainly improve our toxicity. There are many signs by which you can identify if you are in a **state of toxicity:**

**[1] You experience sluggish mental function, especially in the late afternoon.**

**[2] You are in a state of constant stress.**

**[3] Your skin is dull and damaged. You suffer from**

rashes, eczema or breakouts.

[4] There are deposits of cellulite on your body.

[5] You have bouts of constipation, loose bowels or both.

[6] You feel bloated and gassy.

[7] You are prone to depression.

[8] You have numerous food allergies.

[9] You have trouble sleeping – in severe cases you have sleep apnea and must wear an oxygen mask.

[10] You are cranky and irritable.

[11] You have a flaky scalp.

[12] You have abnormal body odor.

[13] You experience frequent headaches.

[14] Your skin and hair are flaky.

[15] You are always tired.

[16] You have terrible cravings.

[17] You sweat profusely.

If you experience any of these symptoms, then you should Eat Clean to help detoxify.

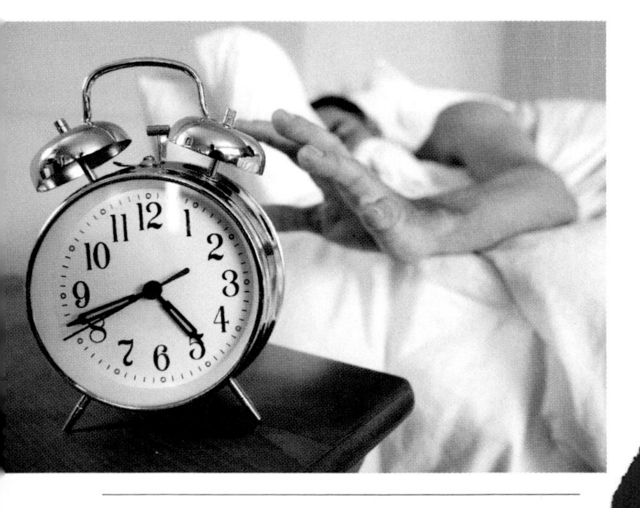

[1] Ref: *The Body Restoration Plan*, Dr. Paula Baillie-Hamilton, 2002

## EAT-CLEAN PRINCIPLES

- Eat 5 or 6 small meals a day.
- Eat every 2 to 3 hours.
- Combine lean protein and complex carbohydrates at every meal.
- Drink at least 2 liters, or 8 cups, of water per day, more if you are active.
- Never miss a meal, especially breakfast.
- Carry a cooler loaded with Clean-Eating foods to get through the day.
- Avoid all over-processed, refined foods, especially flour and sugar.
- Avoid artificial sugars.
- Avoid all preservatives, colors and other chemicals.
- Avoid all saturated and trans fats.
- Avoid sugar-loaded colas and juices.
- Consume adequate good fats (EFAs) each day.
- Avoid alcohol – another form of sugar.
- Avoid all calorie-dense foods containing no nutritional value.
- Depend on fresh fruits and vegetables for fiber, vitamins and enzymes.
- Stick to proper portion sizes – give up the super sizing!

# EATING HABITS OF MODERN MAN VERSUS PRIMITIVE OR INDIGENOUS MAN

## THE DIET OF MODERN MAN

- Concentrated feed-lot meats
- Nitrates
- Preservatives
- Artificial colors
- Farmed fish
- Plant by-products
- Soy additives
- Trans and modified fats
- Decreased fiber and healthy fats
- Refined sugars
- Refined carbohydrates
- Antibiotics

## WHAT THE CAVEMAN ATE

- Wild meats
- Wild fish
- Plants
- Nuts
- Seeds
- Lichens
- Fruit
- Berries
- Sea vegetables

# TYPICAL DIETS OF VARIOUS INDIGENOUS PEOPLES

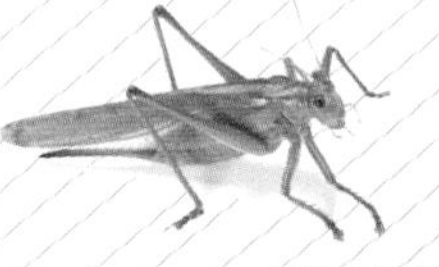

## ABORIGINES

**HUNTER-GATHERERS OF AUSTRALIA**

Kangaroo | Freshwater fish
Turtle | Crocodile | Birds | Insects
Yams | Figs | Bush honey

## THE INUIT

**HUNTER-GATHERERS OF THE ARCTIC**

Seal | Caribou | Whale | Goose
Polar bear | Walrus | Artic hare
Ptarmigan | Berries

## THE MAKU

**RURAL AGRICULTURISTS AND HUNTER-GATHERERS OF SOUTH AMERICA**

Manioc | Wild pigs | Insects
and their larvae | Rodents
Woolly monkeys | Figs
Freshwater fish | Nuts

## THE SAN

**HUNTER-GATHERERS OF SOUTHERN AFRICA**

Mongongo nuts | Tsi beans
Tsa melon | Leaves | Bulbs
Rodents | Snakes | Tortoises
Grubs | Wild game

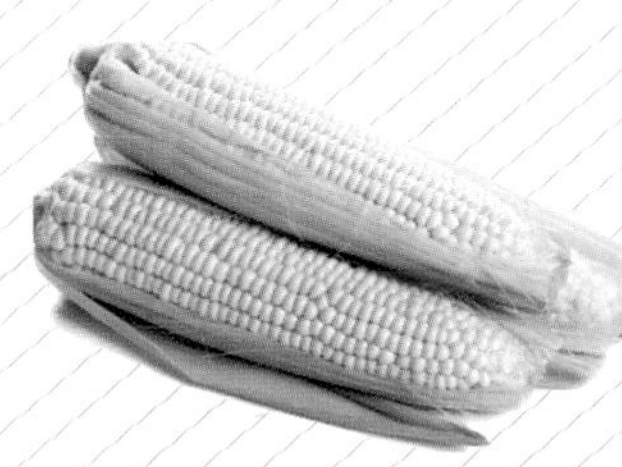

## THE SAMBURU

**RURAL NOMADS OF EAST AFRICA**

Milk | Blood | Corn
Grass-fed cattle, goats and
camels

**Note the prevalence of protein-rich foods in these diets.*

Man has learned to eat what is available to him. For indigenous peoples who knew nothing of sugary simple carbohydrates, carbonated beverages and Twinkies, larvae probably seemed the obvious choice. We don't have to go to those extremes, but it's beneficial to keep in mind the types of foods our bodies adapted to eating, especially in light of the serious health issues facing us today. Eating grass-fed meats, free-range eggs, and natural and wholesome foods in general could certainly assist in correcting some of these problems.

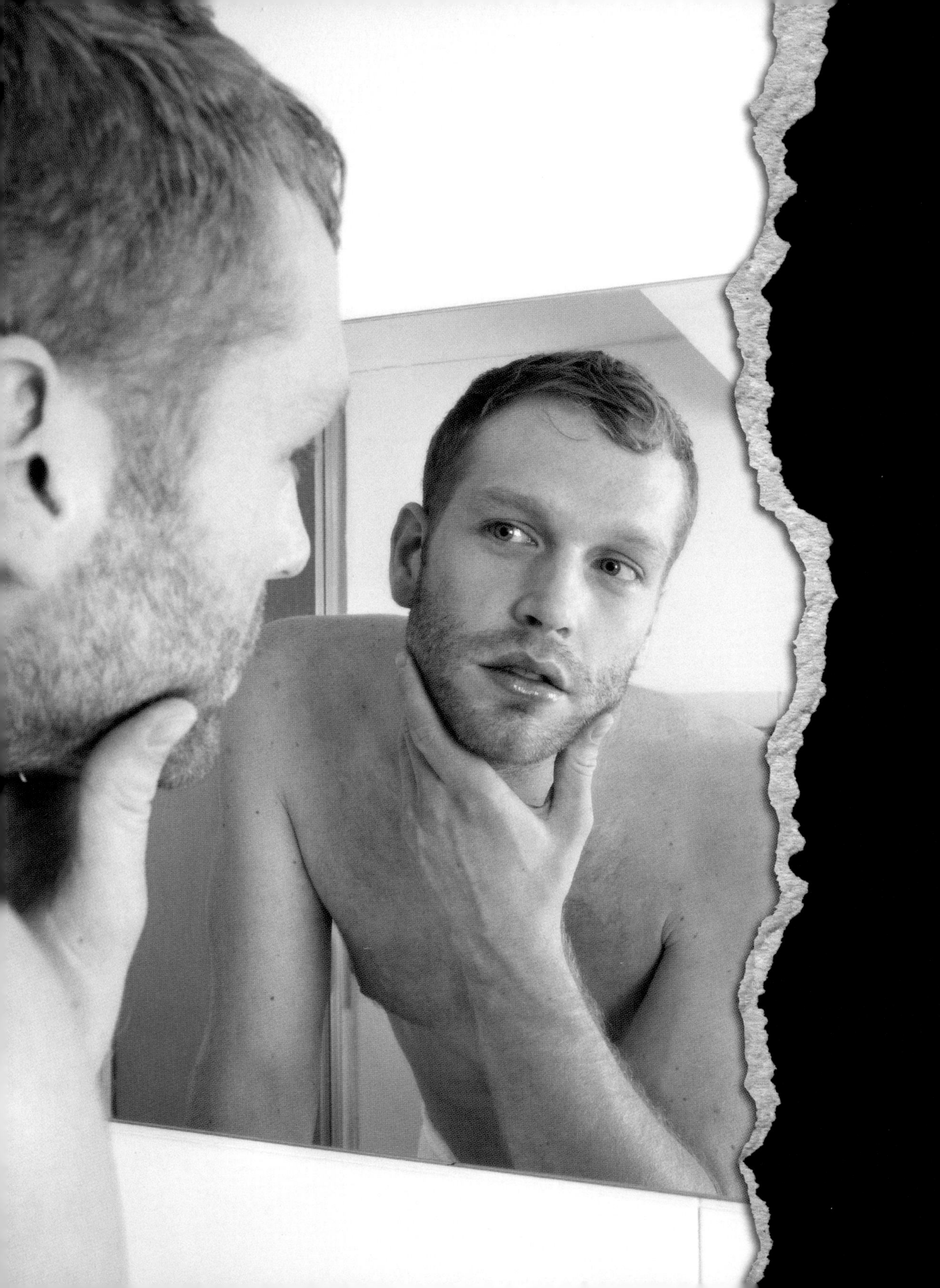

# [CHAPTER TWO]

# TAKE A GOOD LOOK — ASSESSING YOURSELF

## GENTLEMEN, START YOUR ENGINES!

As with anything in life, it's difficult to make a positive change in your physique until you are honest about where you stand right now. Chances are you have this book in your hands because you want to lose some weight. Maybe you want to simply tone up your physique, improve your cholesterol or blood-sugar levels or perhaps just learn about a new healthier lifestyle of good eating – one that will take you well into your later years in good health. Whatever your reasons for making a change, you need to assess yourself right out of the gate. It is virtually impossible to measure your success if you have not taken an initial reading. Your current condition will tell you what you need to focus on for your renovation.

[ Look at the bits you are not happy with and vow to make them look better than ever. ]

## IN FRONT OF THE MIRROR

Have you ever gotten out of the shower soaking wet, only to catch a glimpse of yourself in the mirror and stop dead in your tracks? What you see may not be what you want to see. Is that you in the mirror, or is it someone else who bears little resemblance to the lean, healthy person you once were? Carrying extra weight interferes with the beautiful lines of a lean, healthy body – a body you probably once owned. You stop and stare at the misshapen reflection in the mirror and then quickly gather the towel around you and run out of the bathroom.

Photographs have the same effect. You may never notice your ever-expanding waistline until someone whips out a picture of you at the office Christmas party – Christmas is a wonderful benchmark for measuring change – and in the photo you see the image of someone you hardly recognize. You wonder what happened to the real you.

Instances such as these can act as galvanizing moments, inspiring you to change whatever lifestyle you have been pursuing. We encourage you to seek out that galvanizing moment in order to help you establish your bottom line. Lock yourself in the bathroom and turn on all the lights. Strip off your clothes – all of them! No one is looking but you. Let your tummy hang out. Don't make an effort to locate your best angle. Look at yourself from every position and ask yourself if you are happy with what you see. Look at the bits you love and be okay with them. Look at the bits you are not happy with and vow to make them better than ever. Let this experience serve as a wonderful place to make the commitment to yourself to initiate your physique renovation.

There is no point in getting mad at yourself or sinking into a deep depression about your physical state. It is what it is and you have the power to do something about it. Using the combination of the Eat-Clean principles and a bit of guidance from this book, you will find your way back to improved health and physicality almost as soon as you begin. You can put your clothes back on now!

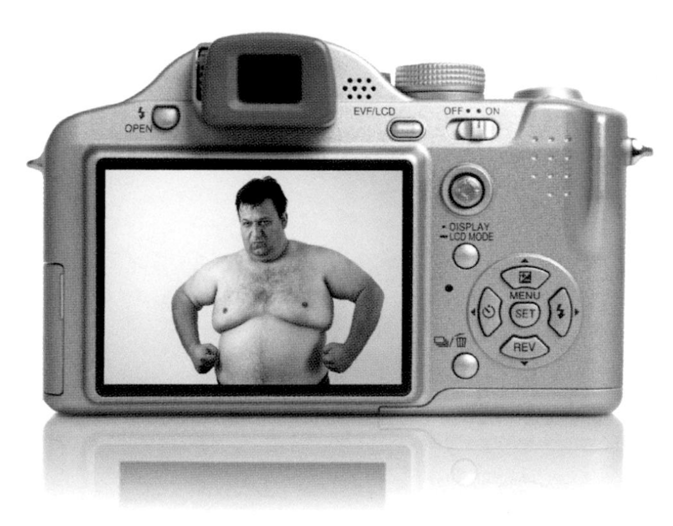


## IT'S A KODAK MOMENT

A photograph records exactly what you look like the moment it is snapped. Photos capture our dynamic history. You may have been a skinny teen and a buff adult, only to realize in your mid 30s or 40s this is no longer so. Many of us lose sight of what we look like because we get so busy with life that we don't take the time to think about it. Still more of us disengage ourselves from our bodies and ignore the consequences of eating and gaining weight.

Photographs have a definitive way of telling us what we need to know, even when we'd rather not know it. This is a little like balancing your bank account. Numbers are black and white and the bottom line tells us exactly where we stand financially. Though we may pretend otherwise, the reality remains the same. Facing this honestly helps us manage our financial lives. Photographs can serve as a bottom line for honestly assessing your physique right now.

In general, a photograph is better than the scale. A scale can be misleading, especially if you gain muscle while losing fat. The image shows you exactly where the excess is and where you need to pay attention to trouble spots. That photo can serve as your motivation every day. If you don't have a recent photo of yourself, have a friend or loved one take a shot of you in a bathing suit or pair of shorts, and then place it on the wall somewhere visible, so you can be inspired to stick to your plan to get started on this healthy new lifestyle – Clean Eating.

## WHAT THE DOC SAID

"Mr. Johnson, the bad news is you now have diabetes. I am afraid we must put you on insulin therapy. I encourage you to consider losing weight." These words are becoming more and more common in today's health-stressed world. For many of you the idea of learning how to eat well by relying on real, Clean foods rather than processed foods is more about your health than your physique. After all, what good is a good-looking body if it is damaged from the inside? Good health going bad is the most important reason for changing to better eating habits. If you are the one being diagnosed with diabetes, cardiovascular disease or any other medical condition, you will feel as if the rug has been pulled out from underneath you. The news gives you an almost physical blow. The gig is up. Mindless eating with no concern for health or other physical repercussions has finally caught up with you and now you will have to pay the price.

Sadly, you are not alone. Millions of Americans and millions more worldwide are facing news just like this from their own doctors about their declining state of health. "That modern man is declining in physical fitness has been emphasized by many eminent sociologists and other scientists. That the rate of degeneration is progressively accelerating constitutes a cause for great alarm, particularly since this is taking place in spite of the advance that is being made in modern science ..." Reference: *Nutrition and Physical Degeneration,* Dr. Weston Price, Price Pottenger Nutrition, 2008

"That modern man is declining in physical fitness has been emphasized by many eminent sociologists and other scientists."

## TEETH – THE INDICATOR OF YOUR STATE OF HEALTH

Some isolated populations on this planet live so close to the earth and eat foods so highly nutritious that they have no need for either a dentist or an orthodontist. This can be seen among the people living in the Loetschental Valley in Switzerland, primitive Alaskans, residents of the islands of the Outer Hebrides and other primitive groups where their isolation from modern foods has been almost complete. Hardly anyone has tooth decay – no cavities and no gum disease! As soon as modern foods are introduced into the diet, the trouble begins.

In North America tooth decay is rampant even with good tooth-brushing habits. Toothpaste and toothbrushes alone are not enough to protect against decay. Solid nutrition is what is needed. It may surprise you to learn that as soon as our family started Eating Clean, our dentist noticed the difference. Our teeth had hardly any plaque buildup and our mouth tissues were healthy and robust. According to Dr. Weston Price, DDS, "This absence of tooth decay among primitive races has been so striking a characteristic of humankind that many commentators have referred to it as a strikingly modern disease." Reference: *Nutrition and Physical Degeneration,* Dr. Weston Price, Price Pottenger Nutrition, 2008

## BOOK A PHYSICAL

Another excellent place to become acquainted with your current state of health is at your physician's office. Call him or her and request a physical check-up During a routine physical you can expect any or all of the following to take place:

- You will need to fill out forms that ask you detailed questions about your medical history.
- The doctor will take a medical history.
- The doctor may examine your skin.
- The doctor will listen to your heart and lungs.
- The doctor will palpate, or feel, your belly.
- A nurse or doctor will take your blood pressure.
- You will have your height and weight measured.
- The doctor will listen to the arteries in your neck, checking for sounds that indicate narrowing.
- The doctor may examine your eyes with an ophthalmoscope – he/she is actually looking at your arteries.
- You will provide blood and urine samples to be tested for sugar, cholesterol, liver and kidney function, infection, anemia and other concerns.
- Blood tests are now recommended for adolescents and adults to screen for HIV.
- Smokers may require a CT scan of the chest.

# PHYSICALS BY DECADE

**30s** – Have a physical every three years, particularly to screen for heart disease, high blood pressure, cancer or other disease.

**40s** – Have a physical every two years. This is when routine testing for cholesterol is essential, especially if you have a family history of heart disease. This is also a good age to undergo a rectal exam – perhaps a little uncomfortable, but highly necessary since colon cancer is a silent killer.

**50s** – Have a physical every year to screen for heart disease, high blood pressure, atherosclerosis, diabetes, other disease, behavioral changes, depression, and weight gain or loss. The colorectal cancer test is a good idea as well. A colonoscopy will screen for unusual growths in the colon. The PSA blood test should be done to screen for prostate cancer.

**60s AND UP** – Visit your doctor regularly and stay on top of all the conditions listed above. You may want to include a hearing and vision test.

## WHY SHOULD YOU DO IT?

A physical will give you and your doctor a good idea of your current state of health. Getting a regular physical helps the doctor track your history and look for changes. The doctor may be the first person to let you know you need to lose weight. Once you decide to take him up on the recommendation, your doctor will also be the first person to give you a clean bill of health (or not) so you can begin to make those healthy changes. While improving your diet is always called for, adding strenuous physical exercise to your regimen if you have always been a sedentary person may not be a good idea until you have gotten the go-ahead from your doctor. This physical will serve as yet another benchmark, or marker, to let you know where you stand right now with respect to weight and health. Once you have this information in hand you can go ahead and plan how to improve things.

## HOW ARE YOU FEELING?

Beyond the visual assessment and the visit to the doctor, you can assess yourself by paying attention to how you feel. If every day is a physical struggle to get through, if you are completely exhausted just walking up a set of stairs, if you can't breathe properly or sleep through the night because you are overweight, if your sex life is waning because it is too uncomfortable to be romantic ... these are indicators that life is not much fun and you don't feel the way you should. The human body is designed to be vital, robust, active and brimming with physicality – that urge to run, fly, swim and simply *do* is part of the joy of being human. The tragedy comes when the body is no longer capable of completing these actions. It does not make sense to reject the simple logic that consuming more nutritious foods will help you turn your life around, enabling you to once again feel the expression of joy rather than sorrow. How are you feeling? Is your body the gleaming, brilliant instrument you want it to be right now? How *are* you feeling?

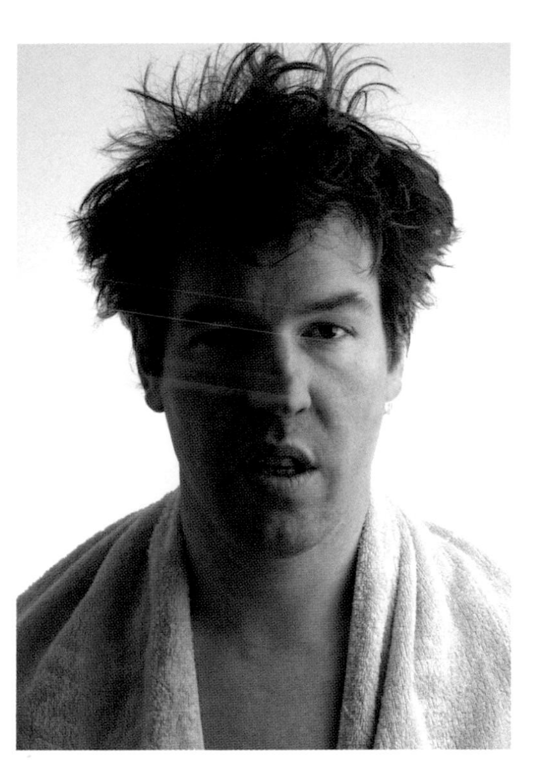

# YOUR MOTIVATIONAL TOOLBOX – The tools you need to get the job done.

If what you have read so far has cemented your desire to become the healthiest ***you*** possible, you will need a few tools to help you get exactly where you want to be. Motivation is that significant element you must have in order to push through every day, good or bad – and you can expect both when on this journey. A big part of the reason we Eat Clean is that we want to live long, happy and healthy lives and be there for our families. Too many children and young adults have their parents ripped from them because of avoidable diseases. We want to make sure we are there not only for our children, but also for our grandchildren.

You will have your own motivation. Your loved ones might be the primary inspiration for you to get back on track and stay there, but reasons are plenty to take better care of yourself. At this point you may want to consider making a "dream board." This sounds corny, but the exercise will certainly be thought provoking. Look for images that represent the changes you want to make happen. Glue them onto a piece of Bristol board or foam core and put a date on the board. Write captions beside the images as a verbal cue to support the visuals. Look at the dream board regularly to assess your goals and decide if you are on track.

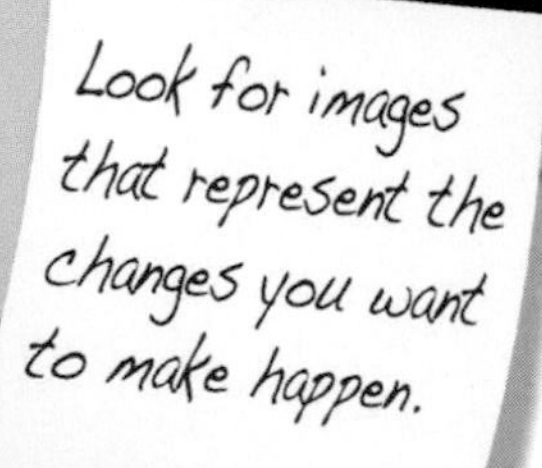
Look for images
that represent the
changes you want
to make happen.

We recently worked with a young man who was significantly overweight. While he created the dream board as part of his motivation-setting process we learned many things about him that he had not shared during our previous meetings. He had always been a fan of sailing but had never done it because he was afraid his excess weight would prevent him from being as flexible and limber as he would need to be while on the boat. He also wanted to get back into running again, something he had not done since his college days. He had placed numerous images of athletes on his dream board and also several images of men in well-tailored suits. When we asked him why he had put these pictures on the dream board he said he was tired of shopping in the fat-guy stores and really wanted to wear a well-cut suit again. He loves to wear suits and had not done so for many years since gaining weight. By placing these images on a board he was able to create a visual reminder of what his goals were. Use images of your own goals and dreams to help you stay committed to the plan of achieving a healthy, lean physique.

## EAT-CLEAN SUCCESS STORY!

**Bryan Hamilton**
From an email dated August 1, 2008

*I just bought your book. So far what I have read makes a lot of sense. I have been overweight most of my life due to bad eating habits and poor exercise habits. The lightest I have ever been is 153 pounds. That was back in high school in 1975. When I got married in 1982 my weight was around 185 pounds. I looked and felt great! I now weigh around 365 and my heaviest was around 425 pounds about two years ago. I have tried all kinds of diets! Diets are a joke! It's got to be a lifestyle change! I have joined a spin class since October and spin between two and four times per week. I walk when it is not 105 degrees outside. I quit cigarettes around six months ago and man that has made a big difference in the way I feel. Anyway I think the biggest factor is that a person must eat as natural as possible and stay away from anything processed. Drink lots of water! I like your book so far. I have type-2 diabetes, an underactive thyroid and high blood pressure, which I keep in check with pills that I want to get rid of. Well today is the day. It is time for a change. A clean change! I like the*

## JOIN IN

Another way to get and stay motivated is to gather positive support around you. The more you surround yourself with others who are interested in pursuing a healthy lifestyle, the more likely you will be successful. Loved ones and family members are the natural place to begin looking for that support. Let them know you are planning to make positive lifestyle changes and that you will want their support in helping you reach your goals. This can come in the form of preparing nutritious meals, a push out the door when it is time to exercise or a hug in recognition of your success when you have lost the first three pounds. Conversely, if you find yourself in the company of folks who love to eat unhealthy foods, try to tempt you into eating foods you know are not good for you and are themselves overweight, you will have a great deal of trouble swimming against that current.

Look for clubs, teams or organizations that involve a healthy, active lifestyle. If one of your dreams is to run a marathon, for example, then find a running club and join in. Many people find that when they train with others they feel a sense of responsibility to their teammates to show up and train with them. Joining a club or team also helps to generate both a friendly competitive spirit and camaraderie. Dragon boating has become enormously popular lately. Men and women join teams to power these huge boats through the water. Being with people who are performing similar activities validates your purpose, too. Your new friends are looking for healthy exercise and working on improving their particular skills and perhaps even winning, and this atmosphere will spur you on to new heights. Another aspect of being part of a team is the sense of responsibility you develop when you are now expected to contribute. These are all positive ways to become and stay motivated.

You can also join a gym where members have similar philosophies on toning up. Gym owners and trainers often establish training groups. Tosca says: "At the local gym where I first began to train I joined an Around the World running group. The idea is to jump on the treadmill or track, road or wherever you love to run, and clock your mileage. You chart a course around the world and use towns and cities as waypoints on your journey. This is a fun way to keep moving while you add up miles and miles of activity."

## WHAT LIES BENEATH

Perhaps the biggest source of motivation is the idea that there is a wonderful, unbelievable person hiding underneath the one you are now showing to the outside world. Weight gain creates disconnect between the size you have become and the person you truly are. When we talk about Clean-Eating success stories we don't just mean success in weight loss, but also in becoming that person you were always meant to be.

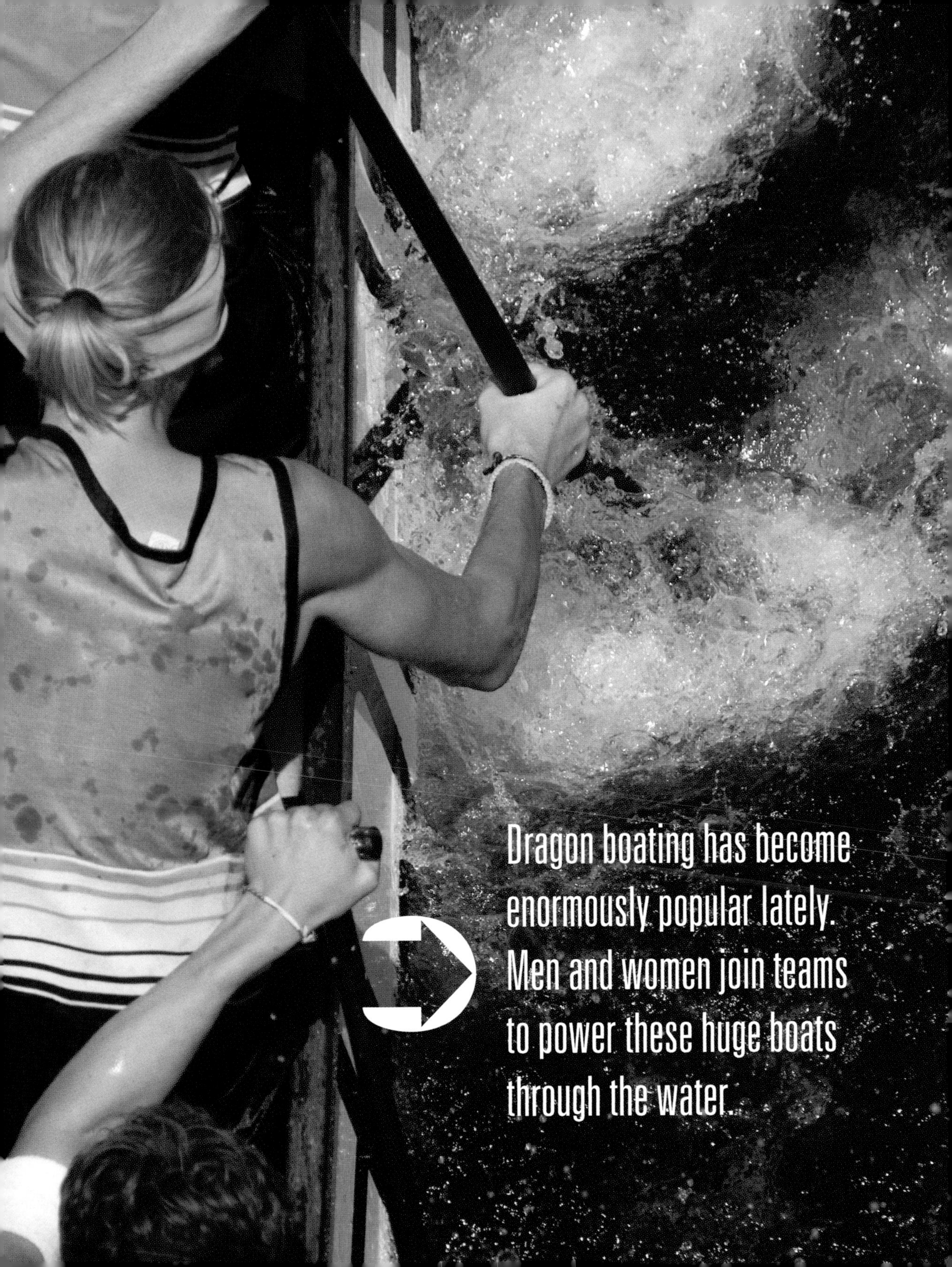

Dragon boating has become enormously popular lately. Men and women join teams to power these huge boats through the water.

# EAT-CLEAN SUCCESS STORY!

**Steve Jackson**
From an email dated August 21, 2008

*I had my first meeting with my trainer. We talked about goals to lose weight and build muscle. She told me to buy your diet book and cookbook. I started on July 30th, 2008. In the locker room I stripped down and stepped on the scale, weighing in at 280 pounds. I took photos of myself earlier that morning so I could track my progress. I cleaned out my fridge and went shopping. I bought fruits, vegetables, some plain old-fashioned oatmeal and started reading labels. Careful! There is garbage in almost everything. Did you know that there is a gram of sugar in one small envelope of regular instant oatmeal? It's true! My fat-free salad dressing contains sugar too. Ketchup? It has lots of high fructose corn syrup.*

*Tosca I can tell you I have now been inspired to eat clean for life. I don't have to ever worry about gaining back the weight I have lost. On August 19th I weighed in again at 267 pounds. That's 13 pounds gone forever in 20 days. I made a big pot of black bean turkey chili and brought some to work. My coworker Carla loved it. She is reading your book now.*

*I started my desk job a little over a year ago. I also have high blood pressure. It has gone down dramatically. I even feel so much better. I went out last Friday to go dancing!*

*Thank you Tosca.*
*P.S. I now have lowered my blood pressure medications too.*

## KEEPING TRACK

What better way to keep track of your success than to write it down? You don't need more than a few lines in a record book to jot down your weight-loss progress, training efforts and even eating details. For those of you who have never recorded progress like this before, please consider it as the best, cheapest and simplest way to keep yourself going in the right direction. Even the smallest details like why you ate pizza when you have been Eating Clean all week will help you understand your eating habits. Some of us eat out of boredom, others out of habit, and there

[ What are you teaching your children about respecting their health and body? ]

are hosts of other reasons we do what we do. Telling your story every day is cathartic and amazingly helpful. It is a way for you to validate your hard work and to testify – even if only to yourself – how you are doing.

Loads of people are using the Internet to post blogs about their physique renovation. If you are good with technology keeping a blog is satisfying because you can see your results and others will see them too – and that gives you more incentive to succeed.

## SO WHAT IF I DON'T EAT CLEAN?

What will happen if you don't switch up your no-no foods for more nutritious options? Good question! If you never make the change you will simply face more of whatever it is you are struggling with now – overweight, obesity, diabetes, high blood pressure, cancer, atherosclerosis, fatigue and so on. If you are already overweight you may continue to gain weight. Worse yet, your health will probably decline if it hasn't already. This not only affects you but also your loved ones. Children in particular will lose out big time. Not only might they lose you before they should, but they need strong role models. These role models should be their parents. What are you teaching your children about respecting their health and body? What strength do you have in your position when you make poor eating choices but command them to eat their broccoli?

If we don't soon make amends to our nutritional patterns the human race faces a radical decline. "Elimination of the 'empty calories' in sugar and white flour would result in increased resistance to infection, a marked reduction in the bizarre and disabling symptoms of reactive hypoglycemia, fewer attacks of so-called 'viruses,' a renewed supply of energy, more zest for life and a gradual reduction in the incidence of degenerative diseases which seem to be the hallmark of our civilization. A healthy body should have increased resistance to chemicals – as well as to invasion by viruses and bacteria." Reference: *Nutrition and Physical Degeneration,* Dr. Weston Price, Price Pottenger Nutrition, 2008

From here on in you should take full strides out toward your new goals of renewed health and vitality! It would be far too uncomfortable for you to stay where you are now, wearing XXXL pants and shirts and struggling to make your body move through daily living. The motivation you needed to get you thinking about making lifestyle changes is a different kind of motivation than what you need every day to sustain change making. Make small changes: eat oatmeal for breakfast rather than eating either nothing at all or sugary, nutrient-depleted foods. That is a simple and easy-to-make change that costs virtually nothing. Once you have gotten the hang of that, make another small change – drink water instead of colas and other sugar-loaded beverages. Even these small changes will bear very significant fruit for you. With a few small successes under your belt you will feel motivated to stick with Clean Eating and go for more. This is the kind of motivation you need for the long term – motivation with staying power.

Never have North Americans been so consumed with health and nutrition yet at the same time so ill. At the turn of the last century – a relatively short time ago, evolutionarily speaking – illnesses such as heart disease and cancer were uncommon. Today "one person in three dies of cancer, one in three suffers from allergies, one in ten will have ulcers and one in five is mentally ill. Continuing this grim litany, one out of five pregnancies ends in miscarriage and one quarter of a million infants are born with a birth defect every year," this according to Sally Fallon in her powerful book, *Nourishing Traditions*. These are among the most powerful reasons of all to Eat Clean starting today. Health is not yours if you don't respect it. As Jack LaLanne, authority on health and nutrition and still living a vigorous life well into his 90s, states: "Would you give your right leg for a million dollars? Of course not. The greatest possession you have is your body, so take care of it."

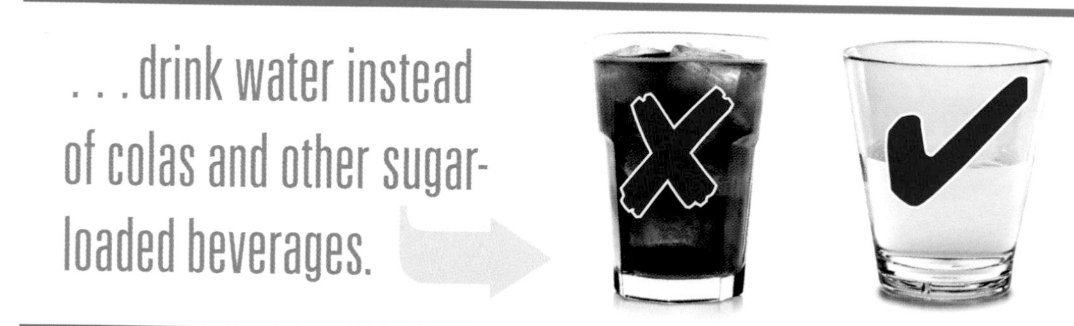
. . . drink water instead
of colas and other sugar-
loaded beverages.

# MOTIVATIONAL CHECKLIST

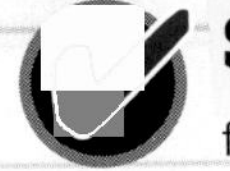

**Set your goals –** Write them down for the long term; write them down for today and for next week. Make your intentions a reality by reviewing your goals and doing something to ensure they happen. Create a dream board to help you visualize your goals.

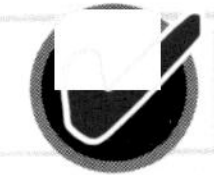

**Record your work –** Photos show the changes you have made even if sometimes you feel you're going nowhere. Writing is validating. It's also useful for letting you discover your stumbling blocks and coming to terms with how your feelings affect your habits. Use a journal or create a blog to help you stay motivated and share your experience.

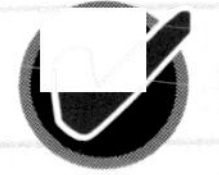

**Celebrate the small stuff –** Treat yourself to a small reward for getting the job done today – go to the movies, buy a new book, or go shopping for a pair of pants that actually fit now that you have lost weight.

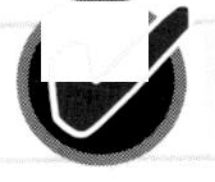

**Celebrate the big stuff –** You have done it! Take a celebratory photo of you and your new physique. Take loads of pictures of you doing the things you set out to do.

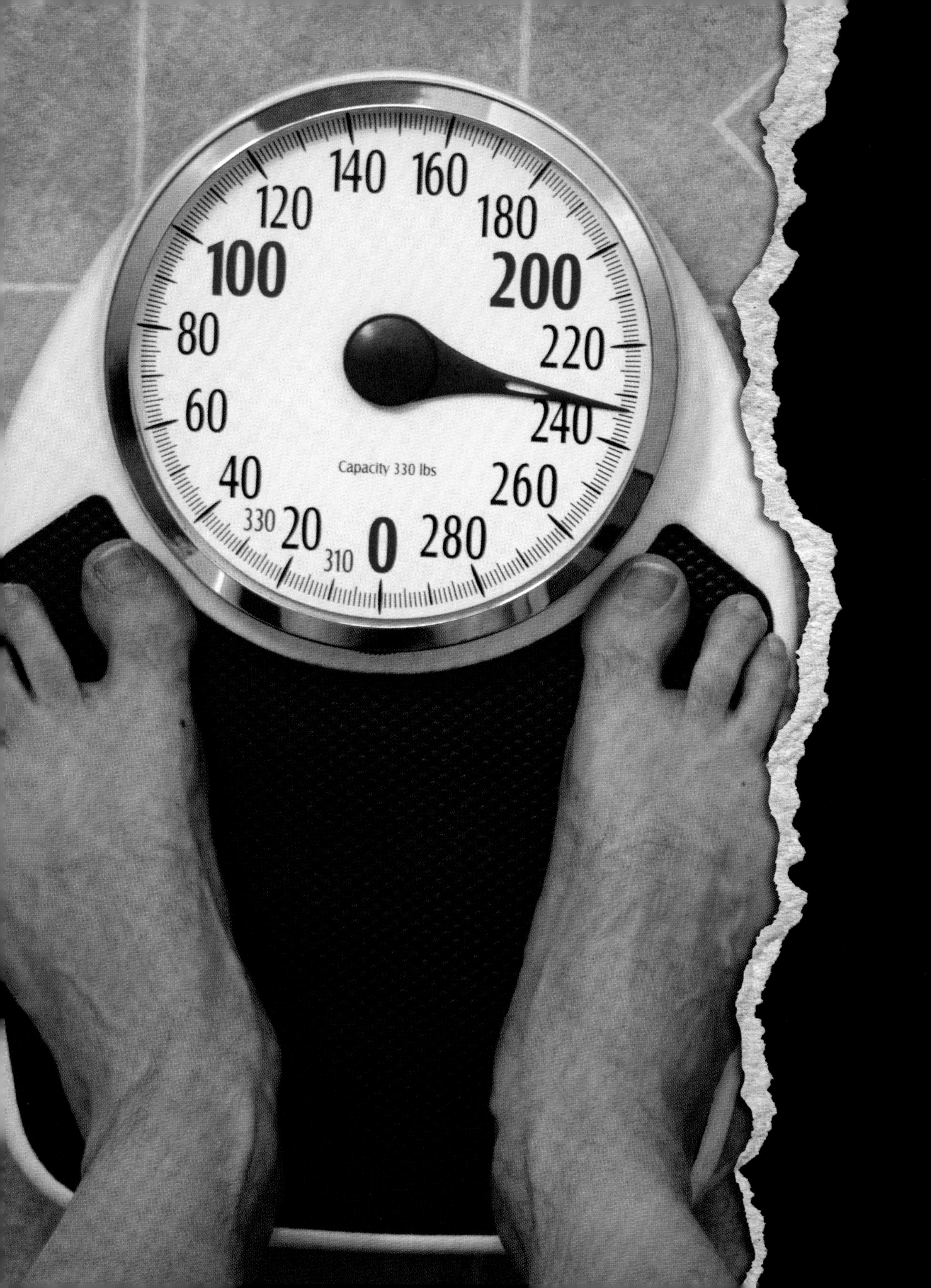
140
160
120
180
100
200
80
220
60
240
Capacity 330 lbs
40
260
330
20
310
0
280

# [CHAPTER THREE]

# DEVELOP YOUR PLAN

## LOOK AT THE NUMBERS– What do you weigh? What is your waist circumference? What is your BMI?

Here you are, standing at the beginning of your journey to renewed health and vitality. You've checked yourself out in the mirror and possibly got some photographs taken. You've hopefully been to your doctor. Now let's take a few measurements to help us get a clearer picture of where you are now. Health and fitness practitioners use one of three methods to measure your weight and body-fat content. These are important tools that give a certain black-and-white quality to your current status and a hard number for medical and fitness practitioners to gauge you by. Numbers help everyone get a clearer picture of where you are at this specific point.

## YOUR WEIGHT

Taking a weight measurement is an obvious place to begin this process. You have to know how much you weigh and how tall you are for a basic starting point. Health care and fitness professionals always make you stand on the scale during a physical in order to assess just that. The technical term is a Body Mass Index or BMI. Your weight is plotted against a chart with standard weights. A BMI under 25 is considered healthy, 18.5 or less is underweight, and a BMI of 25 or more is overweight. Pay attention if your BMI is 30 or more – then you are obese. Take a look at the BMI chart following to figure out where you are.

THE AMERICAN HEART ASSOCIATION

# BODY-MASS-INDEX CHART

| Height | **Minimal** risk *(BMI under 25)* **(lbs.)** | **Moderate** risk *(BMI 25-29.9)* Overweight **(lbs.)** | **High** risk *(BMI 30 and above)* Obese **(lbs.)** |
|---|---|---|---|
| 4'10" | 118 or less | 119-142 | 143 or more |
| 4'11" | 123 or less | 124-147 | 148 or more |
| 5'0" | 127 or less | 128-152 | 153 or more |
| 5'1" | 131 or less | 132-157 | 158 or more |
| 5'2" | 135 or less | 136-163 | 164 or more |
| 5'3" | 140 or less | 141-168 | 169 or more |
| 5'4" | 144 or less | 145-173 | 174 or more |
| 5'5" | 149 or less | 150-179 | 180 or more |
| 5'6" | 154 or less | 155-185 | 186 or more |
| 5'7" | 158 or less | 159-190 | 191 or more |
| 5'8" | 163 or less | 164-196 | 197 or more |
| 5'9" | 168 or less | 169-202 | 203 or more |
| 5'10" | 173 or less | 174-208 | 209 or more |
| 5'11" | 178 or less | 179-214 | 215 or more |
| 6'0" | 183 or less | 184-220 | 221 or more |
| 6'1" | 188 or less | 189-226 | 227 or more |
| 6'2" | 193 or less | 194-232 | 233 or more |
| 6'3" | 199 or less | 200-239 | 240 or more |
| 6'4" | 204 or less | 205-245 | 246 or more |

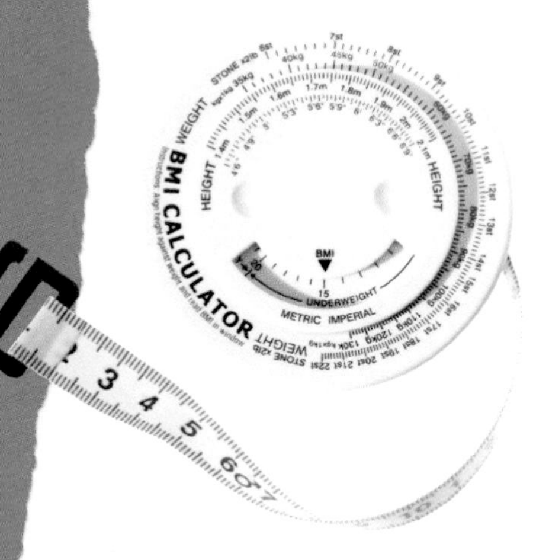


**YOU CAN ALSO CALCULATE YOUR OWN BMI BY DOING THE FOLLOWING:**

- Multiply your weight in pounds by 703
- Divide by your height in inches (5 feet = 60 inches)
- Divide again by your height in inches

The BMI chart can help you set your goals for weight loss. Just look for your height on the chart. Beside it you will find the number for your ideal weight range. For example, if you are 5'10" tall your BMI for a healthy weight should be under 174 pounds. The range reflects different statures for small-, medium- and larger-boned individuals. It may also reflect more muscularity, since muscle weighs more than fat. However, if you have a large degree of muscularity (i.e., if you are a bodybuilder) you may find this chart does not work for you.

## YOUR WAIST CIRCUMFERENCE

Lately physicians have begun to use another measurement to help them decide if you are at risk for certain diseases commonly associated with overweight. This measurement is called the Waist Circumference, or WC, which is the distance measured around your waist just above the navel. Stand with your feet about shoulder width apart and, using a soft measuring tape, start just above the belly button. Bring the tape around your back and to the front again. Don't cheat by pulling the tape tight. In fact, the best way to do this is to have someone else take the measurement. Round to the closest half-centimeter or quarter-inch. On average, men should strive for a WC of less than 40 inches, or 101.5 centimeters, for health reasons. Men should take the measurement about one to two inches above the navel. For a more accurate number, have someone else measure your waist.

## YOUR WAIST-TO-HIP RATIO

Another useful measurement is the Waist-to-Hip Ratio. This measurement involves finding your WC, or Waist Circumference, as described above. Next you will need to find your Hip Circumference, or HC. This is the measurement taken around the widest part of your hips at the lowest part, including the buttocks.

### The Waist-to-Hip Ratio is then calculated as follows:

- **Measure your waist at the smallest part.**
- **Measure your hips at their widest part.**
- **Divide your waist measurement by your hip measurement.**

Men will strive for a number less than 1.0. If your ratio is greater than 1.0, you are at a greater risk for various health conditions including heart disease, stroke, diabetes, cancer and arthritis. If you store your fat in the upper part of your body around your abdomen and chest, you collect your fat around your internal organs, and you have what is called an apple-shaped body. If you store your fat on the hips and thighs below the skin you have what is called a pear-shaped body. Apple-shaped people are at a far greater health risk than pear-shaped people.

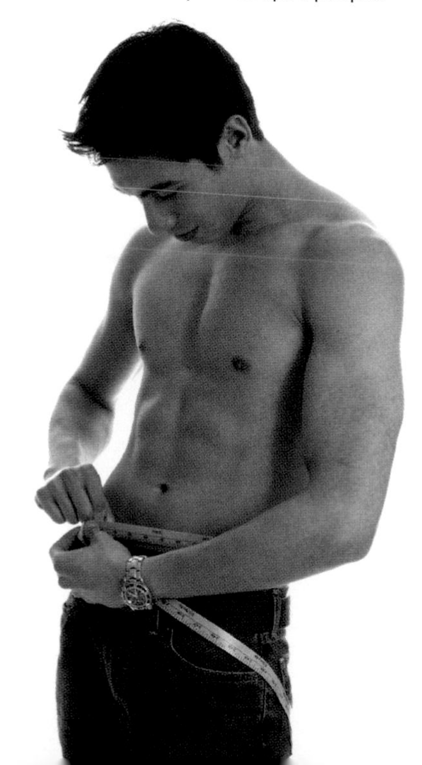

## KEEP THIS IN MIND

The various numerical values you have just worked out are indicators of your general pattern of collecting fat, and can predict your risk for disease. But sometimes numbers don't help you at all. If you are a solid, well-built and muscular person you will probably weigh more than the standards indicated on the BMI chart. You will know for yourself if this is true. Lean, metabolically active muscle weighs more than fat, so do not fear if this describes you. However, if this is the case you will find that your waist-to-hip ratio should be good. If your BMI and waist-to-hip ratio are both off, you likely have some extra fat around your internal organs.

## THE EAT-CLEAN HEALTHY-BODY FORMULA

A fabulous body comes from more than just training, although many people think this is not so. Countless people think the answer to losing weight lies in doing more cardiovascular exercise, but a fabulous body is built from excellent nutrition more than training. You could run for an hour every day, but if you don't follow up with proper, lean, clean nutrition it won't make much difference. Women and men who follow Clean Eating already know this to be true so we hope you will trust us when we say that in order to build the lean body you have always wanted you will have to dedicate yourself to training and eating as follows:

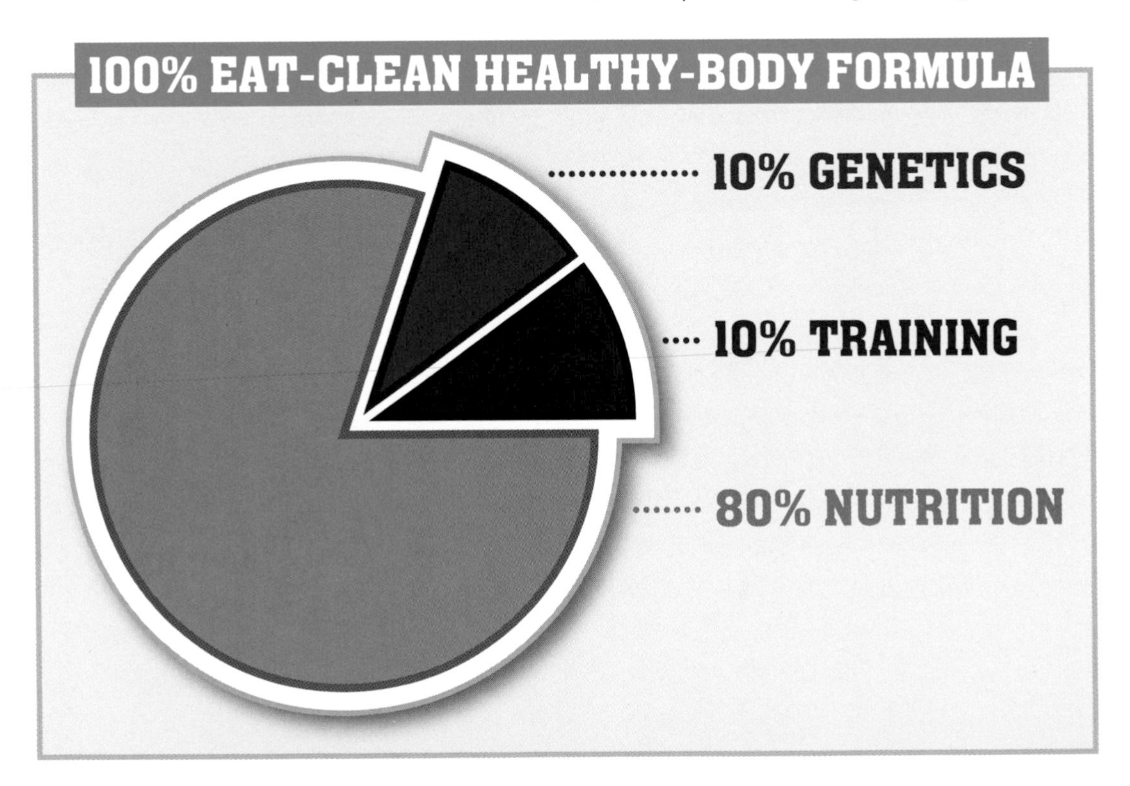

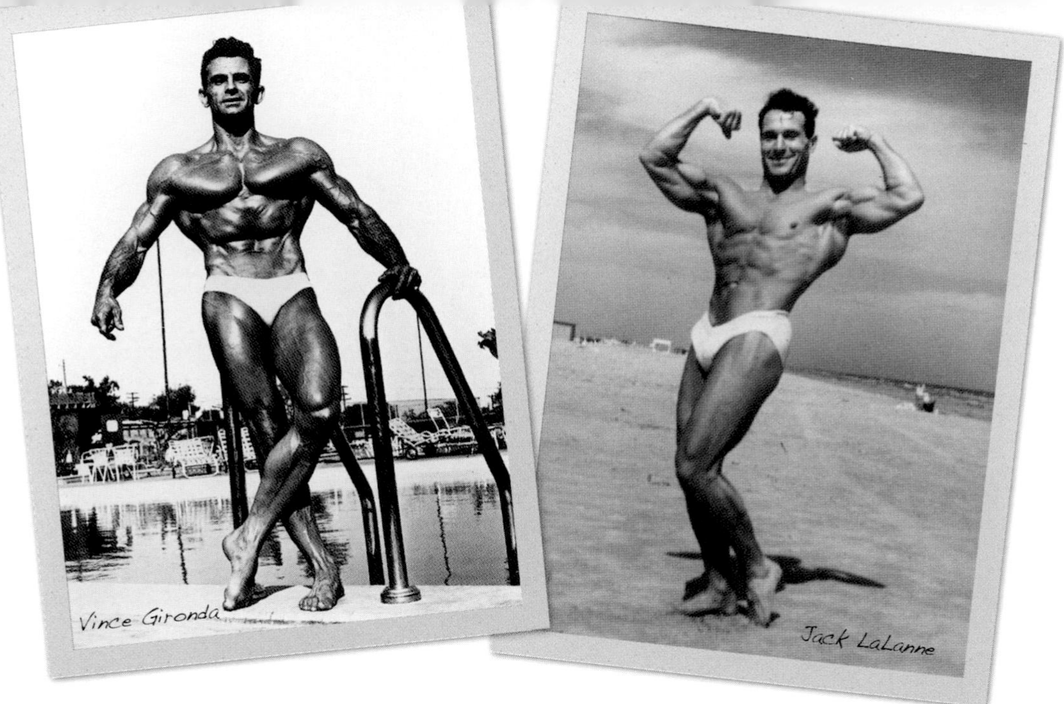


## IN GOOD COMPANY

This formula has served the needs of all physique athletes in their quest to build a lean, fit body. Anyone who has ever competed in big bodybuilding shows, the most noteworthy example being California's current governor Arnold Schwarzenegger, has used this formula to slim down and develop a hard, muscled physique. Arnold knew full well the value of consuming lean protein partnered with complex carbohydrates at every one of his several meals each day. Bill Pearl variously held the titles of Mr. Universe, Mr. World and Mr. America, so fine was his physique. People used to say he was the world's most beautifully built man. This champion happily ate the same Clean-Eating regimen we are about to recommend to you – lean protein and complex carbohydrates many times each day. He eventually went on to become the nutritional advisor for NASA's astronauts. Other competitors in the physique industry, including the current Mr. Olympia, Dexter Jackson, and those who went before him use the Eat-Clean Healthy-Body Formula to get in razor-sharp shape too. They know that everything they eat will end up somewhere in or on their body, so they make every mouthful count. Not a single one of them would ever consider eating a big, greasy burger and an accompanying plate of fries.

Old-time trainer-to-the-stars Vince Gironda trained many an out-of-shape celebrity to get them ready for film parts. When producers gave him six weeks to whip an actor into shape, he would joke, "Six weeks! I can hardly get them sobered up in that time." He preferred to have three months to do the job correctly. Vince would place them on a Clean-Eating food regimen which, when combined with training, would have the actor ready to go. Frank Zane, born in 1944, is another old-time bodybuilding champion

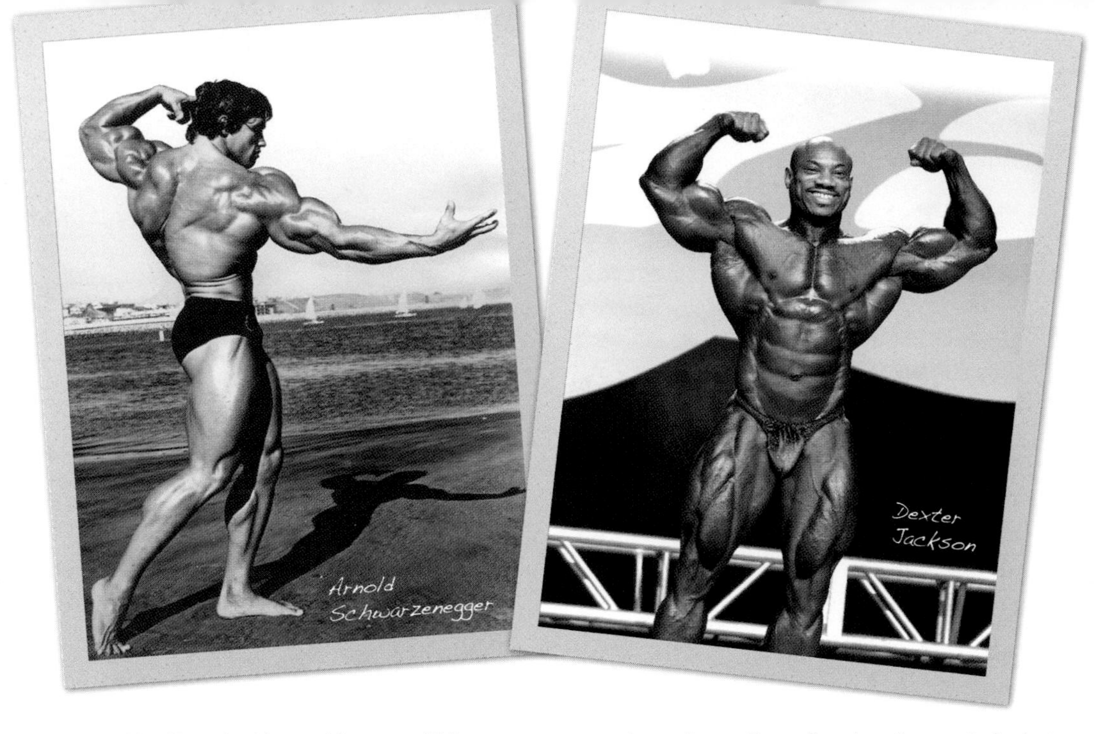


with three Mr. Olympia titles to his name. This man follows the same regimen now that he has followed for most of his life – Clean Eating – and he still looks amazing. You can find him any day working at Zane Haven, his gym in San Diego.

And what about the granddaddy of fitness, Mr. Jack LaLanne? Born in 1914, Jack was one of the first to adopt Clean Eating. This way of eating changed him from a sickly, pimply, scrawny, sugar-addicted young boy with a nasty temper to the world's greatest fitness expert. Jack had a fitness-based television show for 35 years and can still do chin-ups, push-ups and swim like a fish, all with a body fueled by only the leanest, highest-octane nutrition.

Although men like these have taken Clean Eating to the extreme, you won't have to. The regimen of eating six smaller meals each day based on solid, lean protein and excellent slow-burning carbohydrates will work for you too, but you don't have to be as tight on nutrition as a bodybuilding athlete or a movie star (unless you want to of course). Don't waste another minute wondering if Clean Eating is for you. As soon as you begin to eat this way you will notice changes. Nutrition plays a far bigger role in helping you shape a lean physique and improving your health than you previously might have imagined. One hundred years of empirical data from thousands of physique athletes support this claim and you have to admit, they look pretty amazing, don't they? Now it's your turn!

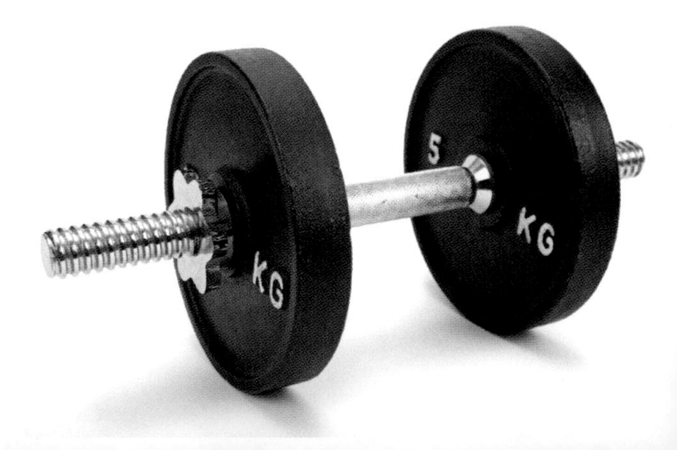

# A GLORIOUS PHYSIQUE

## LEONARDO DA VINCI'S VITRUVIAN MAN – THE IDEAL

- The palm is the width of four fingers, or three inches.
- The foot is the width of four palms and is 36 fingers or 12 inches.
- A cubit is the width of six palms.
- A man's height is four cubits, or 24 palms.
- The length of a man's outstretched arms is equal to his height.
- The distance from the hairline to the bottom of the chin is one-tenth his height.
- The distance from the top of the head to the bottom of the chin is one-eighth his height.
- The maximum width of the shoulders is a quarter of his height.
- The distance from the elbow to the tip of the hand is one-fifth his height.
- The distance from the elbow to the armpit is one-eighth his height.
- The length of his hand is one-tenth his height.
- The distance from the bottom of the chin to his nose is one-third of the length of his head.
- The distance from the hairline to the eyebrows is one-third of the length of his face.
- The length of his ear is one-third of the length of his face.

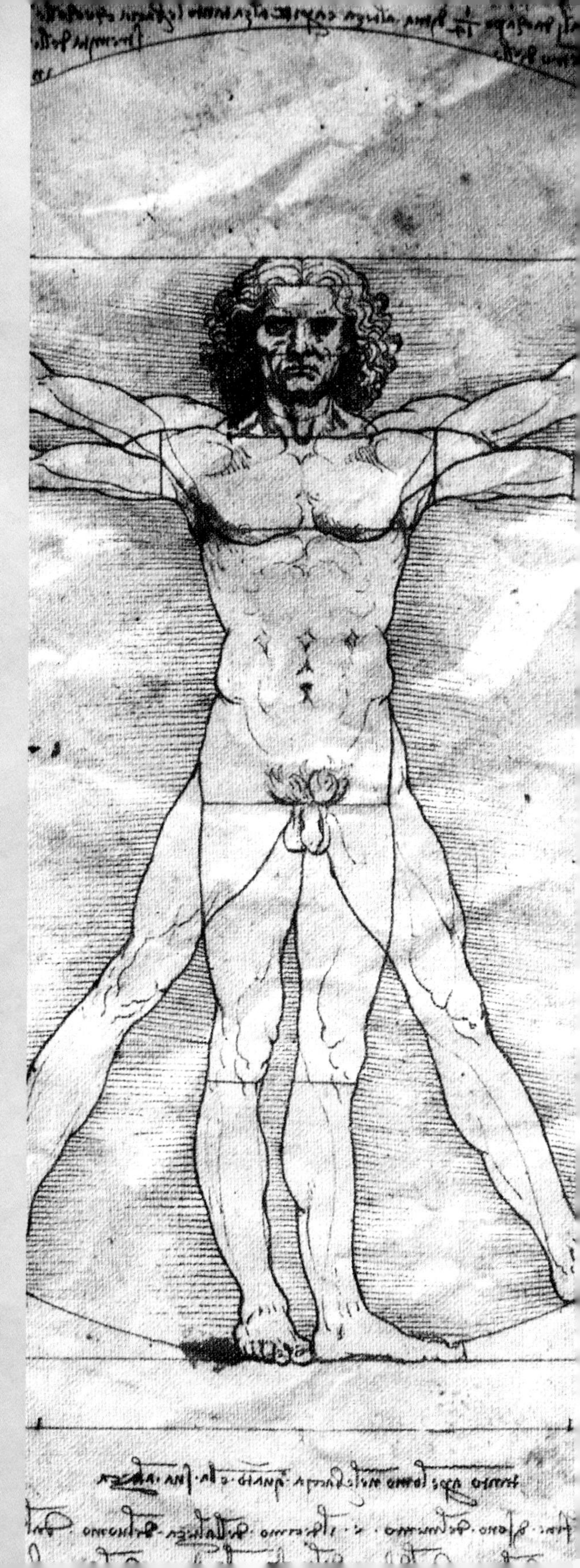

## WHAT DOES AN IDEAL PHYSIQUE LOOK LIKE?

Vitruvian Man came from the brilliant mind of Pythagoras, the Greek philosopher, who was among the first to describe what was considered the ideal physique. It was a body that displayed symmetry and balance with arithmetic precision, the same principles that apply to architecture. Later Leonardo da Vinci drew that ideal in what is known as Vitruvian Man, which has become among the most recognized drawings in the world. This image suggests a precise set of requirements for the perfect physique. Many of us do not possess such pristine genetics, and so we have to work with what we have got!

## COMPONENTS OF A GREAT PHYSIQUE

In general here is what you should be trying to build into your new, lean body:

- **Wide shoulders**
- **Wide lats**
- **Narrow hips**
- **Narrow waist (which means tight abdominals)**
- **Flowing quadriceps, or thighs**
- **Tight, uplifted glutes**
- **Tapering, straight legs**
- **Diamond-shaped calves**
- **Erect posture**

# CLEAN-EATING SUCCESS GUARANTEED

Going forward with your own plans for physical and health improvement, you know that Clean Eating is the only reliable strategy. You are in the company of many excellent examples, as we have already seen. It should make you feel good knowing that Arnold is probably having oats for breakfast and Jack is enjoying fish and greens for supper just as you are. Both of these people went from being ordinary to exemplary for many reasons, not the least of which is they paid strict attention to their nutrition. Let these men be examples for you as you embark on uncovering an exemplary version of yourself. Make every mouthful count. Don't fall back on eating sugary donuts and cream-laden coffee for breakfast ever again.

## HOW
## Tosca's story

When I was first introduced to Clean Eating I did not know what it was, I just knew what it wasn't. The new regimen, which I had promised to adhere to in preparation for my first bodybuilding contest, involved eating more. More!! This was a total departure from what I always believed was the correct way of dieting: food restriction and calorie counting. Okay, so there was more to eating than I'd thought! I was curious and skeptical all at once. What else? A meal had to be eaten every two to three hours. Once again, I was from the old school of eating three squares a day. This was new, eating more often. Now, I already made a point of eating a good breakfast, but I soon discovered I wasn't even getting that right. I was not eating protein and I was eating far too many refined carbs. My new information helped to explain why I felt so lethargic not long after eating. I found I was hypoglycemic, and simple carbs eaten without protein was about the worst thing I could eat. With Clean Eating the deal was that I had to eat lean protein and complex carbs each time I ate – six times per day. So far I was learning many new things about how to eat. Here I had thought eating was so very simple. Not!!!

These details were enlightening and encouraging. Why? Because I felt then and feel now that virtually everyone in North America, including myself, is waiting for someone to tell them what to eat and when. Once I learned about these principles and a few more (see page 25), I felt a great sense of relief. I was stunned by my ignorance about food, but even more stunned to discover how easy it was to Eat Clean, how much better I felt and how soon after I started eating this way my body reflected positive changes. Early on in the process of renovating my eating lifestyle, I was hooked.

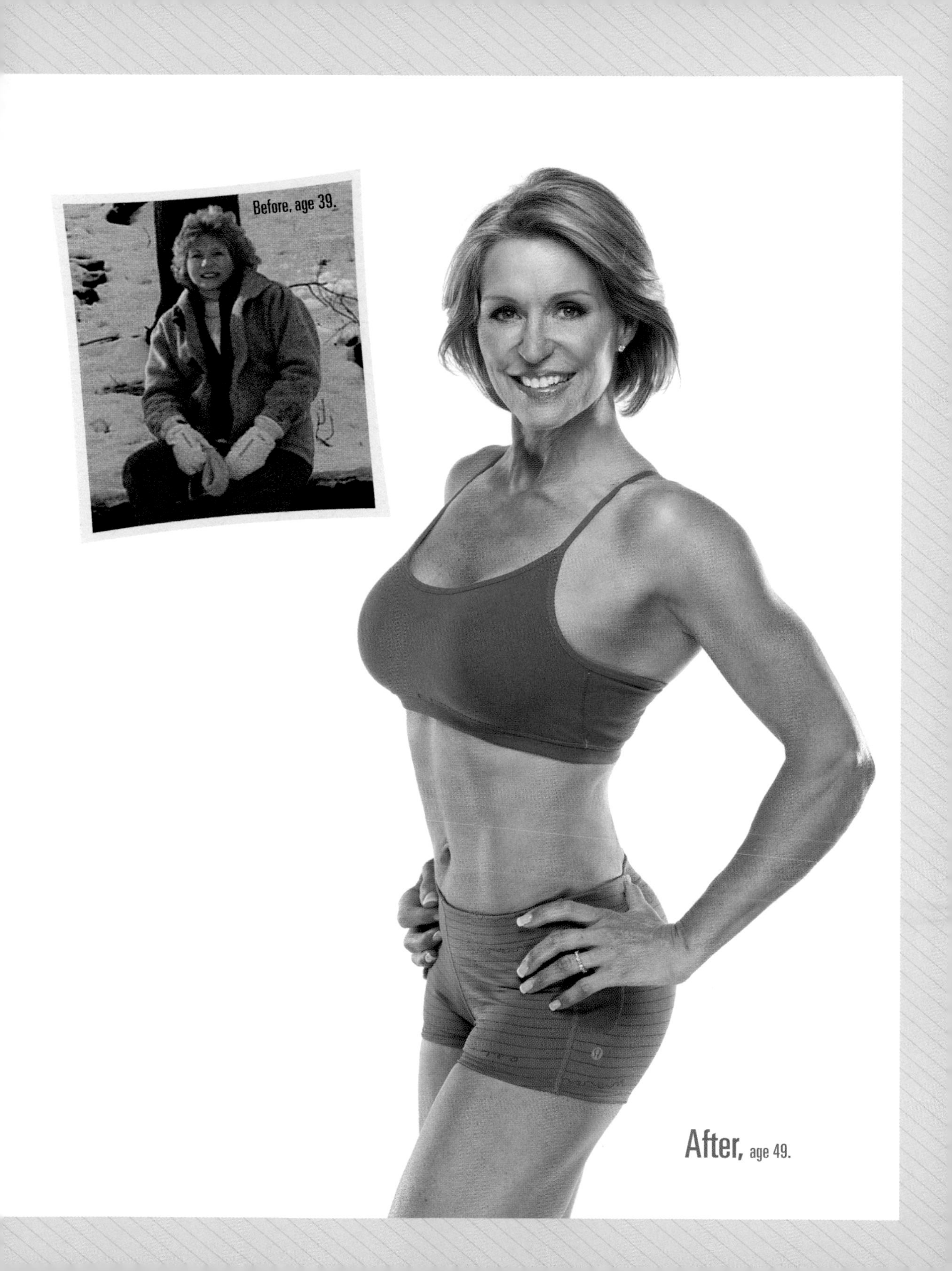

Before, age 39.

After, age 49.

## OOPS! I DID IT AGAIN!
## What to do if you go off course.

You might as well go ahead and plan for those days when sticking to the tightest eating is either difficult or impossible. These times will happen and it helps to know that up front. That does not mean you should make a habit of it! Clean Eating should be your lifestyle eating plan. However, on certain occasions including your birthday or someone else's, weddings, parties and even big sporting events such as the Super Bowl, Eating Clean can be difficult. You can make celebratory occasions like these work in your favor by making the food yourself – Clean-Eating options for wings, ribs, burgers and accompanying dishes can be found in the recipe section of this book – so you don't have to struggle every time.

We live in a food-centered world. Some have too much and some don't have enough, but food filters into every aspect of our lives from work to school to play. Be prepared for those occasions by accepting the prevalence of food in daily life. Don't be afraid of saying "no" to helpings of birthday cake at the office. In one *Seinfeld* episode Elaine gets so fed up with birthday cake she goes on strike against it and screams at her coworkers to get the cake out of her office. You may feel that way too if you are unprepared for these occasions. Handle situations wisely by being prepared to say: "No thank you." You don't have to shout and scream. A firm, polite voice will do nicely.

[ Don't be afraid of saying "no." ]

You can also create scenarios like these in your mind and practice what you might say or how you will handle them. How will you eat when your mother-in-law is serving up a fully loaded Thanksgiving dinner, complete with mashed potatoes whipped with cream, served alongside deep-fried turkey? How much if any cake will you have when it's birthday time? You have been invited out to a neighbor's house for dinner and you don't want to be rude, but … have your answers ready. If there is an obvious healthier option available, request it instead. That goes for beverages, also. Alcohol has only a limited place in a Clean-Eating regimen, since it is largely sugar and besides, it lowers your resistance. Have a glass of wine or a beer on occasion, but not more and not often.

In the event that you can't change the situation, accept it for what it is, and don't worry. Eat small portions and know that tomorrow you will go back to regular Clean Eating – the eating that delivers results. If you go completely off the rails overdoing chips, soda and other not-so-clean foods, use the experience as a teaching tool. That is exactly what it is. The odd time one of us munches on something like a brownie after keeping our eating tight we invariably feel so rotten the next day we recommit to Clean Eating with a vengeance. You can treat yourself once in a while and enjoy it, but it feels best to go back to tighter, Clean nutrition.

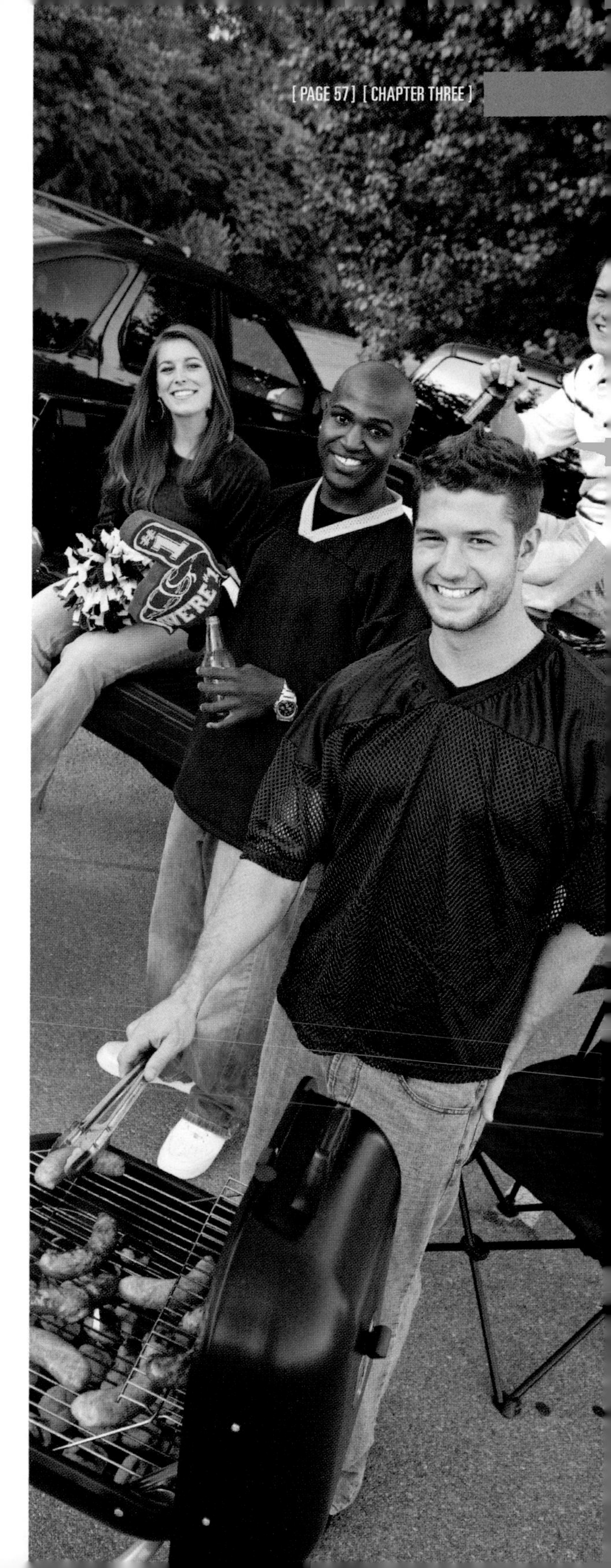

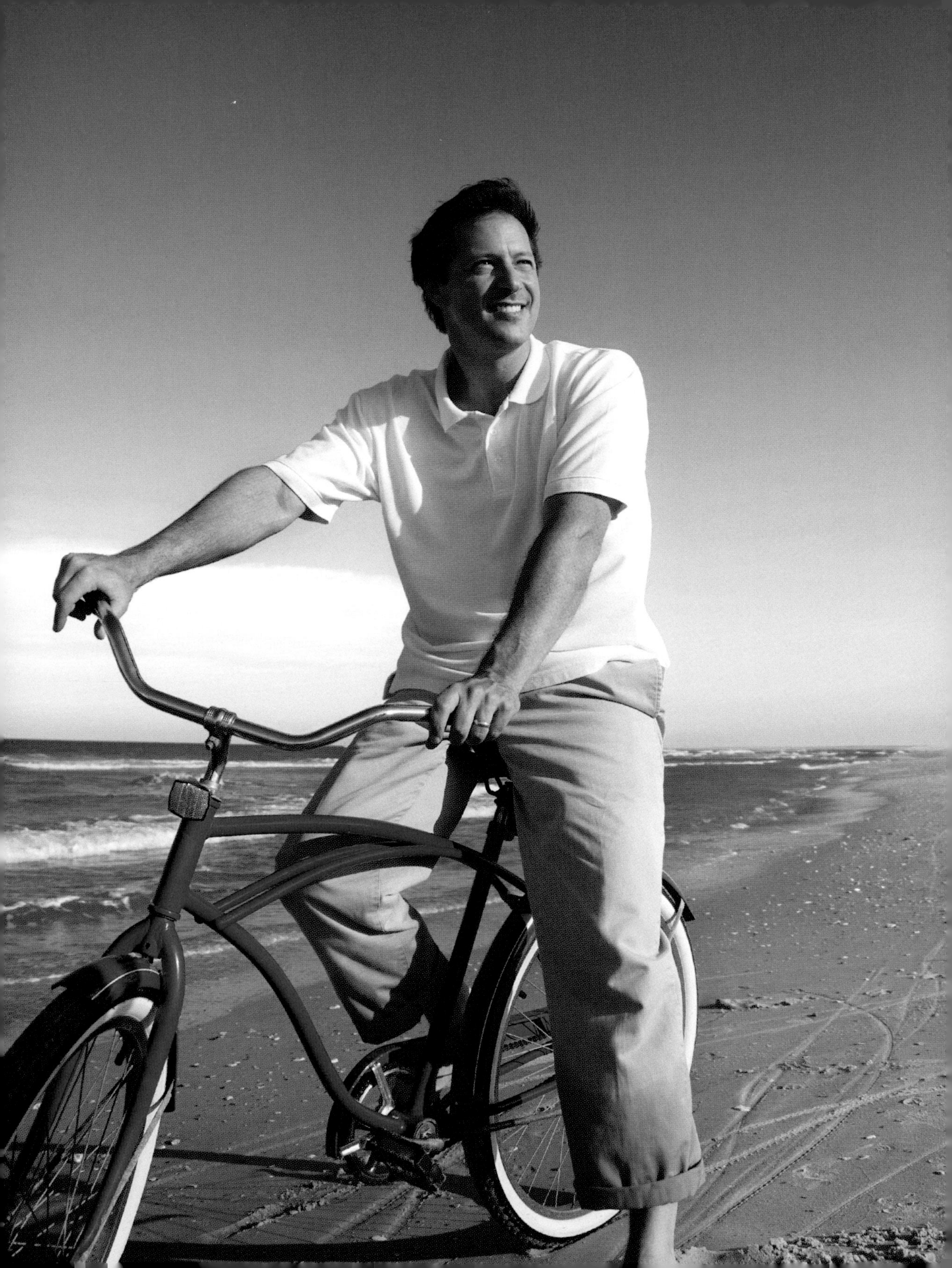

# LOOKING GOOD!

Now that you have decided to Eat Clean, now that you have committed to the lifestyle by firmly accepting the principles of Eating Clean, you are on your way to something totally unexpected. Success! Traditional diets based on eliminating certain macronutrients from your food intake cannot guarantee long-term success. As soon as you reintroduce that macronutrient into the diet, you will most likely regain the weight you have lost – and then some. Restrictive dieting doesn't work for the same reason. It works in the short term but not for life.

You cannot deny your body the essential nutrients it needs to build and maintain a robust physique. That is why Clean Eating is so different. Once you make the lifestyle changes of eating more frequently, eating slightly smaller portions, eating lean protein and complex carbohydrates at every meal, drinking more water and avoiding prepackaged and other quasi-foods, you will have learned a new set of eating skills that will take you long into your life, a life filled with health and vitality, which is how it was meant to be for each of us. By reading this book you are making an excellent choice. You will be glad you did. Now you can reveal the You that has been longing to get out from underneath the questions, the excess weight, the doubt and unhappiness that may have been plaguing you. Our wish is for you to discover your brilliance and live your life with so much energy that others will have a tough time keeping up with you. We know this will happen for you because it has happened for so many others once they began to Eat Clean. The same way the diet has been stripped of unfavorable pseudo-foods, harmful chemicals, unnecessary garbage – in short, all the waste that has been preventing you from being your best – you too will be stripped of the rubbish that may well be killing you.

[ You cannot deny your body the essential nutrients it needs to build and maintain a robust physique. ]

Now go put on your best suit, run the race of your life, play with your kids, make a flavorful wholesome supper, dance with your soul mate or dive into the nearest pool. Make your body an expression of joy. Make your life an example.

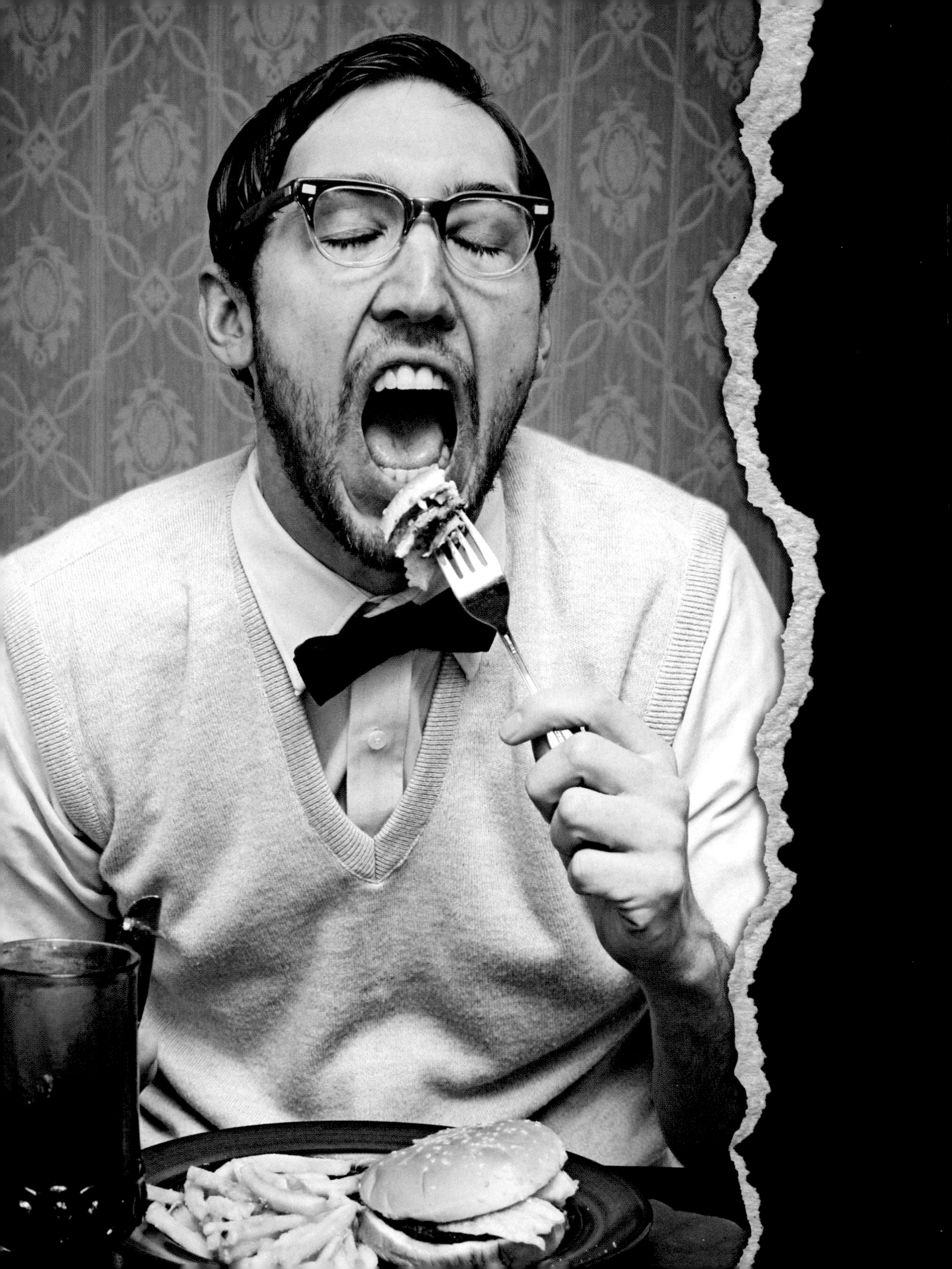

# [CHAPTER FOUR]

## 2,190 MEALS EACH YEAR!

## 2,190 MEALS

Familiarizing yourself with the habits of Clean Eating will help you adopt this wonderful lifestyle. One of the most important habits is eating more food but of better quality. You have to eat every day – that's 365 days and at least six meals per day – or 2,190 meals over the course of a year. It doesn't hurt to figure out how to get it right.

## PROTEIN – FIRST FOOD!

Looking down at a gorgeous piece of steak you are probably not thinking about how it holds one of the most essential keys to creating a stunning, streamlined physique. All you can think about is the delicious aroma wafting into your nose. The grill marks look beautiful, the smell is divine and you just want to devour it. Maybe it's easier to think about protein, the hardworking building block responsible for creating YOU, in the form of egg whites – you know; the runny, uncooked, white part of an egg. This inane-looking stuff is loaded with readily assimilated protein that helps turn you from flabby to tight and lean. Egg whites may not smell or look so good, but along with beef, poultry, fish, game, nuts, some cereals and legumes, they are a source of protein and can transform your body from ho-hum to extraordinary.

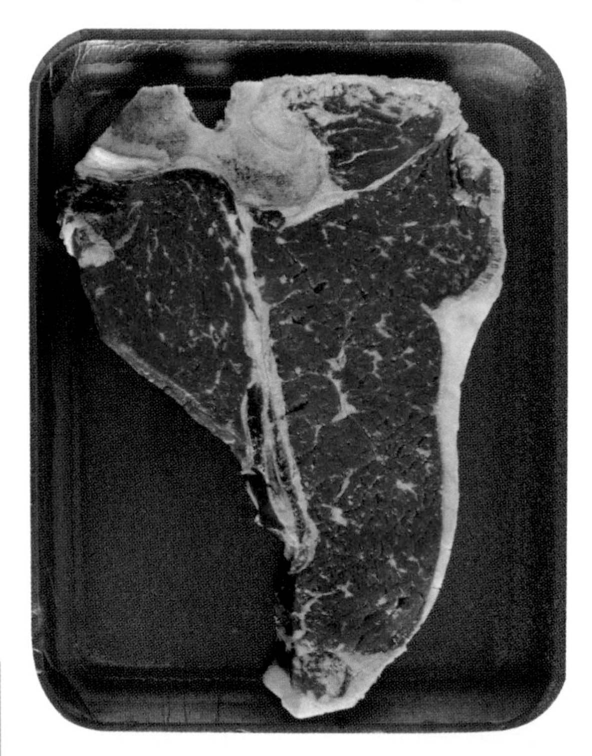

Protein is the hardworking substance that actually builds your body cell by cell, from the moment the egg and sperm meet in utero to the moment you end up six feet under. Every one of the approximately 100 trillion cells in your body uses protein to create muscle, bone and blood, and to produce the enzymes that drive body function. Enzymes are just specialized protein. Without protein, which must be consumed daily because the body cannot store it, we cannot survive. Proteins themselves are made up of 22 amino acids. These combine to form the more than 50,000 various proteins found in organs, nerves, muscles, flesh and bone. Protein is found in every single cell in the body. Humans are predominantly protein – look at your hands, they are made of protein. That steak you are about to eat will eventually end up repairing your eyes, your quadriceps muscles or tiny blood vessels deep in your abdominal cavity. Protein is the glue that binds and the stuff that builds.

## PROTEIN – WHAT IT DOES FOR YOU

- Maintains balanced blood-sugar levels – prediabetics and diabetics, this is important for you
- Encourages cell growth and repair
- Manufactures hormones
- Manufactures enzymes
- Drives cell metabolism
- Balances body fluids
- Strengthens immunity

## ANIMAL PROTEIN – SUPERIOR STUFF

Meat eaters have an easy time finding enough viable sources of protein, because animal protein is the only source of complete protein for humans. However, plants contain only incomplete protein, meaning their protein does not have adequate amounts of each of the eight essential amino acids. Vegetarians have a more difficult time of obtaining complete protein, since to do so they must combine pulses and grains. Think of Mexican food, which often combines corn and beans, Middle Eastern food, which combines wheat and chickpeas and Asian food, which combines rice and soy. Even then it is wise to include some animal proteins in the diet for best health. If your belief system allows it, include at least some eggs, dairy or fish in your diet.

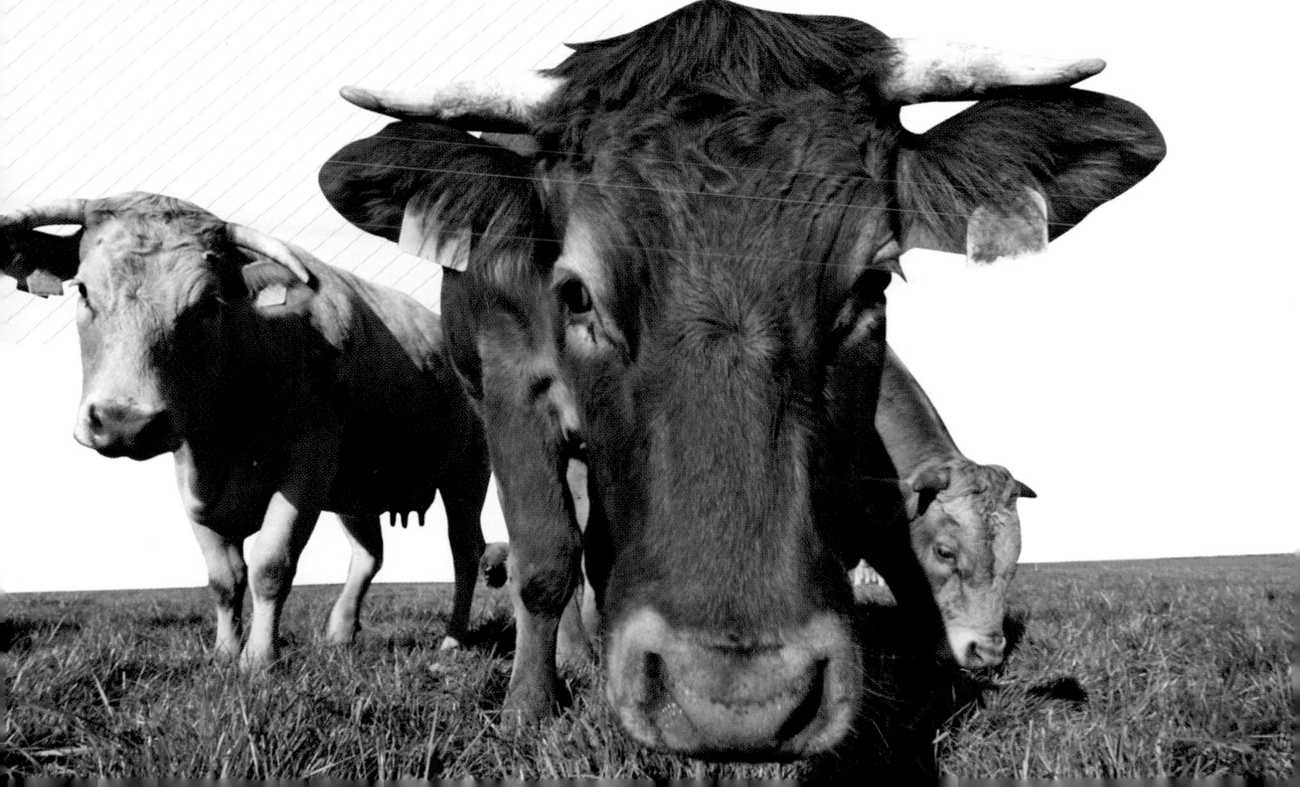

## VEGETARIAN PROTEIN COMBOS

| |
|---|
| Corn and beans |
| Soy and rice |
| Wheat and chickpeas |
| Legumes and nuts, seeds or grains |
| Beans on toast |
| Hummus and pita |
| Nut butter (any kind) on multi-grain bread |
| Pasta with beans |

**Protein Content of Some Foods:**

| | |
|---|---|
| **Six ounces fish** | = 45 grams |
| **Six ounces lean beef** | = 37.5 grams |
| **Six ounces turkey** | = 34 grams |
| **Six ounces chicken** | = 30 grams |
| **Six-and-a-half-ounce tin water-packed tuna** | = 50 grams |
| **Four ounces 1% cottage cheese** | = 14 grams |
| **One cup 1% milk** | = 8.5 grams |
| **One egg** | = 7 grams |

## PROTEIN AND CLEAN EATING – THE MAGIC COMBINATION

Why is protein considered essential to creating a lean physique? The reasons are many, but foremost now that you are Eating Clean is that you will need to keep a steady supply of protein in the bloodstream. Protein in your body undergoes a constant state of exchange in and out of body tissues. It is essential to keep plenty of it flowing through you to encourage the removal of flabby fatty tissue and the growth of lean muscle tissue. Protein is digested slowly and therefore helps maintain blood-sugar levels.

Six ounces = 30 grams of protein

# EGGS – THE GOLD STANDARD

The egg is considered the gold standard for protein. It contains readily available, easily digestible high-quality protein, which coincidentally happens to be reasonably inexpensive. An egg can be examined two ways – with or without the yolk. Yolks are loaded with nutrients, particularly lecithin, protein, healthy fats, calcium, phosphorus, iron, sodium, potassium and vitamin A. However, if you are planning to consume more than one or two eggs each day, it is probably wise not to eat every yolk. They contain all the fat in eggs, and there is some argument that they contain too much cholesterol. Several years ago eggs got a bad rap for causing high cholesterol, but these days the debate is open over the validity of this assertion. To be cautious, as is wise, try eating one yolk for every four or five egg whites.

## AHHH! PROTEIN

Protein is critical to shaping that new physique of yours when Eating Clean, because it is the only nutrient that directly feeds your muscles. You may not have had enough protein today, or possibly ever, since most North Americans have an easier time reaching for a sugary snack than a chicken breast or a boiled egg. However, if you don't keep a steady drip of protein running into your bloodstream your body will actually begin to catabolize itself. That sounds scary, and it is. Catabolism is when the body breaks itself down. It is the opposite of anabolic processes, wherein the body builds itself. You don't want to put yourself in a state of catabolism.

Getting enough protein every day is one of the surest ways to build the body and drive the metabolism, which helps burn fat. Certain foods actually feed your metabolism. The body, made predominantly of protein and driven by this thing called metabolism, needs to consume protein to keep the cycle going. Look at the lists of foods our ancestors ate on page 26. They depended heavily on protein. Even societies considered vegetarian, of which there were few, ate bugs and their larvae because they knew the value of protein.

Once in the body, protein stimulates all metabolically active muscle (that is, lean muscle tissue) and the fat-burning hormone glucagon. Something else happens too. When protein is consumed it needs to be digested. Your body works hard to break down protein fibers in the gut and digestive tract, even after you have done a fair job of chewing it.

Now think of a furnace blasting out heat. Thermogenesis is your metabolic furnace throwing out heat in your body by burning up fat stores and tearing up protein molecules. This occurs as your bite of steak travels further into the gut. Highly thermogenic foods include lean chicken or turkey breast, egg whites, fish, grass-fed lean red meats and wild game, including venison and elk. Although protein powders have flooded the shelves in many forms and varieties, the more work you have to do to break the protein down the higher the thermogenic effect. So try to depend on whole-food protein sources for the most part and use protein powders only to supplement your diet or when you are in a pinch.

## PROTEIN AND CARBS – EAT THEM TOGETHER

Carbohydrates have been much misunderstood of late thanks to fad diets suggesting they be omitted entirely from your diet. Ridiculous! Have you ever tried to function on no carbohydrates? It is virtually impossible to perform even the simplest task once this super-nutrient is no longer present. You feel shaky, weak and completely exhausted.

## PORTION SIZES FIT FOR A MAN!

Most diets tell you exactly what to eat in exactly which amounts. No wonder men hate to diet! The portion sizes they give you are usually created for a 5'2" woman. The poor 6'4" man who thinks he can follow these diets will soon be so hungry he'll be stopping for a greasy burger.

One of the many great things about Eating Clean is that your "diet" is tailored to you. You eat the foods you like (as long as you follow the Eat-Clean principles) and you eat them in the portions right for you. How do you know what portions are right for you? Glad you asked! Look to the right for our "handy" portion guide!

## PROPER PORTION SIZES

1 serving lean protein = **palm of your hand**

1 serving of starchy complex carbs from whole grains or starchy fruit and vegetables = **one cupped hand**

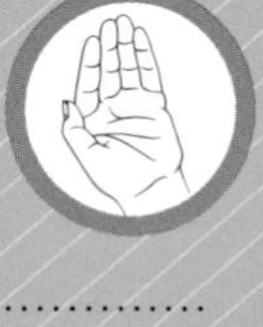

1 serving of complex carbs from fresh fruits or vegetables = **two cupped hands together**

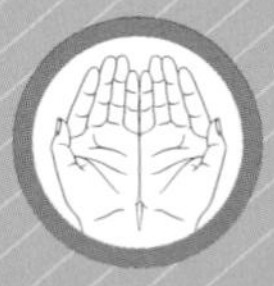

Carbohydrates provide an important source of energy necessary for optimal bodily function and for the maintenance of a lean, healthy physique. Choosing the right ones can mean the difference between weak and strong, overweight and lean or sickly and healthy.

Carbohydrates are found in plants where the sun, along with carbon dioxide and water, created this starch and sugar molecule. When you munch on fresh fruits and vegetables or whole grains and process these foods in your digestive tract, glucose is released into the bloodstream as the primary source of readily available energy. Complex carbohydrates from green plants and whole grains are what you will depend on along with lean protein for your Clean-Eating energy.

Refined carbohydrates are another matter. According to Sally Fallon, author of *Nourishing Traditions,* "Only during the last century has man's diet included a high percentage of refined carbohydrates. Our ancestors ate fruits and grains in their whole, unrefined state. In nature, sugars and carbohydrates – the energy providers – are linked together with vitamins, minerals, enzymes, protein, fat and fiber – the bodybuilding and digestion-regulating components of the diet. In whole form sugars and starches support life, but refined carbohydrates are inimical to life because they are devoid of bodybuilding elements. Digestion of refined carbohydrates calls on the body's own store of vitamins, minerals and enzymes for proper metabolism." Refining carbohydrates strips from food the ingredients most needed for optimal health. The carbohydrates you need are those in their most natural state, including fruits, vegetables and whole grains. Avoid foods such as white breads, sugary breakfast cereals, doughnuts, cakes, cookies, pastries and junk foods if you wish to keep your nutrition lean and clean.

Your energy levels, as well as your muscle-building and fat-burning power, depend heavily on complex carbohydrates since they are the cleanest-burning source of fuel. Your body will always reach for complex carbohydrates first when searching for an energy source – it is the preferred fuel for the body. This is how nature has designed us – to reach for carbs first, leaving protein available to do its main job of repairing and building the body. Eating protein with complex carbs at every meal is the ideal energy combination. It helps to offset the fuel-storage mode – fat – so the body uses immediately available energy – glucose – instead. As Fallon says, "Our physical nature is such that we need foods that are whole, not refined and denatured, to grow, prosper and reproduce. As the consumption of sugar has increased so have all the 'civilized' diseases."

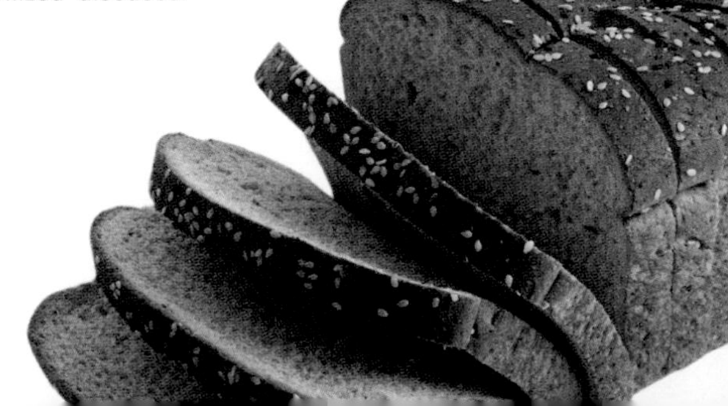

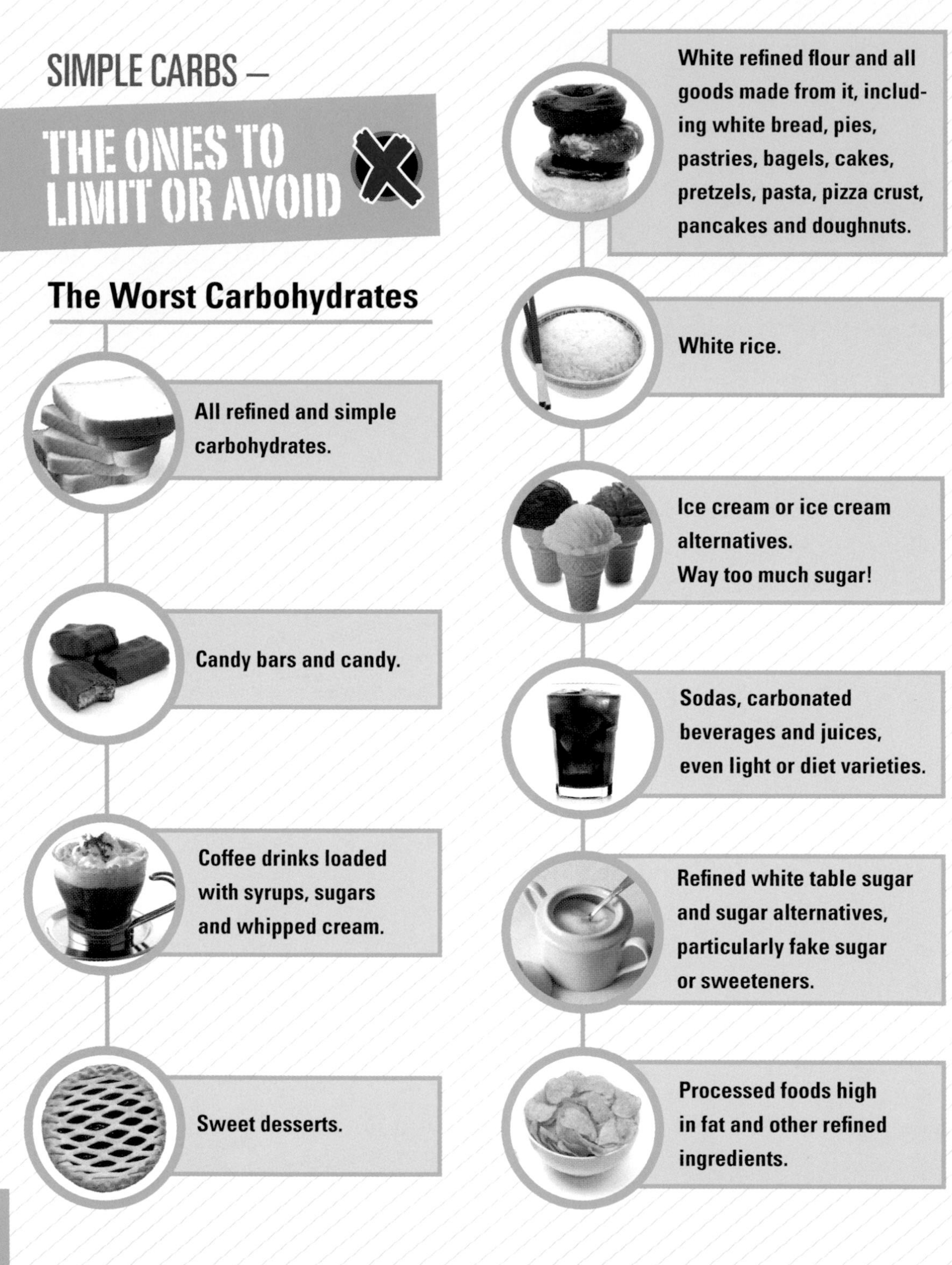
SIMPLE CARBS –
THE ONES TO LIMIT OR AVOID
The Worst Carbohydrates
All refined and simple carbohydrates.
Candy bars and candy.
Coffee drinks loaded with syrups, sugars and whipped cream.
Sweet desserts.
White refined flour and all goods made from it, including white bread, pies, pastries, bagels, cakes, pretzels, pasta, pizza crust, pancakes and doughnuts.
White rice.
Ice cream or ice cream alternatives. Way too much sugar!
Sodas, carbonated beverages and juices, even light or diet varieties.
Refined white table sugar and sugar alternatives, particularly fake sugar or sweeteners.
Processed foods high in fat and other refined ingredients.

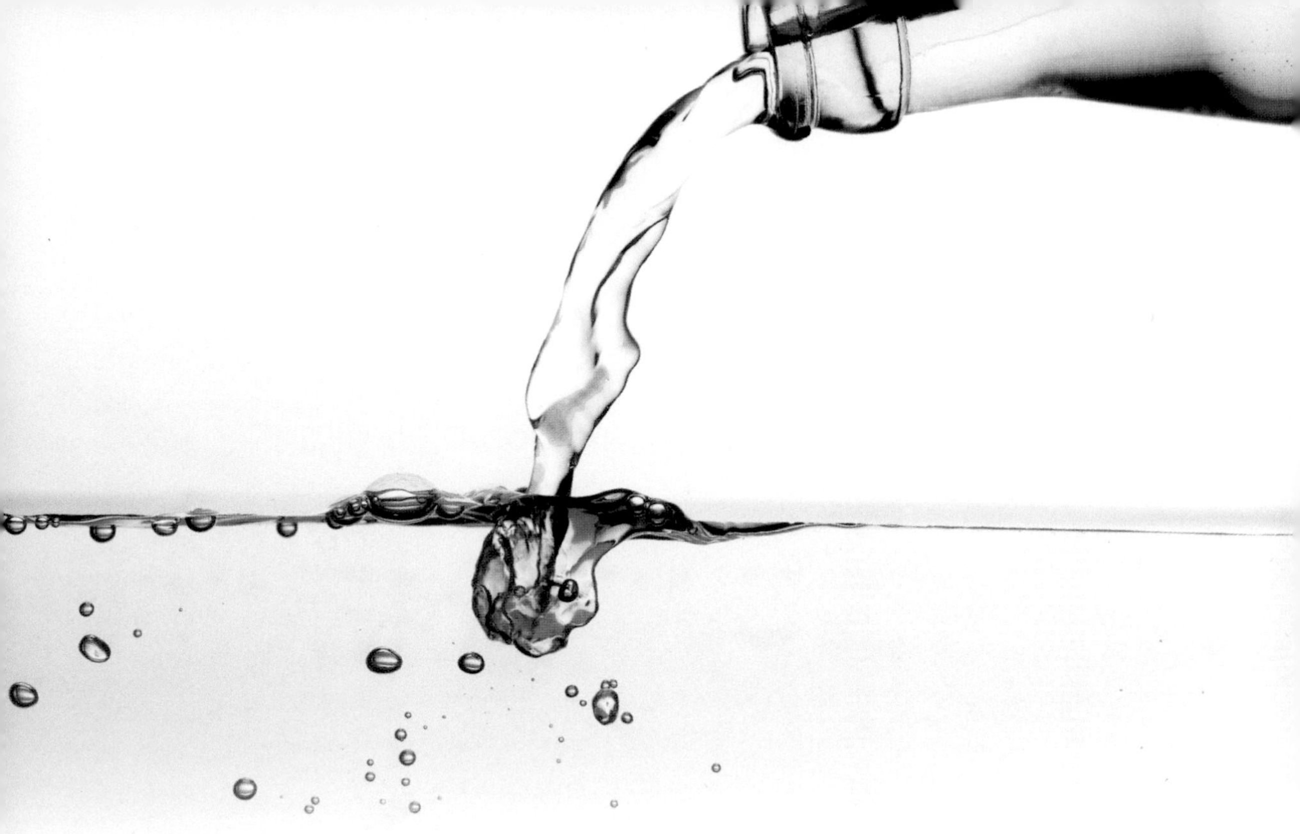

## DRINK UP!

Did you know you can increase your metabolism by three percent simply by drinking lots of water? Yet many of us allow ourselves to become dehydrated, which slows the metabolism by 10 percent. The reason is that your kidneys do the job of filtering waste from the body, but if you have shortchanged yourself on water and the kidneys run out they will borrow from the liver. Then the liver must multitask and cannot properly do its primary job, which is fat burning. All this can be avoided by drinking sufficient water. This is the simplest, smartest thing you can do for yourself today. Switch to water over the soda you have been drinking!

Water is almost too simple an ingredient to think about for most of you. However, if you were in the unfortunate situation that you didn't have water you would die within a week. Then you would realize how necessary the clear liquid is.

## WHAT KIND SHOULD I DRINK?

What kind of water should you drink? You have mineral water, hard water, soft water, distilled or purified water. There are dozens to choose from lately, but what about good old tap water? Hard water, which is what we find pouring out of the tap at our home, contains loads of minerals, necessary for good health. If you can't get enough minerals out of the ground

FACT

Two-thirds of the body is water, so it makes sense to maintain adequate hydration.

due to poor soil quality, then you can drink your minerals right out of a glass. Soft water has no value to you except for keeping your pipes clean and free of calcium and lime deposits. It contains no minerals whatsoever but loads of salt. Studies show there is a greater risk of cancer, heart attack and stroke in those who drink softened water.

And then you have to worry about pollutants and toxins in the water. With the increased use of chemicals of every description in virtually every human activity it is difficult to get away from polluted water. It seems that drinking something as simple as water may indeed be very complicated. It turns out that the best water you can drink and possibly the least expensive is the water out of your tap. But it is a good idea to attach a carbon or ceramic filter to the nozzle to remove heavy metals, chlorine and other chemicals.

## THE QUESTION IS, "HOW MUCH?"

The debate over how much water to drink each day has raged long and hard. An active person needs to replace at least what is lost in a given day, which tends to be around two to three liters, or eight to twelve 8-ounce cups of water. In our house we drink eight ounces of warm water mixed with the juice of one lemon each morning before consuming anything else. Then with breakfast we drink another eight ounces of water mixed with six ounces of wheat grass. Throughout the day we continue to drink water from a Sigg bottle, especially if we have just done a heavy workout or a cardio session. The reusable Sigg water bottle originates from Switzerland and is made of aluminum. Nothing leaches into the water inside the bottle, and you can readily measure the amount of water you are drinking. We are not paid to endorse the container, we just like the idea that it is both healthy and environmentally friendly. Lots of other aluminum and stainless steel bottles are being produced these days, so you should be able to find one pretty easily.

Two-thirds of the body is water, so it makes sense to maintain adequate hydration. If you are a big tea, coffee or carbonated beverage drinker you should be drinking more water than most, since these all deplete the body of water. Water in good supply in your pipes will keep your body working properly on all levels, including elimination of waste material, both solid and liquid, regulation of your body temperature, production of digestive enzymes, distribution of nutrients to all parts of the body and maintenance of healthy organs, skin and hair.

# THIRSTY? TOO LATE!

**Pay attention to these signs of thirst:**

- Fatigue
- Dark urine
- Loss of appetite
- Poor concentration
- Skin flushes
- Clumsiness
- Dizziness or light-headedness

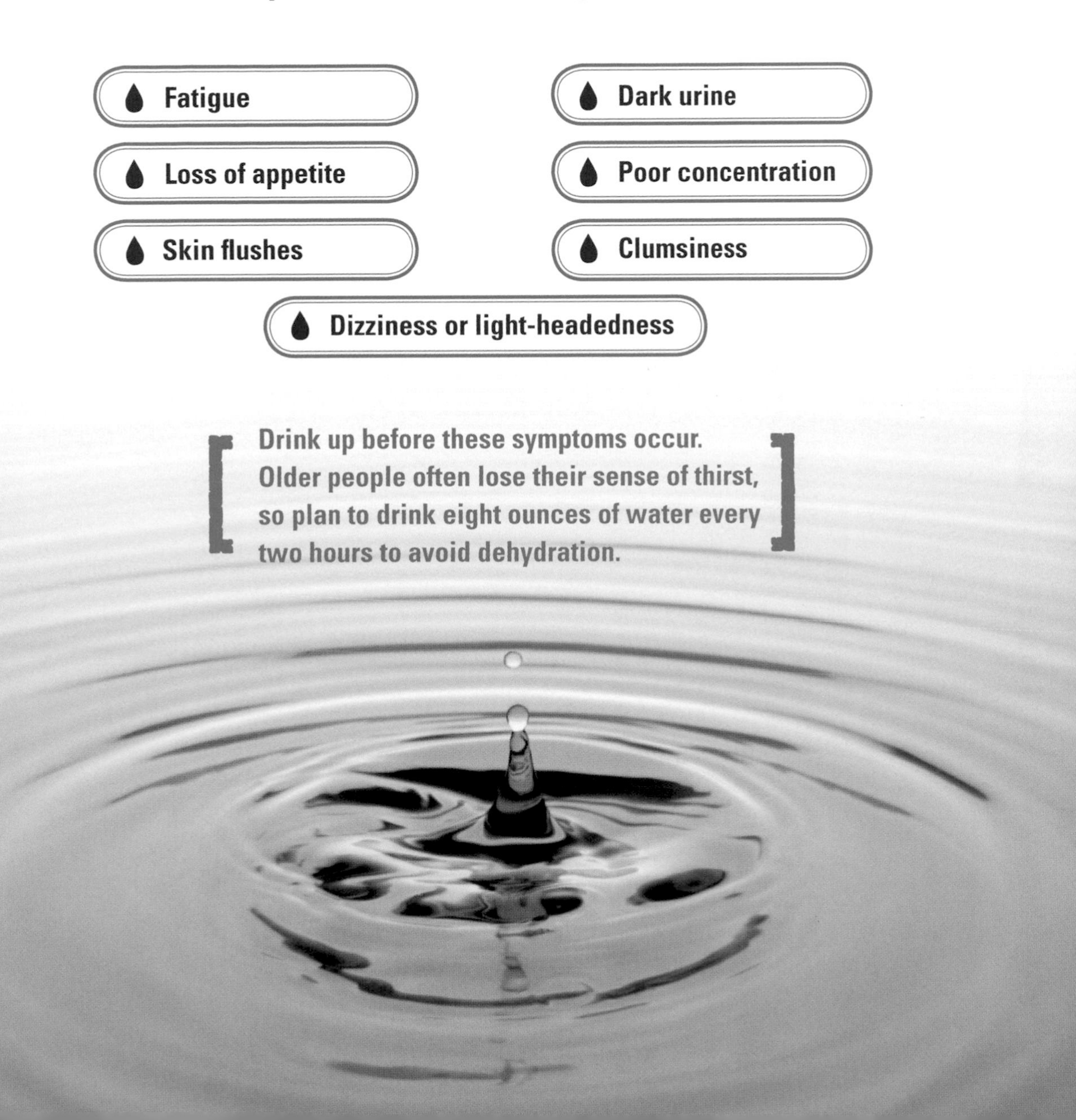

[ Drink up before these symptoms occur. Older people often lose their sense of thirst, so plan to drink eight ounces of water every two hours to avoid dehydration. ]

Lean protein eaten with complex carbohydrates will fuel the transformation while water completes the job.

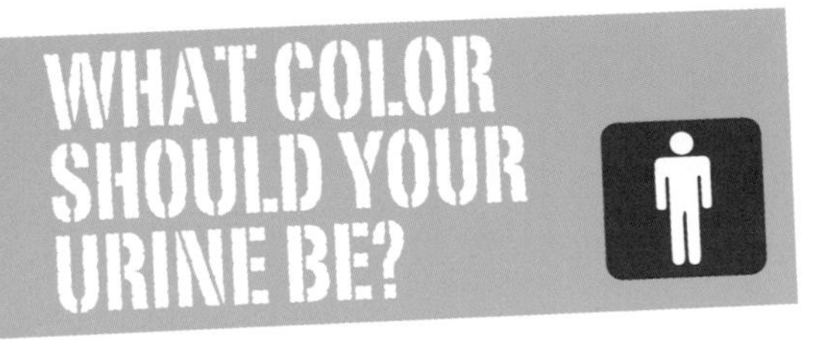


- The ideal color for urine should be light yellow with no smell.
- Dark or golden urine with a strong smell is a sign you are dehydrated.
- Eating beets or asparagus can throw off both the smell and color of your urine, so don't be fooled.

## EAT CLEAN FOR YOUR BEST HEALTH!

Now you have a good idea of which foods are best for shaping this new, chiseled physique you have always wanted to own. Lean protein eaten with complex carbohydrates will fuel the transformation while water completes the job. Next, we will show you how to set yourself up with the best foods to accomplish the task.

## EAT-CLEAN SUCCESS STORY!

**Christine Johnson**
From an email dated July 23, 2008

*My husband Bryan is Navajo and has been battling diabetes since gaining weight in his mid-20s. Shortly before his father died of the disease, Bryan was close to 340 pounds. Because of his father's ailing health Bryan took it upon himself to try to teach his father, as well as himself, about eating healthy. You must understand that the Navajo diet consisted of fry bread (cooked in lard), mutton (not lamb, but greasy sheep), corn stew (loaded with leftover sheep meat and fat) and potatoes – in other words, very unhealthy! Bryan began living on chicken and steamed veggies every day with oatmeal in the mornings. With this diet Bryan lost just under 100 pounds! Clean Eating was his method, even though he had not heard of your concept. After the death of his father, he continued to walk twice a day, which turned into jogging up to three-and-a-half miles. (He was never able to do this as a kid.) He*

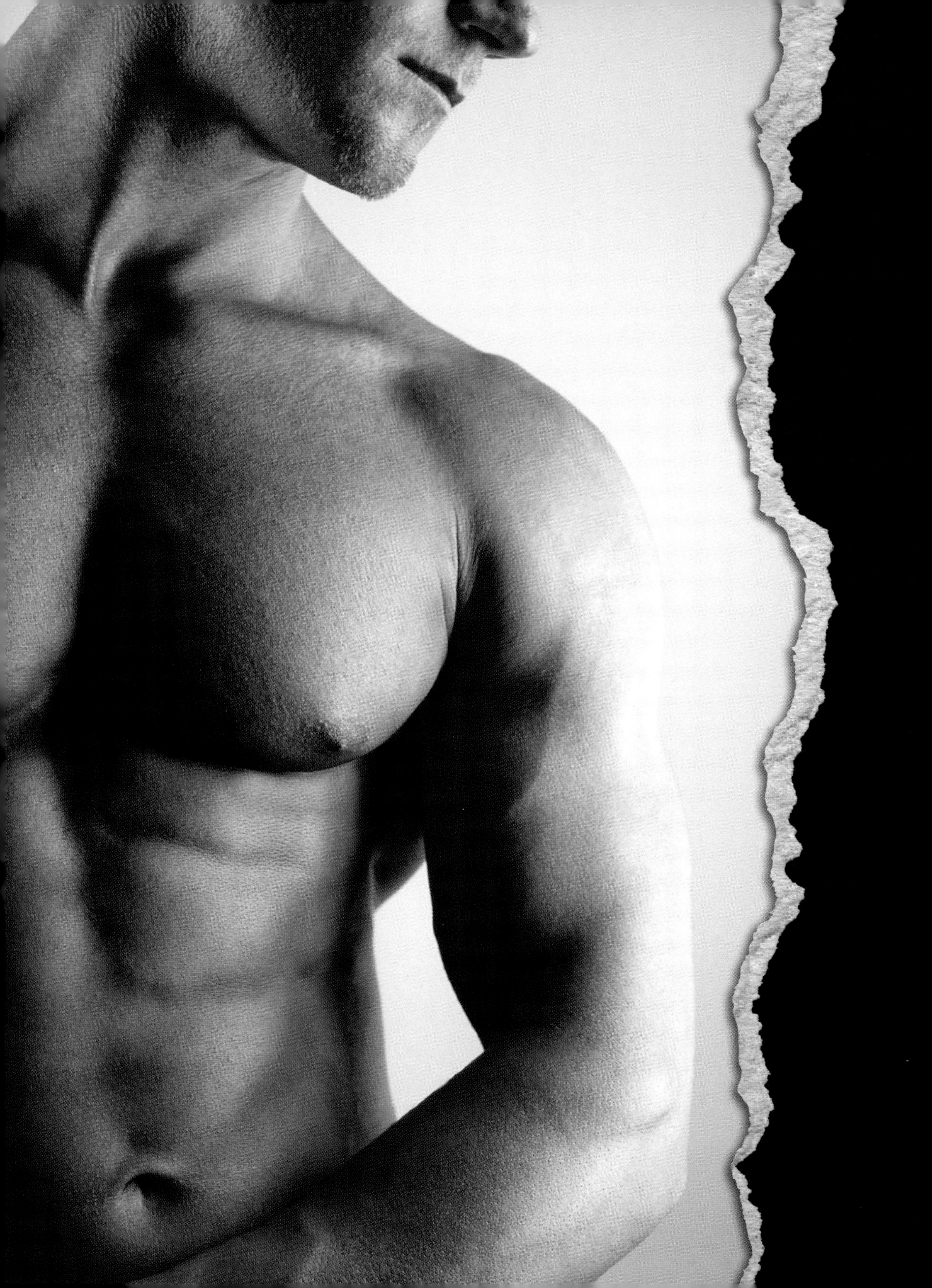

# [CHAPTER FIVE]

# CLEAN-EATING RESULTS

## WHAT WILL I SEE?

When embarking on a diet, most of us want the visual results right away. It's as if you have made up your mind to run the race of your life, putting all your energy into it right then, only to discover you will have to train for a month – or longer – before you run it. Unfortunately, dieting is a lot like that – hurry up and wait. How will starting the Clean-Eating lifestyle be any different? If you are expecting dramatic results you won't be disappointed; but they will probably not arrive tomorrow. The process of becoming overweight and unhealthy took some time. Years and years of poor eating habits and lack of exercise helped you get that way. To lose weight in an intelligent manner you will need to be patient and let the little changes add up to big change.

## EAT-CLEAN SUCCESS STORY!

**Stephanie's Dad**

From an email dated July 10, 2008

*This story is not about me – it is about my 68-year-old father. I purchased a copy of your* Eat-Clean Diet *book for my stepmother (who is really into health and fitness) and she subsequently purchased a copy of your* Eat-Clean Diet Cookbook *for herself. She has been cooking from your book exclusively for the past two months. I would like to share a bit of news I got today from my stepmother with respect to my father.*

*She said that when he had his three-month checkup at the gym he goes to regularly (he likes to keep active now but didn't always eat the best) the trainer was astonished to find that he had lost seven percent body fat since his last checkup. She was very curious to find out what he was doing differently. He said that he had just been eating different foods his wife had been making from your cookbook and that he had changed nothing else. My father has never been fat per se, but just not in the best shape.*

*I am so proud that a man of 68 years of age is able to lose seven percent body fat in a matter of months. He looks great, feels great and is leaner and more cut. Obviously your strategies work very well for people of all ages. See what a little common sense can do?*

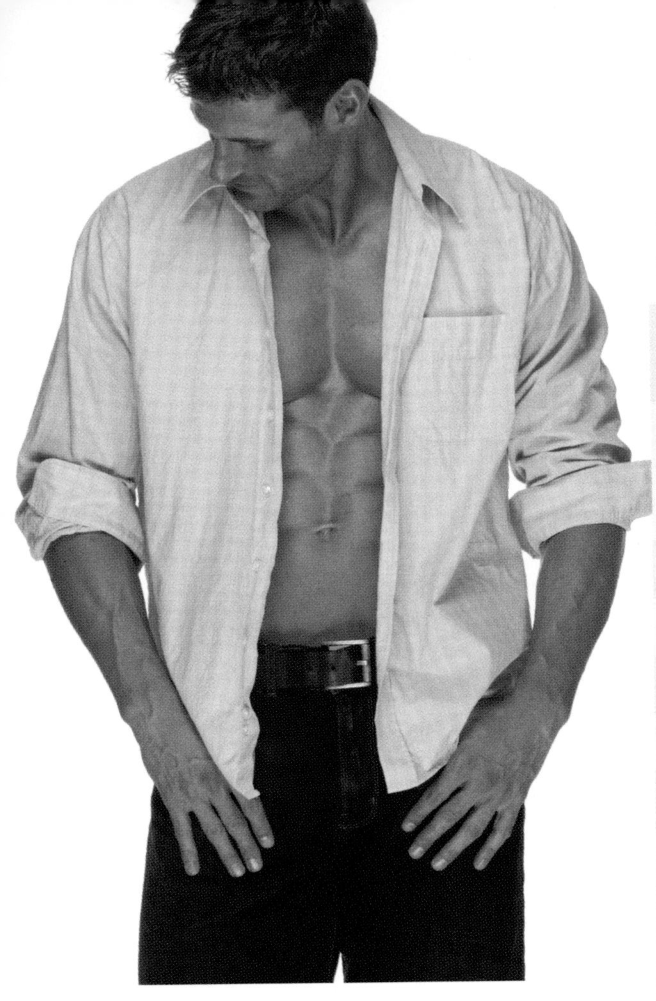

In general, once you begin to Eat Clean you can expect to see any or all of the following results:

- **An average weight loss of three pounds each week until you get to your ideal weight.**
- **Some people who have a great deal of excess weight will lose as much as 10 to 15 pounds in the first week.**
- **Increased energy.**
- **Increased libido.**
- **Fewer headaches.**
- **Fewer cravings.**
- **Improved sleep.**
- **Radiant skin.**
- **Stronger fingernails.**
- **Lustrous hair.**
- **Improved elimination.**
- **Stronger immune system.**
- **Improved fertility.**
- **Stabilized blood-sugar levels.**

## THE RESULTS

So you see, there is much to expect from beginning to Eat Clean. An older man changed his whole body simply by changing what went into his mouth. He can expect to live a full, active life rather than be chained to machines and equipment. Another younger man altered his entire physique from being obese – the medical definition of obesity is having 30 pounds or more excess weight in fat – to ripped and lean. Your own expectations may fall somewhere in between these two, but certainly you have expectations.

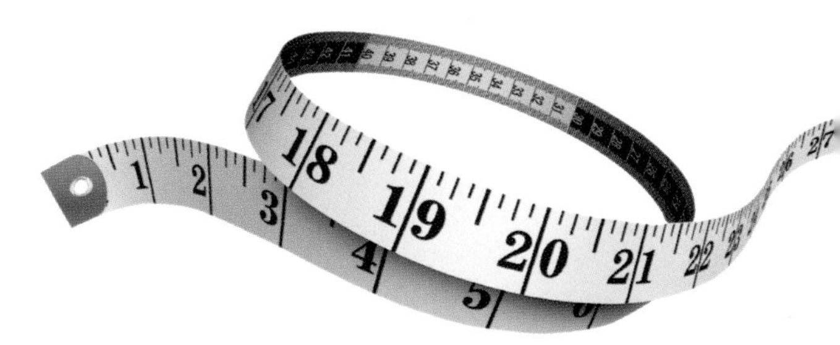

# EAT-CLEAN SUCCESS STORY!

From an email dated October 7, 2008

**Josh Levy**

*Dear Tosca,*

*My family, friends and coworkers have often asked me, "How did you do it? What's the secret? How did you lose all that weight and build all that muscle all at the same time?" My answer is simple: "*The Eat-Clean Diet *by Tosca Reno."*

*My journey began about a year ago when I weighed 180 pounds and measured 28 percent body fat. I was the heaviest I had ever been and was eating more than I had before. My pants size peaked at 36 in the waist. I was depressed that even with all the exercise I was doing five days a week I was not shedding any fat. Through the loving kindness of my wife, I stumbled across two of your books,* The Eat-Clean Diet *and* The Eat-Clean Diet Cookbook. *We began reading your ideas and theories behind what Clean Eating really was, and clearly what we were doing was nothing of the sort. It only took less than a week to realize breakfast, lunch, dinner and snacks were not only easy to make, but fantastic to eat!! I felt like I was never hungry, eating four to five meals a day. In fact, at times I questioned how this could even help me lose weight.*

*My transformation was such that literally within a month of Clean Eating my coworkers were already recognizing that I had trimmed down and looked better than ever.*

*I am now 140 pounds, with 10 percent body fat and at the age of 31 never looked better in my entire life. I thank you, Tosca, for providing me with the tools to aid me in my transformation and lifestyle change I live by each and every day. Oh, did I forget to mention that my pants size is now 30 in the waist?*

*Sincerely,*
*Josh Levy*

# EATING CLEAN YIELDS MORE THAN JUST WEIGHT LOSS

## THE RESULTS I CAN'T SEE

Neither of us are doctors, nor do we claim to be. But we know from the many letters and emails we receive that Eating Clean helps in many medical ways too. Many people have told us that they were able to minimize their diabetes medications when they began to Eat Clean. Others still have told us they were able to go off their medications completely. Such is the power of the Eat-Clean diet.

Making wholesome, natural foods your first choice at mealtimes will also affect many changes in the body that you cannot see. At a microscopic level body chemistry is dramatically altered once these nutrients are introduced. Where blood was once thick it can flow more freely, bringing nutrients to every cell of your body.

## WHAT WILL YOUR SUCCESS BE?

No matter what your goals are, when Eating Clean you will reach them in a healthy, long-lasting way. Many fad diets depend on dangerous restrictive eating methods or ask you to omit entire food groups. Clean Eating embraces all healthy food groups – lean protein from animal and vegetable sources, complex carbohydrates from fresh fruit and vegetables and also from whole grains, in addition to healthy fats. Eating foods like these in their most natural forms will virtually ensure improved health as soon as you start eating them. So not only will you lose weight if that is your goal, but you will also gain the most desirable goal of them all – excellent health. Without it, you have nothing!

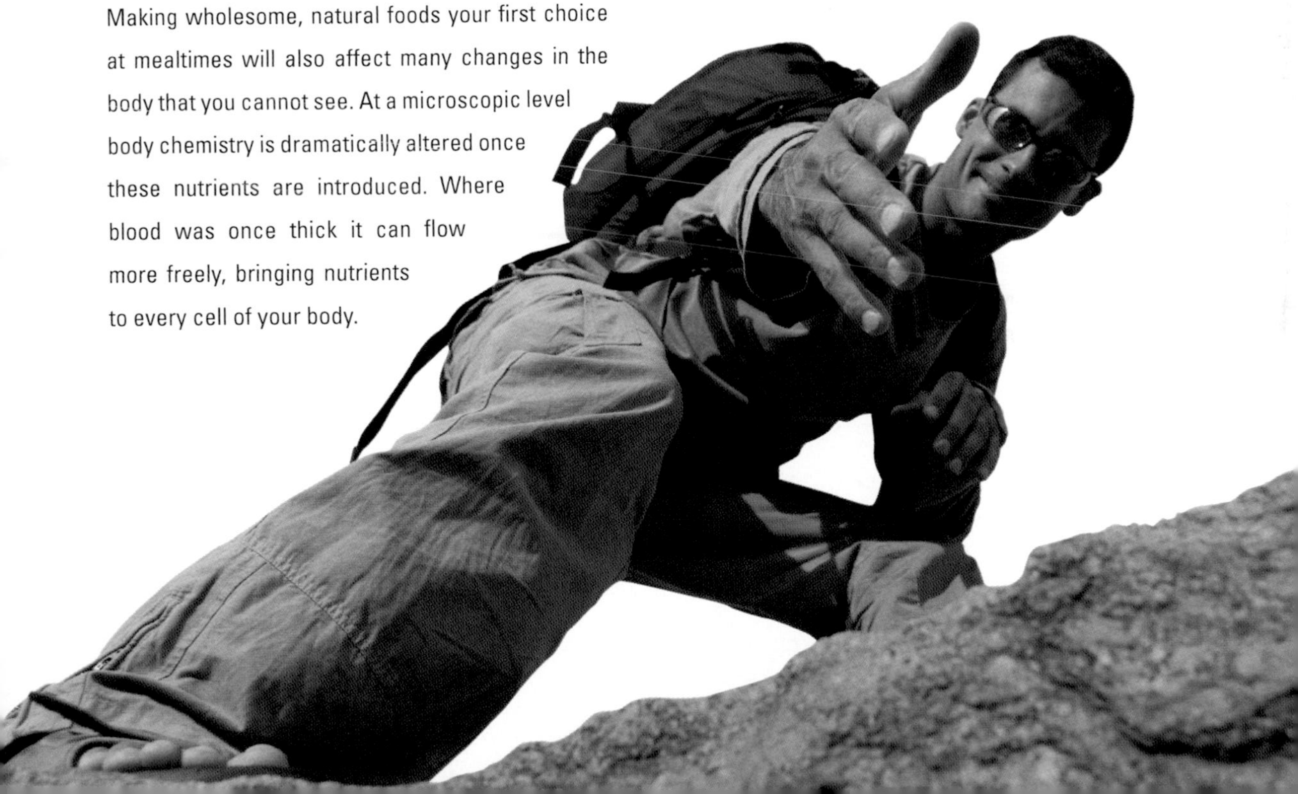

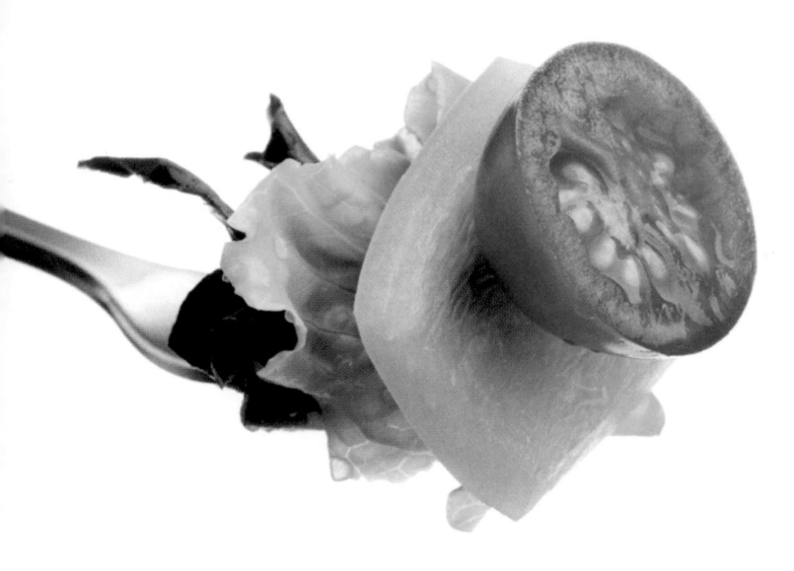

Your best life is yet to come and it's as simple as choosing powerfully nutritious, Clean foods.

## HOW WILL I FEEL?

Most of you will feel wonderful right from the start. The increase in energy levels alone is enough to make you jump for joy. You should get through the afternoons easily instead of hitting a wall. You may notice that you feel less irritable. Often food additives make us grouchy and uncomfortable. Once you begin to eliminate these from the diet it can be totally amazing! Your thoughts become clear. You can remember things more readily. You begin to feel like your old self – the one that used to be healthy and vibrant.

Some of you will find the first few days somewhat uncomfortable. You will be the fellows who have had steady dates with chips, nachos, beer, fries, pizza, fast food, giant burgers and all those other foods that don't qualify as Clean foods. Should we call them dirty foods? Exchanging junk for treasure – that is garbage foods for Clean foods – will cause you to ultimately feel better, but initially you may suffer some detox woes. When your body works to rid itself of chemicals, fat, preservatives, refined foods and other toxins, you may experience more headaches, more irritability and more discomfort. But be patient and stick with the plan because these minor discomforts will pass very soon. Then you will be on your way to the best that Eating Clean has to offer you.

If you have been struggling with other health issues, the new lifestyle of Eating Clean will help you regain your former robust health. Many health problems, including cardiovascular disease, impotence, stroke, hypertension, certain cancers, metabolic disorders, diabetes and more are positively affected by feeding yourself with higher quality, natural foods. Your best life is yet to come and it's as simple as choosing powerfully nutritious, Clean foods.

# EAT-CLEAN SUCCESS STORY!

**Bradley Rauscher**
From an email dated August 3, 2008

*My story: It started when I was a junior in high school. I was diagnosed with epilepsy. The doctors put me on a medication to control my seizures and the effects of the medicine were hard on my health. The medicine they put me on also doubled as an anti-depressant. Since I was not depressed my attitude and my emotional state was that of a log. All I wanted to do was lie around and watch television and eat. The meds increased my appetite and I gained 65 pounds in less than 15 months. With no one coming alongside me to advise on diet and exercise, it was plain to see the path of weight gain that I headed down. After five years I started new medicine and a new life when I began to prepare for college. When I transferred to the school I also lived in a dorm where food was very accessible. I made a decision to eat right and exercise. And I did. I lost 45 pounds and was doing great until I moved out the next year. Food was no longer convenient and healthy but convenient and unhealthy as I began to eat out for almost every meal. Needless to say after four years I gained it all back and then some.*

*Before I read your book I was at my heaviest ever at 255 pounds and I began to think, "It's all over; I am on the closer side to 300 pounds." I thought that no matter what I did I would always be fat. Now if it wasn't for my wonderful wife who encouraged me every step along the way I don't know where I would be today. She and I picked up a copy of your* Eat-Clean Diet *book and began to read it together. It was important information; not just to improve our looks, but we wanted to be healthy and happy for as long as the Lord would allow. I was very happy with the layout and how easy it was to follow. My wife started to implement Clean Eating a little over two months ago and I feel better and am dropping fat – 15 pounds and my clothes are loose and I can't wait for the end goal of having all the confidence. It's just around the corner. This also could not come at a better time for my wife and me because we are newly expecting. Thanks again, Tosca!*

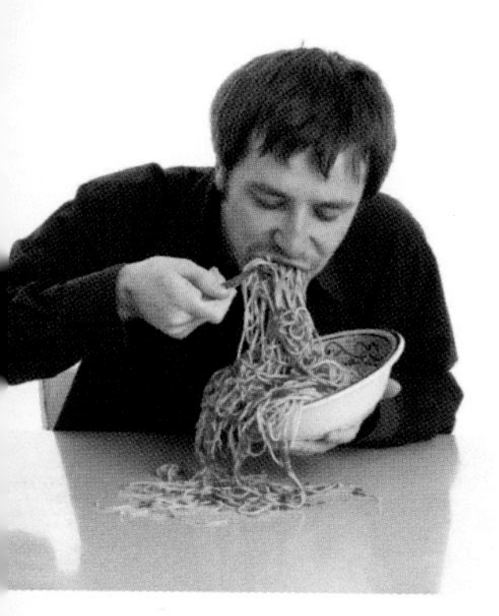

## HOW TO GAIN – NOT LOSE

Some of you wish to gain rather than lose pounds. While you may not garner much sympathy from the portly crowd, we understand what that feels like. We both tend to be the ectomorphic, skinny types who are always running around doing things. Our metabolisms seem to always be running at full speed. It is extremely difficult for us to sit and chill. But take our word for it – you will need to learn how to relax and stay still in order to gain some good muscular weight.

We often take a time-out after a workout. We mix up a couple of protein shakes and sit down to *Seinfeld* or *Frasier* reruns with our feet up. Rest helps your body take the protein you are drinking straight into the trillions of muscle cells you have broken down during your workout. While the protein and rest are feeding these cells, you are recuperating. Your heart rate comes down and your metabolism settles into a less frenetic pace. Such rests are not to be considered wussy or wimpy. They are musts!

You may also be surprised to learn that in order to gain weight you must do some of the exact same things as to lose weight. Yes you must! Here is where Eating Clean comes in handy. Using the structure of this healthy lifestyle helps you program regular feedings into your day. Every three hours you are required to nosh on high-quality foods. You may even have to eat every two-and-a-half hours, depending on the rate of your metabolism.

The other component that completes your weight-gain strategy is to eat only the best-quality foods. That doesn't mean the most expensive steak. It means eating foods that deliver the highest quality nutrition. You can't afford to fill up on empty, refined, white, over-processed foods. That won't work. Your body will gain weight on foods densely packed with fiber, nutrients, healthy fats, complex carbohydrates and protein. This is true body-building stuff! It is folly to think a bag of Doritos is going to do the trick. That is like sending a boy in to do a man's job. Depend on whole grains such as brown rice, oatmeal, quinoa, wheat germ and other grains of that ilk along with plenty of vegetables of all colors (especially green); they will work wonders for you. Fruit also delivers a load of enzymes and nutrients that round out proper nutrition.

When considering your approach to training, you might have to do things a little differently. In general you will need to increase the intensity of your workouts but decrease the number of sets and reps. This translates into lifting heavier but doing only 6 to 8 repetitions of an exercise. Also, rather than doing 10 sets for any one body part, perform 6. The point here is to break down enough muscle tissue during your workout that your muscles will be rebuilt bigger than they were before, but not break down so much that your rebuilding process can't keep up.

After each workout it's essential to down 20 to 30 grams of lean protein – animal, vegetable or otherwise – in order to begin the cell-rebuilding process. Developing this habit of loading up on protein immediately after training is probably your most effective strategy for laying on healthy lean muscle tissue. Who wants to put weight on in the form of a dozen Dunkin' Donuts? That is not the way to go!

Are you a smoker? Do you jiggle your legs when you are sitting? Always nervous and restless? Even peculiarities like these will need to be minimized in order to allow the body to generate size. Ideally smoking would be best left to the remains of a campfire. Smoking destroys a body in numerous ways, including increasing your risk of developing disease and in many other ways we don't fully understand. Drop the habit if you can.

**In summary, if you own a "rocket metabolism" thanks to genetics you will need to do the following:**

- **Eat more frequently.**
- **Eat nutrient-dense foods.**
- **Increase the intensity of your training by lifting heavier but doing fewer reps and sets.**
- **Eat 20 to 30 grams of good-quality protein immediately after your workout!!**

## HEALTHY BLOOD NUMBERS

Your blood is a complex mixture of cells, fluids and plasma. In order for blood to flow properly through your body into the minutest places it needs to be an ideal consistency. Our diet absolutely affects blood consistency. Sugars, fats, protein and other nutrients give blood a viscosity that is either healthy or not. Sticky blood is detrimental to health. Blood fats, or lipids, are components we can measure to determine how healthy our blood is. Lipids in the right numbers tend to manage certain functions in the body. If too many lipids are present, then you can expect trouble in the form of high cholesterol and high triglycerides. A yearly visit to your doctor and regular blood testing will help you track where you

**According to the American Heart Association, healthy blood numbers should look like this:**

**Low LDL cholesterol levels, ideally with a large LDL particle size:**

- Optimal: less than 100 mg/dL
- Near optimal: 100 – 129 mg/dL
- Borderline high: 130 – 159 mg/dL
- High: 160 – 189 mg/dL
- Very high: 190 or higher mg/dL

**High HDL cholesterol levels (this is a good cholesterol)**

- High: greater than 60 mg/dL
- Low: less than 40 mg/dL

**Low triglyceride levels**

- Normal: less than 150 mg/dL
- Borderline high: 150 – 199 mg/dL
- High: 200 – 499 mg/dL (medical treatment may be needed)
- Very high: greater than 500 mg/dL (medical treatment may be needed)

# GENERAL HEALTH STATS FOR MEN

## LEADING CAUSES OF DEATH IN MALES

1. Heart disease • 27.2% • 321,973
2. Cancer • 24.3% • 286,830
3. Stroke • 5.0% • 58,800
4. Chronic pulmonary diseases 5.0% • 58,646
5. Diabetes • 3.0% • 35,267

*References:*
*2004 US statistics courtesy of the CDC.*

# PREVENTIVE MEASURES

## HEART DISEASE

❶ **Don't smoke!** If you smoke make it a priority to quit. If you don't smoke, don't start. Avoid smoke-filled areas, as ingesting second-hand smoke is just as dangerous to health as first-hand smoke.

❷ **Exercise regularly.** Regular physical exercise strengthens the heart and lungs while controlling your weight and your stress – both significant contributing factors in heart disease.

❸ **Eat Clean.** A diet rich in fresh fruits and vegetables, whole grains, legumes and lean proteins and low in saturated and trans fats is the best diet for your heart. Make sure to consume enough omega-3 fatty acids and other healthy fats in a healthy balance. Minimize alcohol consumption.

❹ **Stay lean.** Even a weight gain of as little as 5 pounds means extra work for your heart. The extra weight further increases your chances of developing high blood pressure, high cholesterol and diabetes – all risk factors for developing heart disease.

**#1 CAUSE OF DEATH IN MALES IS HEART DISEASE**

❺ **Schedule a physical.** It's easy to put off going to the doctor when you don't feel anything is wrong, but you may never know you have dangerous risk factors including high blood pressure or high cholesterol until it's too late. Scheduling an annual physical check-up with your physician is a good investment in your health.

## CANCER

❶ **Give up the cigarette habit!** Quitting smoking reduces the risk of developing various cancers. Avoiding second-hand smoke is equally important in maintaining health.

❷ **Eat Clean.** Eat loads of fresh fruit and vegetables, plenty of whole grains and lean meats, and drink enough water every day. Eat the correct balance of healthy fats, but avoid trans and saturated fats.

❸ **Limit alcohol consumption.** The occasional glass of wine or alcoholic beverage – one or two glasses per week – is acceptable. Excessive alcohol consumption, however, is associated with an elevated risk of developing various types of cancer.

❹ **Use sunscreen with a minimum SPF of 15.** The powerful rays of the sun can break through even on a shady day. The sun is at its maximum strength between 10:00 a.m. and 2:00 p.m., so try not to spend too much time unprotected and outdoors during these hours. Be vigilant about your moles – if you see any suspicious changes in your skin or your moles please visit your doctor.

❺ **Avoid carcinogens.** Toxins are everywhere and difficult to avoid, but the more aware you are of them the more readily you can avoid them. Common culprits include pesticides, car fumes, plastics, cleansers, preservatives, and personal care items from shampoo to soap to cosmetics. Avoid these cancer-contributing products when possible. Drink water from an inert metal water bottle and eat plenty of greens to fortify antioxidant levels in the body. Stay abreast of public health messages.

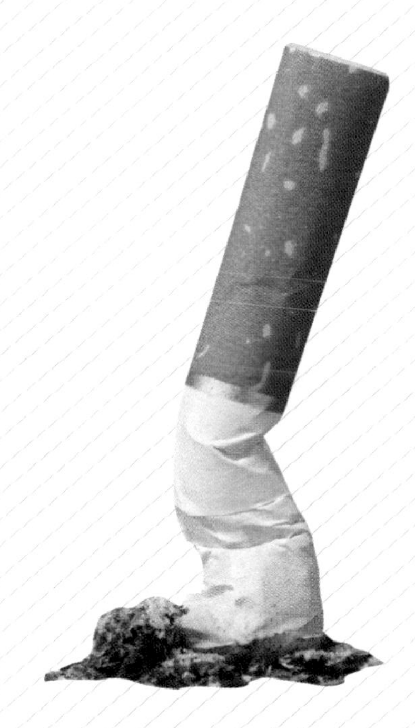

## STROKE

❶ **Limit alcohol intake.** Alcohol consumption is a significant contributing risk factor for stroke. Consuming more than two or three alcoholic beverages each day significantly increases the risk of stroke. This is one instance where less is definitely more.

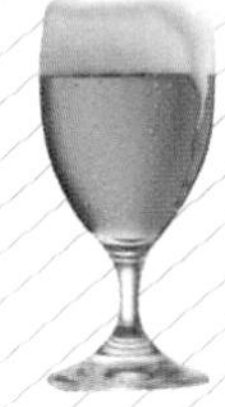

❷ **Quit smoking.** Smoking doubles your risk of developing a stroke.

❸ **Exercise regularly.** Develop the habit of exercising. Strive to perform 30 minutes of cardiovascular or resistance exercise at least three or four times per week.

❹ **Control blood sugar and blood pressure.** Eating Clean helps with both of these, especially if you consume a diet low in saturated and trans fats and limit your table salt intake. Switch to sea salt for a healthier salt option and follow the Eat-Clean principles on page 25.

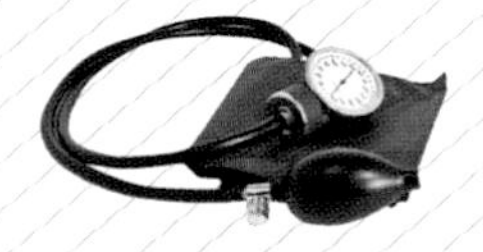

❺ **Schedule a regular annual physical!** If you have a risky lifestyle or a family history of stroke, schedule a regular, annual physical with your doctor. Doing so screens you for potential health issues and provides you with tools to offset illness. Home blood-pressure devices are available to help monitor blood pressure regularly.

## PULMONARY (Lung) DISEASE (COPD)

❶ **Quit smoking.** The number-one way to avoid lung disease is to not smoke. Every cigarette package warns the public of this danger. Second-hand smoke is best avoided as well.

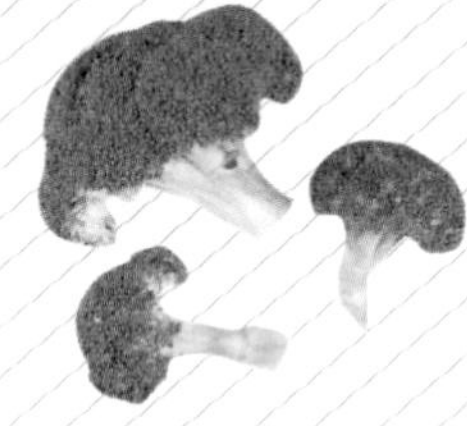

❷ **Eat Clean.** Your diet affects the potential of developing lung disease. Eating a plant-rich diet contributes to your body's ability to fight cancer and COPD with the help of antioxidants – nature's own cancer-fighting agents.

❸ **Exercise regularly.** Cardiovascular exercise strengthens the heart and lungs, making them less susceptible to COPD and other disease.

❹ **Avoid exposure to antagonizing agents.** Radon is the second-leading cause of lung disease and cancer. Check your home and business for radon levels. Don't buy a home before checking radon levels. It is your right.

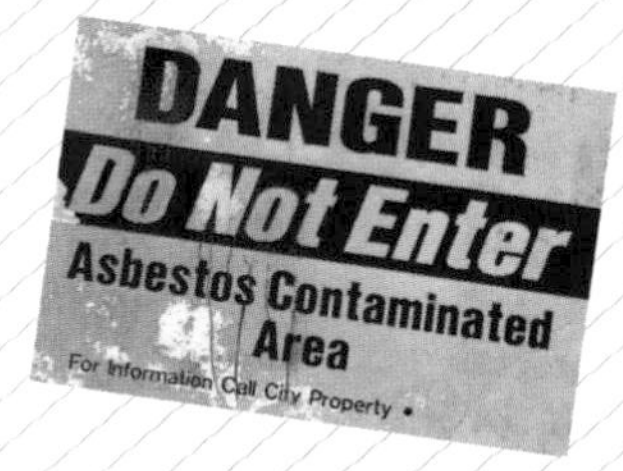


Asbestos is common in many households built before the 1970s. Asbestos is easily disturbed, especially during home renovations, creating toxic dust that seeps into the lungs. A work or home environment that has you breathing in small particles of asbestos may put you at risk for developing disease. Don't guess. Check asbestos levels in your home and office.

Farm workers often breathe in mold from various crops and factory workers often breathe in fibers from cotton, jute, flax and hemp. Wear a particulate filter mask to avoid breathing in toxic particles.

❺ **Avoid pollution.** Pay attention to the air quality each day and follow environmental warnings. If smog is high, don't go for a run outside. If possible, live in an area with cleaner air. Offset toxic accumulation by Eating Clean. Certain plant foods are known anti-toxic agents that help to rid the body of pollutants.

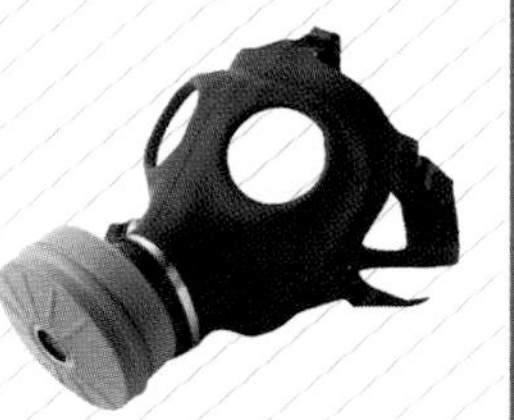

## DIABETES

❶ **Eat Clean!** The most powerful way to prevent type 2 diabetes is to control your blood sugar and body weight through diet. Avoid refined sugars and flours or foods made with these ingredients. Avoid or limit alcohol intake. One or two glasses of alcohol each week is plenty.

Eat small, frequent meals consisting of lean protein and complex carbs eaten together. Eat healthy fats in the correct ratio to help slow digestion and to nourish the brain.

❷ **Control your weight.** Nearly 90 percent of those with diabetes are overweight. That is a staggering number. Weight control is the most powerful preventive medicine!

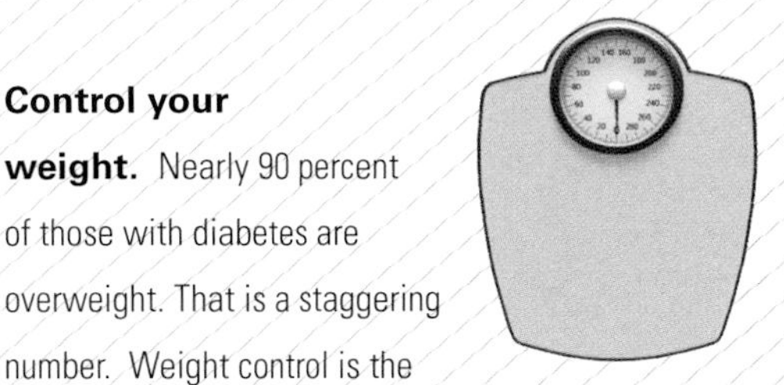

❸ **Build muscle.** A body with less fat and more lean muscle tissue possesses less likelihood of developing diabetes. Body composition is more relevant than just body weight, since where the fat collects is also significant. If your weight is predominantly around your middle your chance of developing disease is much greater. Exchange fatty tissue for lean muscle mass to offset potential illness.

❹ **Exercise regularly.** Both cardiovascular and resistance exercise are important to physical health. Cardiovascular exercise increases circulation, strengthens heart and lungs and promotes a lean physique. Include regular exercise in your health regimen.

❺ **Don't smoke.** The newest research shows that those who smoke are at a greater risk of developing diabetes. Live in a smoke-free environment.

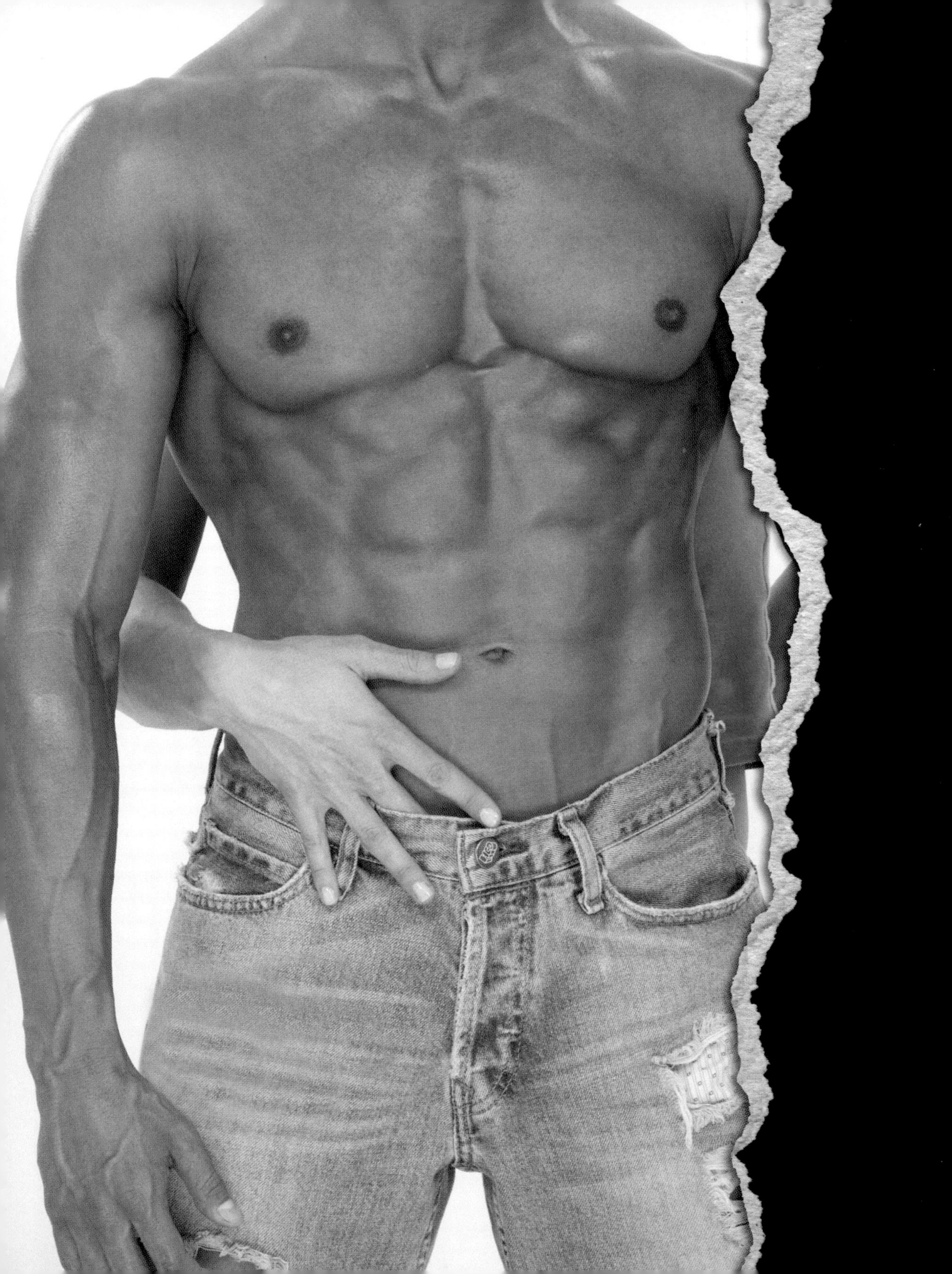

# [CHAPTER SIX]

# EATING FOR INCREASED FERTILITY AND SEXUAL FUNCTION

## DOES FOOD REALLY AFFECT SEX?

Other than the obvious pleasure of eating strawberries and whipped cream à la *9½ Weeks* with Mickey Rourke and Kim Basinger, there really is a food/sex connection. Most of you should be sitting upright in your chairs right now, taking notes. What you eat has more to do with enhanced sexual function than you might have ever imagined. Weak erections, losing an erection during sex and ejaculating too soon are all signals that you may not be getting proper nutrients for normal sexual function. If you knew foods were so directly related to sex then you may never have indulged yourself in so many health-destroying foods, particularly giant, greasy burgers, accompanying fries and gravy and other fast-food team members – not to mention the beer you guzzle alongside. Many natural foods contain sex hormones, so it is easy to eat your way to a better sex life!

## FAT IS A LIBIDO BUSTER!

A study by A. Wayne Meikle, a professor of endocrinology and metabolism at the University of Utah School of Medicine, discovered that blood testosterone (the male sex hormone) plummeted by 50 percent in men after drinking a fat-loaded milkshake containing 57 percent calories from fat. When the same men drank a shake containing 73 percent calories from carbohydrates, 25 percent from protein and 1 percent from fat, their testosterone levels did not drop. Apparently fat is a libido buster! Eat your pasta before bed gentlemen – the Italians have it right.

**LESS FAT = MORE TESTOSTERONE**

## GOOD FOOD, BAD FOOD

More and more researchers are warning of the deleterious effects of consuming powerless foods. Not only do these foods affect your health in a negative way, but they also affect sexual health and performance. Every man wants to be sexually active and potent from the minute it becomes possible and continue this way long into life. Yet research shows a good 52 percent of men struggle with some form of impotence – the inability to achieve an erection. Sex is the number-one indicator of human health. It is a loving act that is the crowning glory of what the human body is capable of, and it requires an animalistic physicality that is pleasurable and awe inspiring. Without it we become less than what is intended for us.

Sexual health is also fragile in the face of what we throw at ourselves today. Humans living on this planet struggle with situations our forefathers did not face. The list includes atrocities like 9/11 and terrorism worldwide, pollution of our entire environment and the incidence of diseases like cancer and diabetes as never seen before. Additionally, our food sources have become suspect, since lately they have been poisoned either by chemicals or bacteria and then laden in man's infinite wisdom with other food evils such as sugars, trans and saturated fats and preservatives. That is why it becomes more important than ever to make more informed food choices.

It is easy to become depressed in the face of this news. And yet the human spirit can triumph. The surest way to defend against this litany of troubles is to take every step possible to be your healthiest. With a healthy body and strong immune system you will also enjoy an enriched sexual life, since the act of having sex is an expression of healthy, human love.

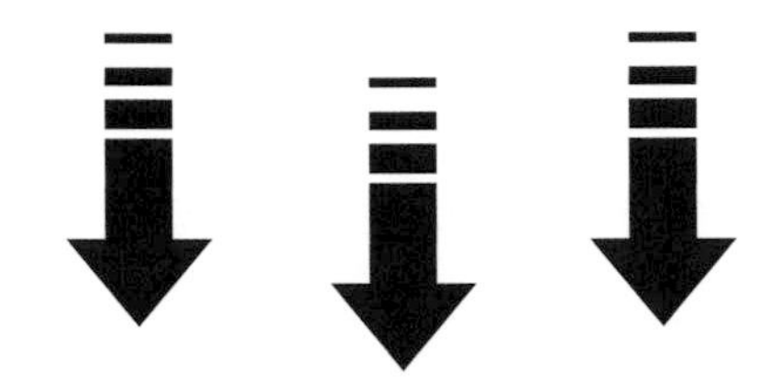

More and more researchers are warning of the deleterious effects of consuming powerless foods. Not only do these foods affect your health in a negative way, but they also affect sexual health and performance.

## THE CULPRITS

The preceding paragraphs may well put you off any bedroom activity, given their depressing nature. Thinking too much about any of it – including your performance – is a turn off. However, the real culprit lies in your cardiovascular system. Anatomy 101 lesson: To become erect a penis requires supple blood vessels that can easily expand and contract; in short, they must be flexible. As a man ages, cardiovascular disease begins to factor into heart health and consequently penile health. Arteries become narrower and harder – atherosclerosis – and blood does not flow as readily. Unfortunately, coronary disease, which is identified by fatty deposits and hardening of the arteries, is the number-one killer among men in North America, so it stands to reason many men also struggle with impotence. That would be why Viagra and other impotence treatments are among the best sellers in the pharmaceutical industry. So if your heart is in good condition your sex life will be too, since you will have plenty of blood flow to achieve an erection.

Any measures you take to improve heart health will also improve penile health. One of these very basic measures would be to embrace Clean Eating. Diet alone plays an enormous part in overall health, including sexual health. The current Standard North American Diet (SNAD) is high in unhealthy fats, particularly saturated and trans fats. These fats cause trouble in blood vessels, where they interfere with their ability to expand and contract, hence achieve and maintain an erection. Eating Clean advocates the consumption of healthy fats, particularly essential fatty acids. Excellent sources of these include flaxseeds (our all-time favorite), fish oils and plant oils (especially olive and pumpkin). Twenty percent of the daily diet should include healthy fats, since male hormones require fat for normal function – as does the brain. You see? "Fats" is no longer a four-letter word. The trick is to know what to avoid and what to eat. That is why Eating Clean is so good for you. The framework of eating several smaller meals loaded with healthful foods along with heart-healthy fats helps you to become the robust, vital man you were always meant to be.

**If your heart is in good condition your sex life will be too, since you will have plenty of blood flow to achieve an erection.**

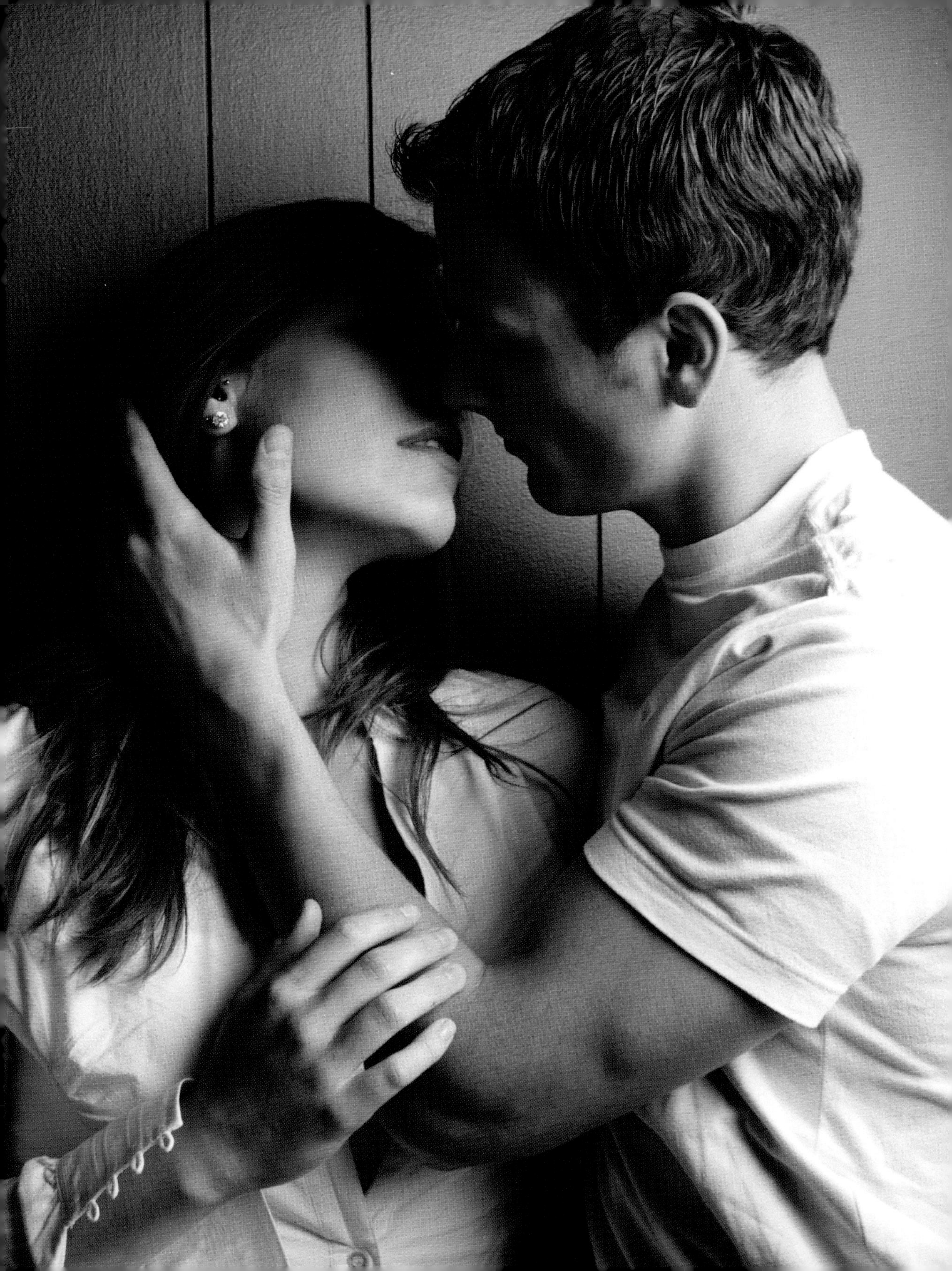

# DIABETES AND SEX

The statistics for men suffering from type 2 diabetes and pre-diabetic conditions are huge. With the increased number of men that are overweight or obese, there is a much greater chance of being stricken with these conditions. Today, approximately one in 17 men suffers from type 2 diabetes. Men with this condition are three times more likely to experience erectile dysfunction than men without.

Additionally, in an evolutionary blink of an eye, humans have dramatically altered their diet by consuming manufactured foods rather than natural foods. Diabetes is not the only outcome of the repercussions this has had on human health. Metabolic syndrome X (MSX) sounds like something from a sci-fi movie. Too bad it isn't. Instead, it describes a cluster of conditions that predispose men to illness.

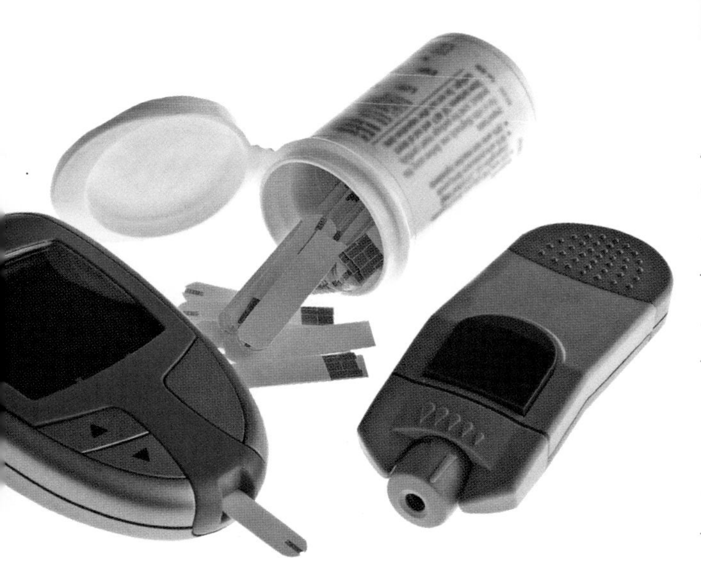

**In that cluster you may find any or all of the following symptoms:**

- **Insulin resistance**
- **Glucose intolerance**
- **Overweight and obesity**
- **High blood pressure**
- **Inflammation**
- **High LDL (low-density lipoproteins)**
- **Elevated triglycerides**
- **Type 2 diabetes**
- **Cardiovascular disease**

Insulin resistance is usually the instigator in MSX. As the body exhibits increasingly greater difficulty in managing it's glucose/insulin equation, it falters, and in doing so triggers MSX. A great deal of the fault lies directly with what you are consuming. The Standard North American Diet is notably lacking in fiber and plant nutrients. Other contributing factors include poor diet, genetics, age, ethnicity, socioeconomic status and lack of physical activity. Gentlemen, it is easy to see how to solve at least some of the problem – Eat Clean!!

# SEXY SUPPLEMENTS

## Vitamin C

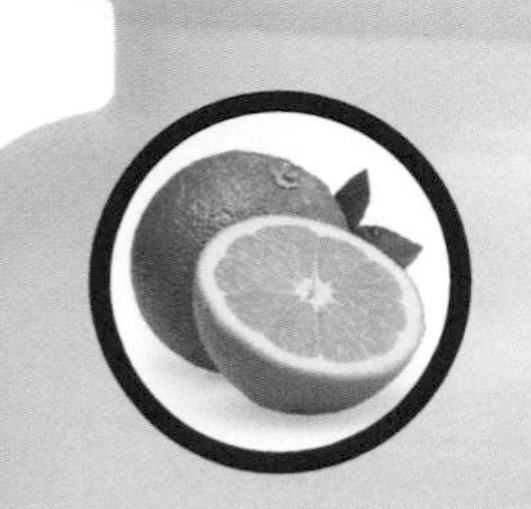

**1,000 mg per day –**

Reputed to revive tired, lackluster sperm.

## Vitamin A (beta-carotene)

**2,300 IU per day –**

A powerful antioxidant.

## Vitamin E

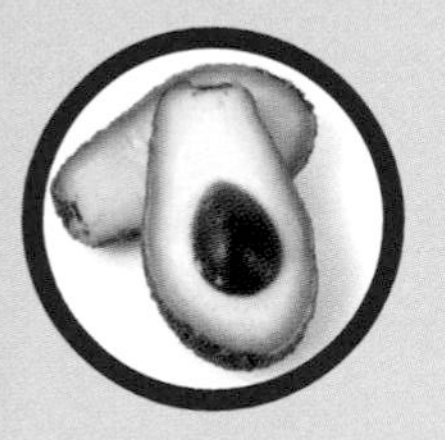

**400–800 IU per day –**

Keeps blood vessels elastic.

## Vitamin B-3 (niacin)

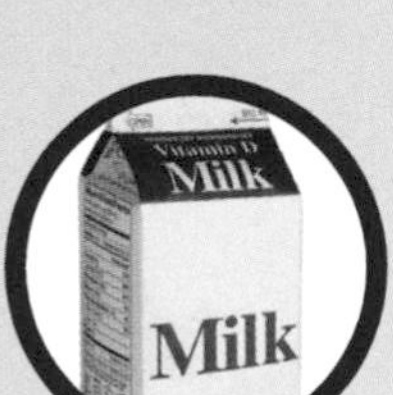


**16 mg per day**

## Vitamin B-6

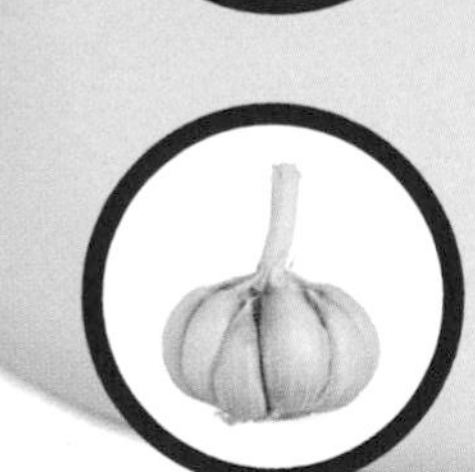

**50 mg per day**

## Vitamin B-12

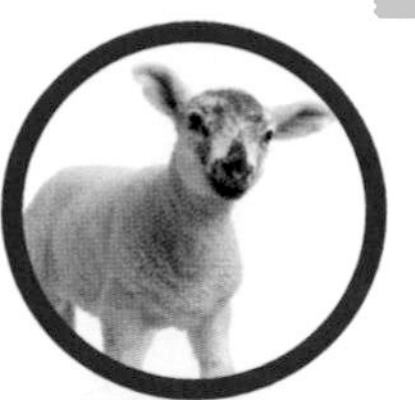

**50 mcg per day**

## Folic acid

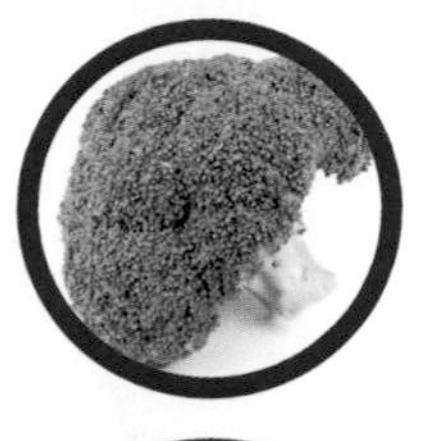

**400 mcg per day –**

Necessary for healthy sperm, hence healthy babies.

## Pycnogenol

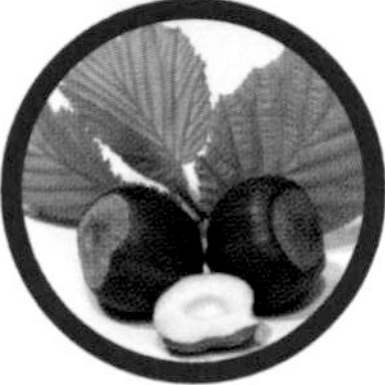

**25 – 50 mg per day**

## Coenzyme Q10

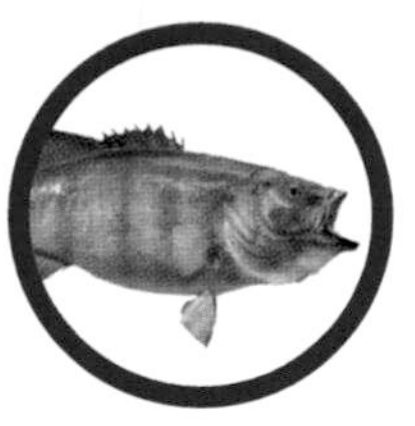

**30 – 60 mg per day –**

Helps increase energy production, especially in the heart

## Zinc

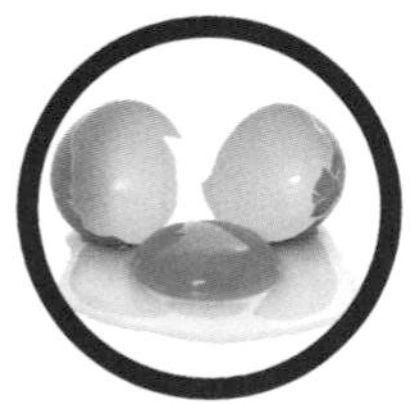

**30 mg per day**

## Selenium

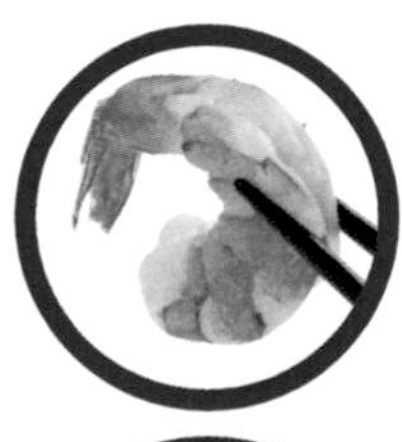

**100 mcg per day**

## Flaxseed oil

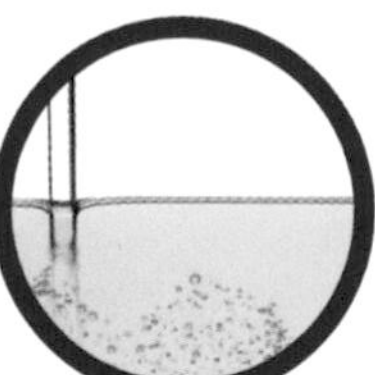

**1,000 mg per day**

## VITAMIN C IS THE SAVIOR FOR TIRED, LACKLUSTER SPERM –

## EAT THESE FOODS TO GET YOUR MOJO BACK.

Each of these contains 200 milligrams of vitamin C – the dose shown to reenergize sperm.

- **1½ red bell peppers**
- **2 cups steamed broccoli**
- **3 kiwifruit**
- **1 cantaloupe**
- **3 oranges**
- **2 x 8-oz glasses orange juice**
- **1¼ cups mixed frozen berries**
- **2½ cups raw strawberries**

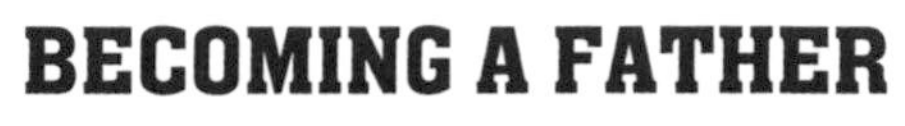

## BECOMING A FATHER

At some point in your life the possibility of fathering a child (or children) may well be a subject of interest for you. If it isn't then feel free to skip this segment, but you might find it interesting anyway. Our ability to conceive is gravely affected by stress, nutrition and exercise. The busier we are the less we manage to take care of ourselves, and consequently the less we seem able to make babies. When your goal is to become pregnant, both you and your partner will need to pay attention to nutrition and physical health – even when the idea of having a baby is but a distant glimmer in either sets of eyes. Becoming a father is a job that starts before you even consider jumping into bed. In other words, there are foods you can eat and habits you can adopt that will increase your chance of conception. A food as lowly as the walnut could be the nut that cracks this problem.

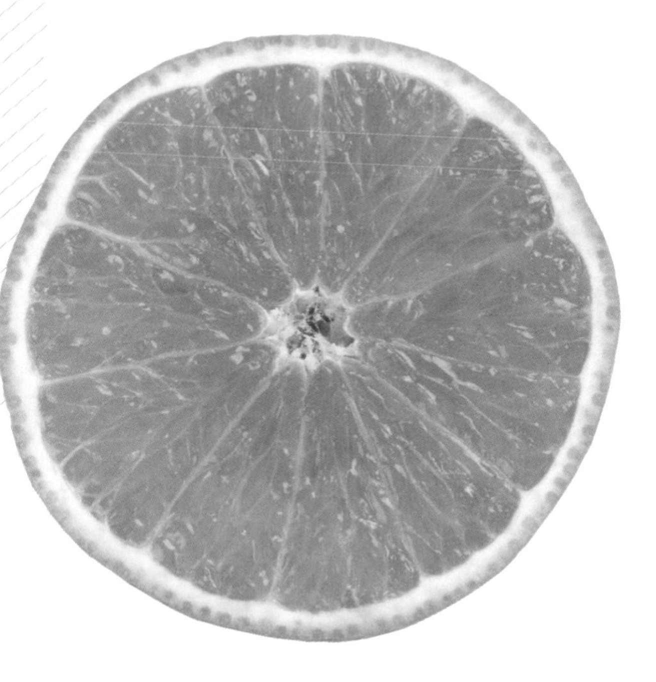

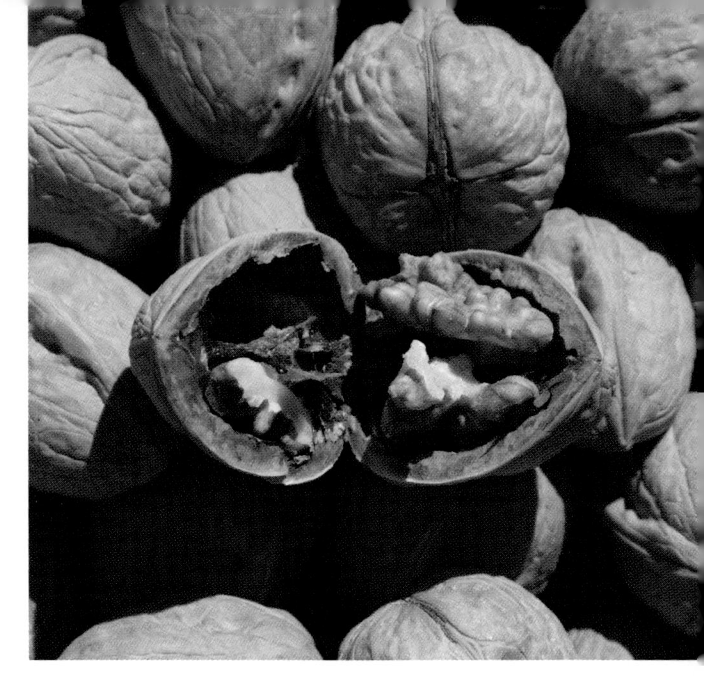

## EAT WALNUTS

Early cultures recognized the fertile time in a couple's life as one requiring more nutritional attention than others. Special foods were reserved for this critical time because those foods were known to increase the chance of fertilization. In many civilizations the man who could father many children was viewed as a kind of god. Ancient Greeks and Romans knew well the reputation of the walnut and its aphrodisiac qualities. That was probably why walnuts were thrown at newly married couples and their guests rather than rice. Stewed walnuts were also traditionally served as part of the wedding feast to bless the couple's fertility. The Chinese recognized the walnut as an important food to help treat impotence as well as boost sperm quality.

What is it about a food that makes it a factor in promoting fertility and often libido? Healthy fats are part of the answer. Many a joke is made about how low the national average for having sex is – some people aren't getting any at all. Could it be that all the brainwashing about fats has turned off the country's collective desire? Healthy fats are critical for lovers because the sex hormones are made from such fats. If we shun all fats then the machine for creating sex hormones shuts down. The walnut could be part of a very healthy solution. Loaded with omega-3 fatty acids and alpha linoleic acids, walnuts offer just the healthy fats needed for the job at hand.

## NUTS AGAIN!

The mineral selenium has been much in the minds of fertility researchers lately. Many studies show that without sufficient amounts of this mineral, sperm motility is decreased dramatically – that means sperm has difficulty swimming toward the desired target, the egg! Conversely, by eating foods containing plenty of this nutrient the situation can be corrected. Once again, nuts come to the rescue. The Brazil nut contains the most abundant supply of selenium of any food. Selenium can also be found in adequate supply in dried mushrooms, walnuts, barley, canned tuna and lentils. Make a note of the fact that too much selenium can be dangerous. Stick to the limits recommended below.

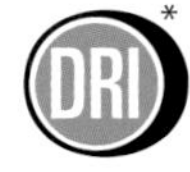


The healthy range is from 55 to 400 mcg per day for men 18 and over.

*DRI: Dietary Reference Intake – the accepted healthy range of a given nutrient.

# LIBIDO-BOOSTING SHAKE

**Make one for the two of you! Toss all these ingredients in a blender »**

1 fresh kiwi, peeled

¼ cup / 60 ml cantaloupe, peeled, seeded and cubed

Juice of 1 navel orange

¼ cup / 60 ml fresh strawberries or mixed berries

1 Tbsp / 15 ml wheat germ

2 Tbsp / 30 ml walnut butter

1½ cups / 355 ml coconut water

1-2 Tbsp / 15-30 ml agave nectar, depending on your sweet tooth

Blend all ingredients until smooth. If you need to add more liquid, then orange juice, coconut water or even ice cubes will do. Make it the way you like it. Pour into two glasses, garnish with a fresh, happy-looking strawberry and sip over candle-light. Oh yeah!

# FOODS RICH IN SELENIUM

| SELENIUM-RICH FOODS | MICROGRAMS | PORTION (g) |
|---|---|---|
| Brazil nuts | Up to 1,500 | 100 |
| Wheat germ | Up to 300 | 100 |
| Brewer's yeast | Up to 260 | 100 |
| Kidneys | 250 | 100 |
| Liver | 150 | 100 |
| Tuna | 90 | 100 |
| Other oily fish | 25-60 | 100 |
| Shellfish | 20-40 | 100 |
| Sunflower seeds | 45 | 100 |
| Lentils | 30 | 100 |
| Cashews | 30 | 100 |

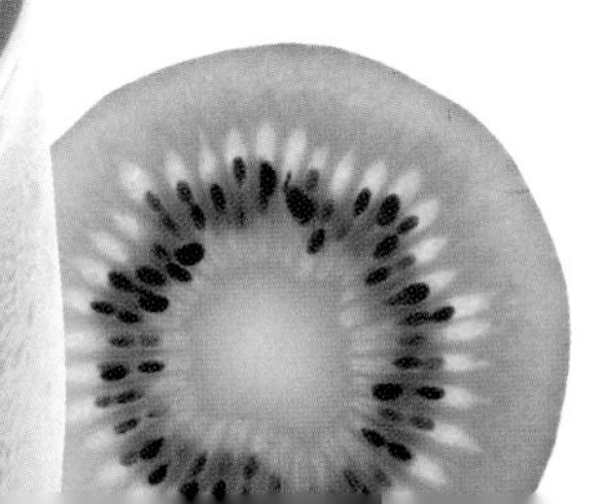

## ZINC IS NOT JUST FOR YOUR NOSE

You know zinc as the active ingredient in heavy, white, surfer-dude sunblock. It does protect the skin from overexposure to sun, but zinc is not just for the exterior. Along with the many roles zinc plays in the body, including assisting in wound healing, participating in metabolic processes, protein and blood formation, and general growth and maintenance of all body tissues, it is also an essential ingredient for optimal sexual health. Low zinc concentrations reduce sperm production, cause low sperm counts and reduce sperm motility (that means the little buggers don't swim well). For anyone trying to get pregnant a lack of zinc or zinc deficiency could be devastating to your plan.

Zinc is most often obtained from the diet by eating poultry, fish and whole grains, but most of you don't get enough of this potent mineral. Recent studies suggest men do not consume enough of this mineral.

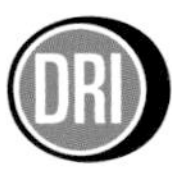


**FOR ZINC** – 11 to 40 mg per day for men between the ages of 18 and 50.

**Boost your zinc intake with any of these zinc-rich foods:**

| ZINC-RICH FOODS | MILLIGRAMS | PORTION (g) |
|---|---|---|
| Oysters | 25 + | 100 |
| Shellfish | 20 | 100 |
| Brewer's yeast | 17 | 100 |
| Wheat germ | 17 | 100 |
| Wheat bran | 16 | 100 |
| All-Bran cereal | 7 | 100 |
| Pine nuts | 7 | 100 |
| Pecans | 6 | 100 |
| Liver | 6 | 100 |
| Cashews | 6 | 100 |
| Parmesan cheese | 5 | 100 |
| Fish | 3 | 100 |
| Eggs | 2 | 100 |

# Vitamin C – The Multi-Tasking Vitamin

Gentlemen, eat your oranges! Eat anything loaded with vitamin C if sex is on your mind. Vitamin C is the multi-talented nutrient that is critical to creating the hormones needed for sex and fertility. Those hormones include progesterone, estrogen (yes, men have estrogen too!) and androgen. Hormones are the basis for sexuality and hence the act of sex. Vitamin C also plays a role in assisting an individual sperm to get its job done. Sperm have a tendency to clump together – this is called agglutination. If sperm remain in clumps they cannot effectively get to the egg. Men who are deficient in vitamin C are more prone to having sperm agglutination. Vitamin C fixes the problem and lets sperm swim happily on their way to the egg. This potent vitamin also reduces the incidence of defective sperm, especially for smokers. Smoking is not the ideal habit to begin with so quitting would be best, but vitamin C certainly helps improve the quality of sperm.

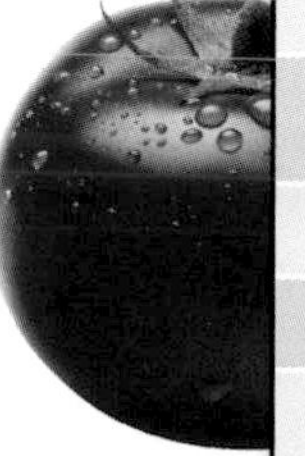

In the presence of vitamin C you will not only feel vibrant and healthy, but also you will want to show your partner that you are. This translates into an increased sex drive which … well, we don't have to explain the rest, do we?

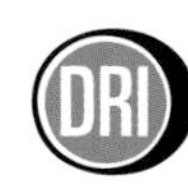


**FOR VITAMIN C** – 90 to 2,000 mg per day for men 19 and older.

**Boost your vitamin C intake with any of these vitamin C-rich foods:**

| VITAMIN C-RICH FOODS | MILLIGRAMS | PORTION (g) |
|---|---|---|
| Rosehip extract | 1,000 + | 100 |
| Black currants | 200 | 100 |
| Guava | up to 200 | 100 |
| Strawberries | 80 | 100 |
| Lemons | 60 | 100 |
| Oranges | 50 + | 100 |
| Kiwi | 50 + | 100 |
| Clementines | 40 + | 100 |
| Grapefruits | 36 | 100 |
| Raspberries | 30 + | 100 |
| Lychees | 30 + | 100 |
| Nectarines | 30 + | 100 |
| Peaches | 30 | 100 |
| Mangoes | 30 | 100 |
| Peppers | 70 + | 100 |
| Spring greens | 70 + | 100 |
| Brussels sprouts | 60 + | 100 |
| Broccoli | 44 | 100 |
| Curly kale | 70 + | 100 |
| Gourd | 35 + | 100 |
| Snow peas | 30 + | 100 |
| Cauliflower | 27 | 100 |
| Tomatoes | 20 + | 100 |
| Green cabbage | 20 + | 100 |
| Potatoes | 15 | 100 |

# VITAMIN E

"E" may well stand for ecstasy since this sexy vitamin factors heavily in getting your engines started in the first place. It is commonly known as the vitamin most responsible for sex drive or libido. Try this little experiment. Eat one cup of lightly steamed broccoli florets every day for one week. See if you don't notice a difference in your desire. We tried this at our house and although this is by no means a scientific experiment, it was a lot of fun and had the desired effect. But you don't have to rely on broccoli to get a little pleasure. You can also eat avocados, wheat germ and other foods listed in the chart to the right to fan the flames in your bedroom.

Vitamin E is thought to make sperm more vital and thus make you more fertile. When given vitamin E, couples who have been going through in vitro fertilization see a marked improvement in fertilization rates.

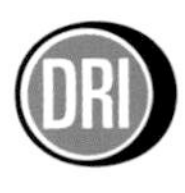

**FOR VITAMIN E** – 15 to 1,000 mg per day for men 18 and older.

**Boost your vitamin E intake with any of these vitamin E-rich foods:**

| VITAMIN E-RICH FOODS | MILLIGRAMS | PORTION (g) |
|---|---|---|
| Sunflower oil | 49 | 100 |
| Cottonseed oil | 43 | 100 |
| Safflower oil | 40 | 100 |
| Hazelnuts | up to 25 | 100 |
| Almonds | 24 | 100 |
| Wheat germ | 22 | 100 |
| Rapeseed oil | 22 | 100 |
| Cod liver oil | 20 | 100 |
| Corn oil | 17 | 100 |
| Soya bean oil | 16 | 100 |
| Peanut oil | 15 | 100 |
| Pine nuts | 13 | 100 |
| Popcorn | 11 | 100 |
| Peanuts | 10 | 100 |
| Margarine | up to 8 | 100 |
| Brazil nuts | 7 | 100 |
| Sweet potatoes | 4.5 | 100 |
| Walnuts | 3 | 100 |
| Egg yolks | 3 + | 100 |
| Muesli | 3 | 100 |
| Avocados | up to 3 | 100 |

## AND THE REST

There are numerous other players in the drama of becoming pregnant. L-arginine is an amino acid found in high concentrations in the head of sperm. Healthy sperm production depends on the presence of this amino acid in good concentration. Eat more cold-water fish such as salmon, tuna, herring and halibut as well as onions, garlic, olive oil, celery, leafy greens, legumes and potatoes for increased L-arginine levels. The DRI for L-arginine is not established since this amino acid is considered non-essential; however, a healthy guideline would be to try to consume at least 0.36 grams of readily digestible protein per pound of body weight. Once you begin to Eat Clean as your new way of life, this kind of consumption will not be a problem for you since you will be eating lean protein at every meal.

L-carnitine is another amino acid necessary for normal sperm function. When L-carnitine is present in adequate levels in sperm there is a corresponding increase in sperm motility and concentration. Eat more meat products, including lamb, beef, pork, rabbit, chicken, cow's milk and eggs, and also peanuts.

There are numerous other players in the drama of becoming pregnant. L-arginine is an amino acid found in high concentrations in the head of sperm.

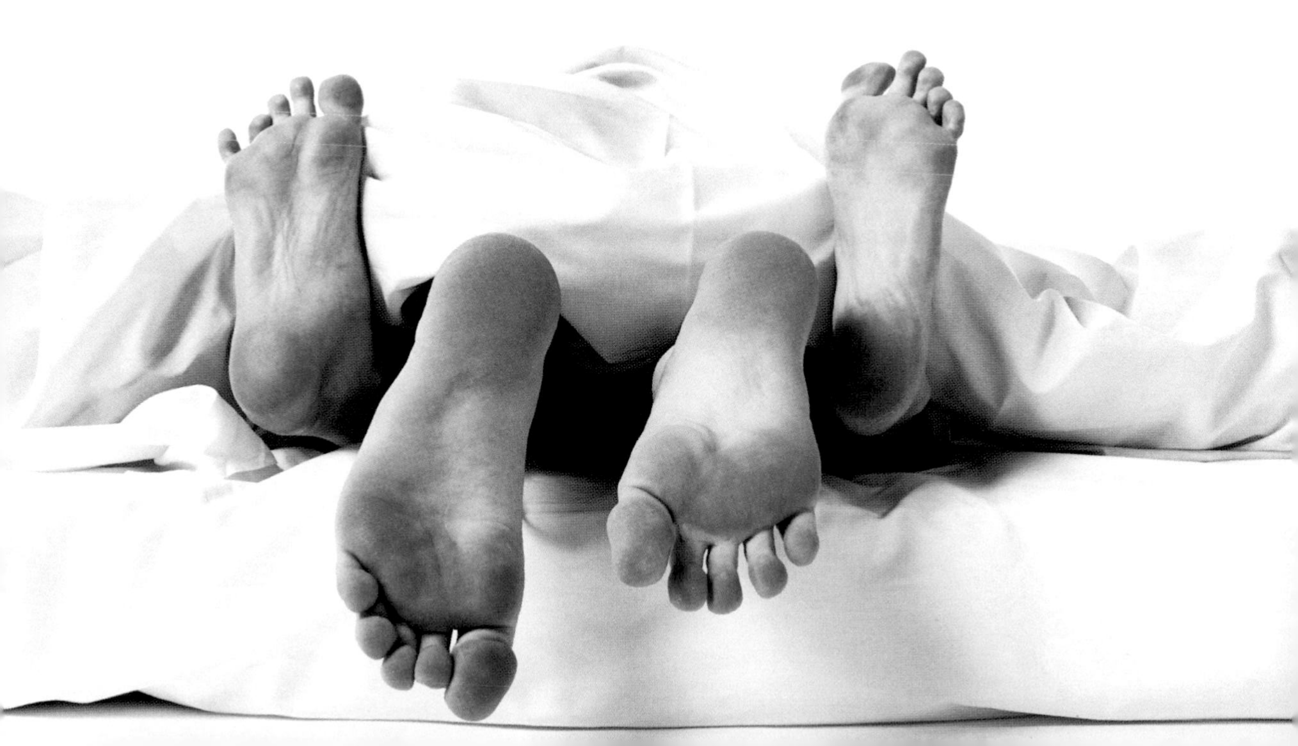

## SUGGESTIONS TO BUILD IMMUNITY AND INCREASE SEXUAL HEALTH

Regular exercise in which the heart rate is elevated for periods of 30 minutes or more should be done at least four times per week.

The diet should embrace the Eat-Clean principles. Choose whole grains, lean proteins and complex carbohydrates from fresh fruits and vegetables.

Keep your living, personal and work environments pleasant and clutter-free. Let the sun shine in, open the windows and drink pure water.

Supplement with a good-quality multivitamin that also contains minerals. You can boost immunity (and sexual health, indirectly) by supplementing with wheat or barley grass and chlorella or spirulina. When you are in the produce section look for sprouts. They contain loads of readily digestible nutrients that fortify the immune system.

Drinking alcohol can reduce fertility by as much as 50 percent. This goes for both you and your partner. Once again, Clean Eating suggests that you minimize your alcohol consumption, which is in line with increasing health and fertility. Erectile dysfunction can come about from excessive alcohol use.

Smoking also decreases fertility because it reduces sperm count. It also makes sperm sluggish, and that diminishes their chances of getting to the egg. In addition, smoking restricts blood flow, which makes it more difficult to get – and keep – an erection.

## THE CLIMAX

Sorry, we could not resist! With the pun aside we would like to emphasize that the more you embrace Clean, whole and natural foods in your diet, which is a natural outcome of Clean Eating anyway, the healthier you will be and the more positive your efforts at conception. This is by no means a medical solution to any serious fertility problems you may have. These will have to be addressed by a physician. But it cannot be overstated how much of an impact nutrition has on the entire human condition.

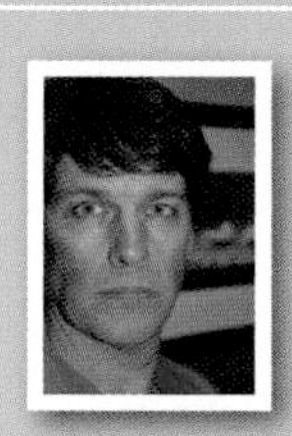

Dr. Lars Thompson, Urologist

## Nutrition and Sexual Function

*When my friend Tosca asked my medical opinion about a link between diet and male sexual function I had a private chuckle. It reminded me of two semi-true jokes I tell my patients. The first is that for every 40 pounds of weight they lose, they gain an extra inch of penis. That could definitely be viewed as a plus, but in my mind it is a secondary, not primary, benefit. The second is that whether or not they lose a day of life for each cigarette they smoke, they probably give up an erection! The same goes for every candy bar or plate of French fries eaten.*

*In my urological practice I routinely see men with erectile dysfunction, and the question of cause always comes up (no pun intended). Unfortunately, when a man has already had difficulty getting an erection, correcting the problem is not an easy fix. This is definitely a situation for which preventative medicine is the best medicine. And the key ingredients of preventative medicine are diet and exercise. The maintenance of male sexual function, including the ability to get a good stiffy, benefits from a healthy diet and lifestyle, as with all other body parts.*

*The main causes of erectile dysfunction are related to damage to the lining known as the endothelium of the blood vessels of the penis. The same processes that put you at risk of erectile dysfunction are the risk factors for heart disease. These include blood-fat abnormalities (high cholesterol), high blood pressure, diabetes and smoking. Erectile dysfunction is considered a marker for the development of heart disease and often predates it, probably because the blood vessels are smaller to begin with.*

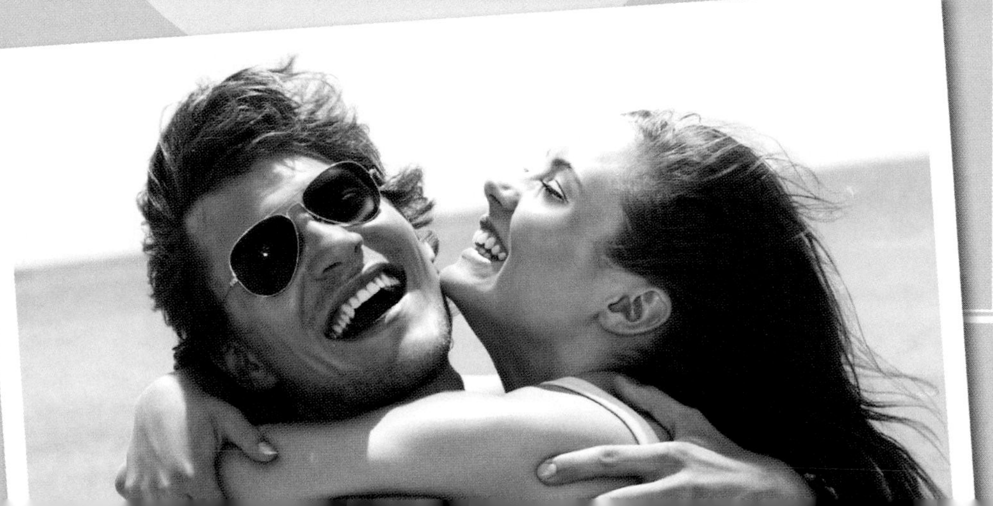

*The diet link is related to body composition – or to be blunt, how fat you are. Obesity is a direct result of what and how much you eat balanced with what and how much you do. The fat that develops in our abdomen is not just a reserve of stored energy. It becomes a metabolically active tissue that produces chemicals that cause harm to the blood vessels similar to the effect of smoking. These chemicals have the effects of lowering good blood fats, raising bad blood fats, raising blood pressure and causing insulin resistance and thus diabetes. The combination of these changes associated with a waist measurement greater than 38 inches is called Metabolic Syndrome. Similar to smoking, Metabolic Syndrome is a major risk factor for the development of endothelial or vascular damage, which causes heart disease, erectile dysfunction and strokes.*

*Obesity not only puts your life expectancy at risk, but also the quality and quantity of your erections. In addition, it can diminish your sex appeal. The sexual response has three phases:*

**1. Desire, or libido**

**2. Arousal, which is the development of an erection**

**3. Orgasm**

*Each of these can be negatively affected by poor diet and lifestyle.*

*My message is to try to stay active, watch what and how much you eat, protect those blood vessels and preserve your body image. By following* The Eat-Clean Diet for Men *you may enjoy better-quality erections for a greater period of time, and if you lose weight that erection may even look longer!*

*Enjoy healthy living,*

**Lars Thompson, MD**

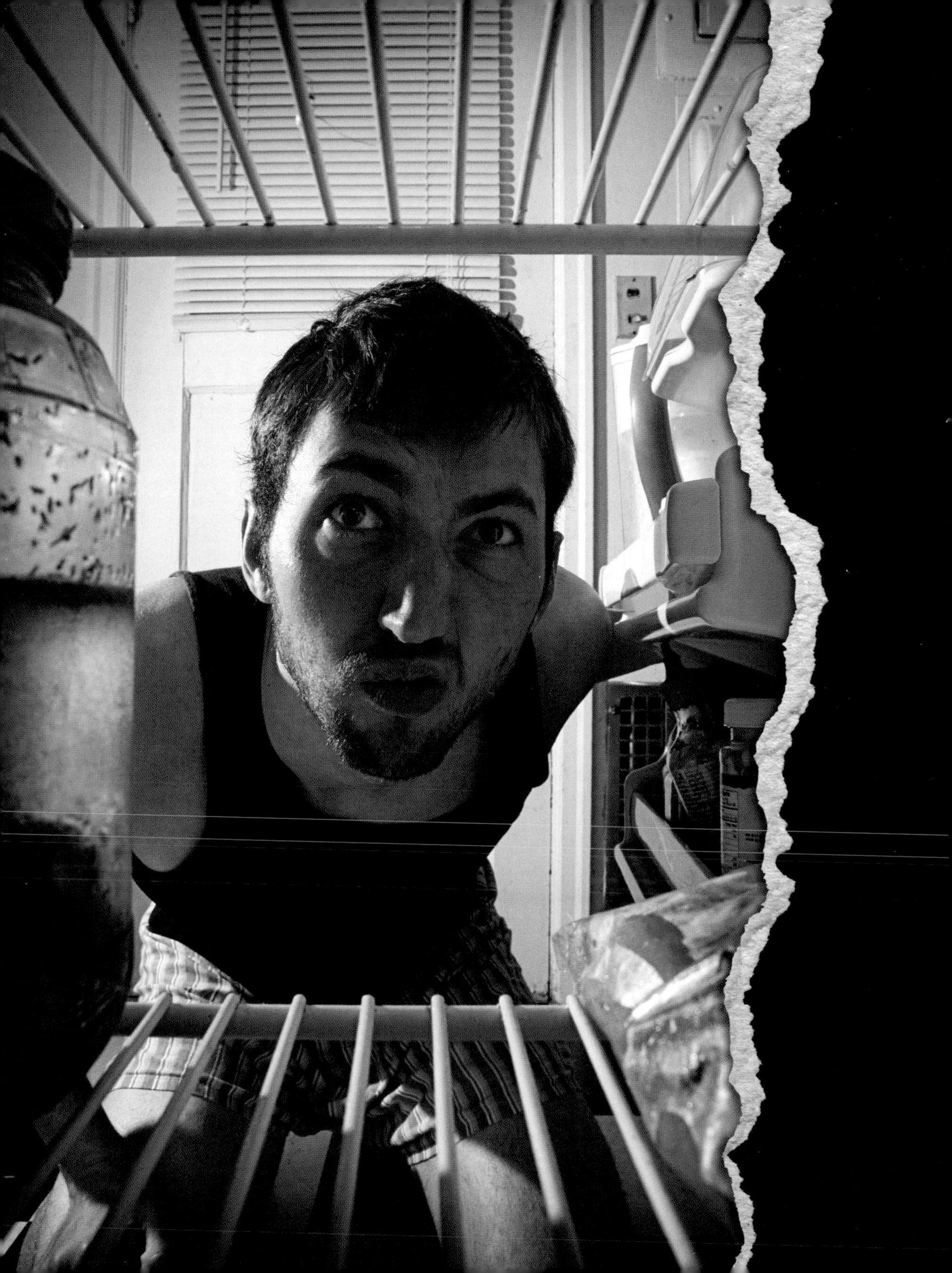

# [CHAPTER SEVEN]

## GETTING CLEAN IN THE KITCHEN

## TOSSING DIRTY FOODS!

Every kitchen has its problem spots. No sense making plans to fix your physique only to let it fall away because your kitchen is booby trapped! Booby trapped with not-so-Clean options. The way to solve this little lemon is to clear out the rubbish while your mind is made up. Make a date with yourself – and a like-minded pal if it helps – to do a kitchen clean up. This doesn't mean rubber gloves and disinfectant, unless of course you get the urge. It means grabbing a few garbage bags and pulling open all your cupboards and drawers, pitching whatever nasty business you may have stashed away in there. Your refrigerator and freezer are part of the job too.

Begin to make better food decisions now by tossing whatever items you have that don't fit the Eat-Clean bill. We suggest starting with the junk-food cupboard. Junk food has little place in your new eating regimen, so out it goes – Doritos, potato chips, salted nuts, candy, cheap chocolate bars, Cheezies, corn chips and any other gems you have stashed away. We know how hard it is to throw away food, but come on guys! This stuff isn't really food, is it? It will only make you sicker and fatter long-term, so ditch it now. If you have pretzels they can stay, but eat them in moderation. The same goes for popcorn, but it has to be hot air popped – not the stuff with goo and salt all over it.

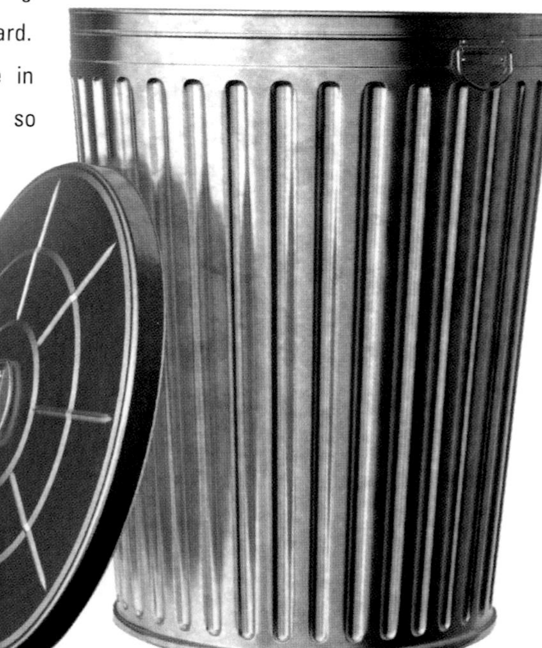

Move on to the cereal cupboard where we are sure to find a minefield of sugary stuff. Here's a simple rule of thumb: if you can't read the ingredients on the package or don't have a clue what they are, then you probably should not be eating them. That makes life really easy. Look for any packages in your cupboard containing only one or two ingredients. If all you have are boxes full of 26-letter words, toss them. All of them! Do the same with other cupboards containing crackers, cookies and canned goods. Many of these are jammed full of the very ingredients that will defeat your physique-renovation goals – refined flour, sugar, trans fats, sodium, preservatives, nitrates and more. *Fuhgeddaboudit!* You don't need the stuff. You need good-for-you bodybuilding foods. Keep going – we are not done yet!

TOSCA ASKS –

# WHAT'S IN A TWINKIE?

The uber-iconic food product, the archetype of all processed foods, the rare food to become part of the popular culture (proof: President Bill Clinton included them in the Millennium Time Capsule): Twinkies. Urban legend has it that Twinkies are so loaded with chemicals and preservatives that they will not decompose in a garbage dump and will take seven years to fully digest. Whatever the case, the little cake contains a laundry list of ingredients that neither you nor I can pronounce, nor should we eat them. For your edification, here is that list:

- Enriched wheat flour – enriched with ferrous sulphate (iron), B vitamins (niacin, thiamine mononitrate [B-1], ribofavin [B-12] and folic acid)
- Sugar
- Corn syrup
- Water
- High fructose corn syrup
- Vegetable and/or animal shortening – containing one or more of partially hydrogenated soybean, cottonseed or canola oil, and beef fat
- Dextrose
- Whole eggs
- Modified corn starch
- Cellulose gum
- Whey
- Leavenings (sodium acid pyrophosphate, baking soda, monocalcium phosphate)
- Salt
- Cornstarch
- Corn flour
- Corn syrup solids and corn dextrins
- Monoglycerides and diglycerides
- Soy lecithin
- Soy protein isolate
- Natural and artificial flavors
- Polysorbate 60
- Dextrin
- Calcium caseinate
- Sodium stearoyl lactylate
- Sodium and calcium caseinate
- Wheat gluten
- Calcium sulphate
- Natural and artificial flavors
- Caramel color
- Sorbic acid (to retain freshness)
- Added color (yellow 5, red 40)
- May contain peanuts or traces of peanuts

Reference:
*Twinkie, Deconstructed* by Steve Ettlinger, 2007

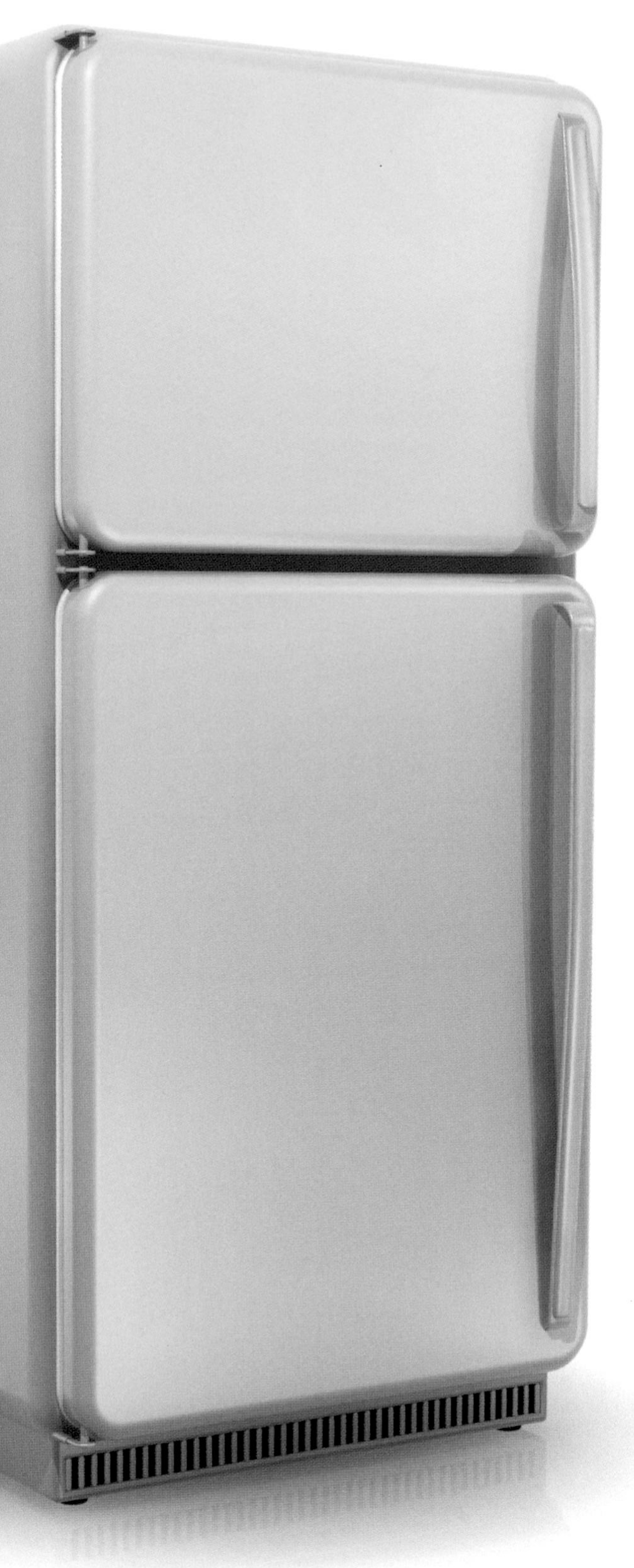

# WHAT'S IN YOUR FRIDGE?

Trouble hides in your fridge and freezer too. Along with the troublesome packages of deli meats, bacon and fried chicken there could also be problem foods such as beer, greasy meats and whatever else your particular brand of sin might be. We get especially grossed out over things like mayonnaise, commercially prepared salad dressings, sodas and commercial sauces. What the heck is in those foods anyway?

In the freezer there will likely be TV dinners, ready-to-eat burritos, enchiladas and other such foods along with ice cream, frozen treats, cakes, brownies and more. We hate to be the bearers of bad news, but these are all going to have to go! Toss it all. If you feel bad about wasting this "food" (if that is what you want to call it), then deliver it to a food bank. Besides, is it any less wasted sitting in your abdomen as fat? Now is not the time to waver. You have made up your mind – this is the last time you will be jiggly, squishy or feeling lousy about yourself. Play hardball and stick to that plan. Get rid of the poisons in your kitchen. Don't worry! We are going to feed you; we will just do it differently. You are going to love the results. Hold on... is that leftover pizza? That has to go too.

## TRIGGER FOODS – GET THEM OUT OF THERE!

Many of us have trigger foods. Once we start eating them we cannot stop ourselves. It is like that with us when we buy ice cream or cheese. We both love ice cream, but once we open the carton we can't seem to stop ourselves from eating the damned stuff. We save that treat for special occasions when we know there will be lots of people around who will help us eat the contents of a carton of ice cream. Cheese is another trigger food. Once the package is cracked open the gloves are off and we saw off great chunks to munch on. Gnawing away at a three-inch-square block of cheese is decidedly not Clean Eating.

You may have the same trouble. Some particular food will start you on an eating binge intense enough to sink your ship. Oh-oh! Now what? The trick is to either not buy the trouble foods or eat them sparingly. Never be alone with your particular trigger food or you may end up eating the whole business and then you are going to feel just awful.

## I CAN'T BELIEVE I ATE THE WHOLE THING!

Once you have gone completely off the rails and eaten both an entire carton of ice cream and a family-sized bag of chips – anything else? Then it is time to stop the madness. We have found that most people eat out of boredom. We tried the experiment ourselves. In our daily lives we are incredibly busy people, but recently we had a weekend when four kids left at the same time – and there were no time obligations for us to meet. We decided to simply hang around and watch classic movies. We poked through a copy of Roger Ebert's *The Great Movies* and chose several that interested us. And that was all we did for two days. But between showings of *Alfie* with Michael Caine, *Bonnie and Clyde, The Shawshank Redemption, Nosferatu, The Silence of the Lambs* and *The Night of the Hunter,* we were bored. Consequently we ate. And ate junky foods! It was mindless eating that did not really serve a purpose of feeding us. Instead it was eating out of boredom. Sure, go ahead and watch some classic movies, but eating junk does you no good.

A movie weekend with your main squeeze is loads of fun! Try it, but have good food on hand so you don't stray. We recommend Clean-Eating snacks from the recipe section of this book to keep you from going astray.

Gnawing away at a three-inch-square block of cheese is decidedly not Clean Eating.

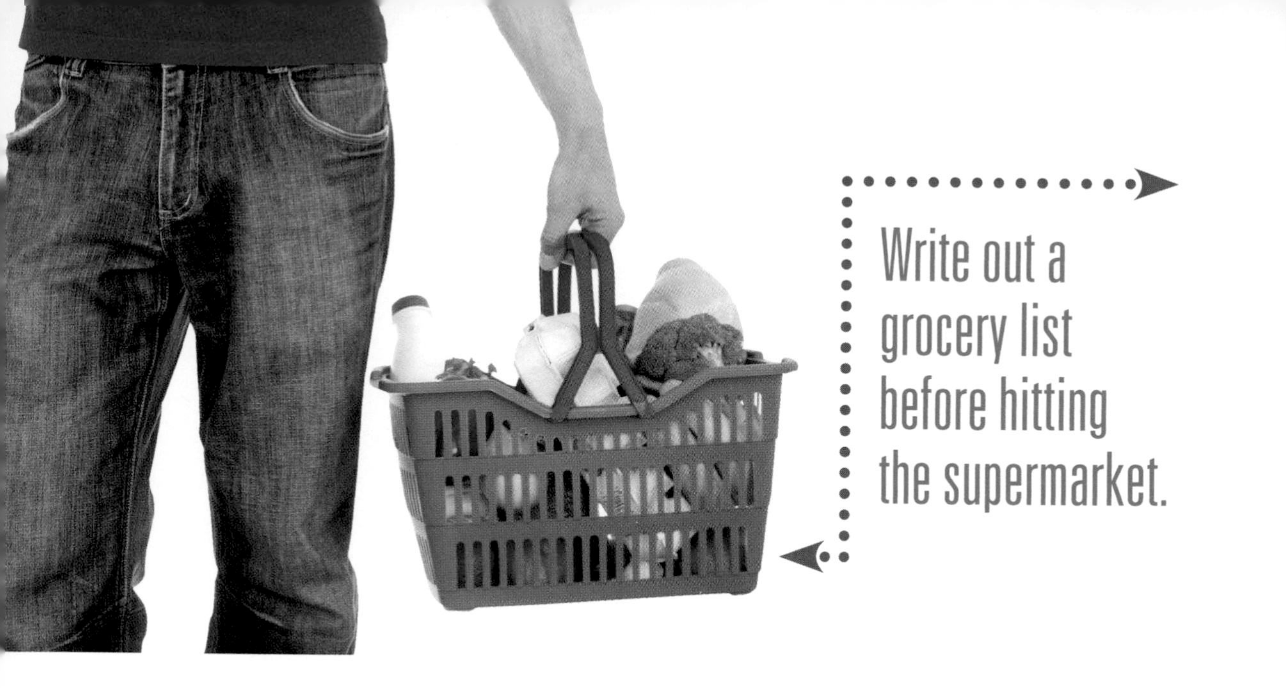
Write out a grocery list before hitting the supermarket.

## GETTING IT RIGHT – Loading up on the good stuff

Now that your cupboards are bare and you are wondering what in the world you are going to eat, it is time to stock up on the good stuff. That is, Clean Eats! We have already described how necessary it is to consume lean protein and complex carbohydrates at every meal. That is not exactly a death sentence, since most men love meat. And if you are a vegetarian, no worries; there are plenty of non-meat options to chow on too. Don't forget to partner those lean proteins with complex carbohydrates. They work better together than individually.

We like to write out a grocery list before hitting the supermarket. It helps to keep us on track with buying the good foods we intend to buy when we set out. Plus, with increasing frequency we forget things if we don't write them down. So make a list – it doesn't take much time, and if you lose your list it just might end up in a future edition of the hilarious book *Milk Eggs Vodka* by Bill Keaggy.

Back to the task at hand. We need to feed you, and fast! When you are just beginning to put Clean foods in your kitchen you will have to do a little stocking up. You will need certain ingredients to get you through the week, and a well-stocked pantry will keep you knee deep in wholesome foods and out of eating trouble. If you doubt the value of creating a pantry-stocking list, just think about all the male chefs in the world who have to do the same. Jamie Oliver wouldn't be without a list when whipping up a little something. Chef Ramsay would probably yell obscenities at anyone unfortunate enough to have forgotten. So you get the point. Don't try to remember what you need; you won't manage it. Just write the list and go shopping.

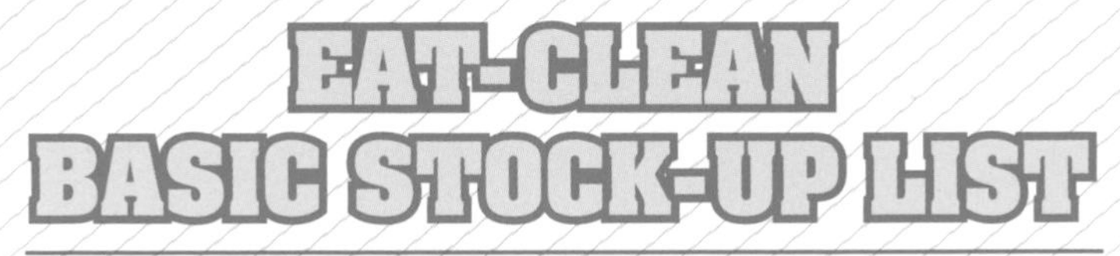


## Here's a list just for you!

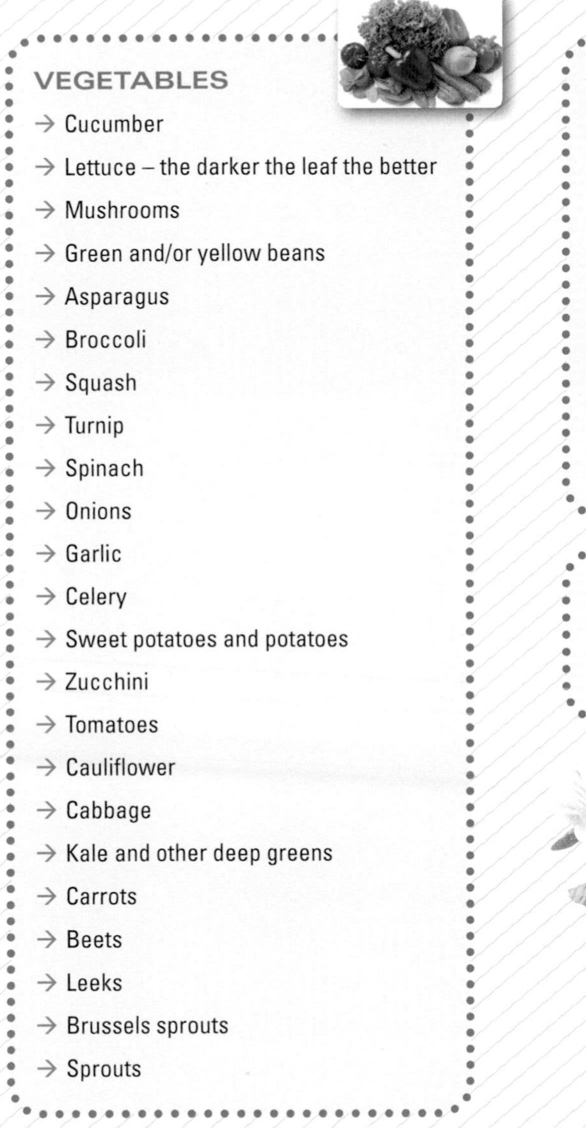

### VEGETABLES

- → Cucumber
- → Lettuce – the darker the leaf the better
- → Mushrooms
- → Green and/or yellow beans
- → Asparagus
- → Broccoli
- → Squash
- → Turnip
- → Spinach
- → Onions
- → Garlic
- → Celery
- → Sweet potatoes and potatoes
- → Zucchini
- → Tomatoes
- → Cauliflower
- → Cabbage
- → Kale and other deep greens
- → Carrots
- → Beets
- → Leeks
- → Brussels sprouts
- → Sprouts

### FRUIT

- → Berries, in season or frozen
- → Apples
- → Bananas
- → Pears
- → Avocado
- → Unsweetened dried fruit
- → Lemons and limes
- → Oranges
- → Melons

### BAKERY

- → Whole-grain breads
- → Whole-grain tortillas

### MEAT, POULTRY, SEAFOOD AND MEAT ALTERNATIVES

- → Boneless, skinless chicken breasts
- → Skinless turkey breast
- → Pork tenderloin
- → Salmon – wild if possible
- → Tilapia, cod, sole or other whitefish
- → Tofu, extra firm and silken
- → Tempeh
- → Miso
- → Textured vegetable protein
- → Beef tenderloin
- → Bison
- → Elk
- → Lean ground turkey
- → Lean ground chicken
- → Lean ground bison or beef
- → Water-packed tuna
- → Eggs – large, free range if possible

### DAIRY

- → Skim milk
- → Soy, almond and/or rice milk
- → Plain yogurt
- → Kefir
- → Butter and/or olive oil-based spread

### NUTS, SEEDS, OILS AND SNACKS

- → Unsalted almonds, cashews and walnuts
- → Unsalted sunflower seeds
- → Natural nut butters – walnut, peanut, almond and cashew
- → Flaxseeds
- → Extra virgin olive oil
- → Pumpkin seed oil
- → Avocado and other exotic oils

### CEREALS

- → Muesli with no added sugar
- → Weetabix
- → Kashi cereals
- → All-Bran
- → Fiber One
- → Red River cereal
- → Oatmeal
- → Oat bran
- → Wheat germ
- → Cream of Wheat
- → Other hot cereals

### BEVERAGES

- → Green tea
- → Regular black tea
- → Coffee

### DRY GOODS

→ Brown rice
→ Quinoa
→ Millet
→ Bulgur
→ Wheat berries
→ Whole-wheat unbleached flour
→ Baking powder and soda
→ Vanilla
→ Sea salt
→ Sugar alternatives – Sucanat, agave nectar, maple flakes
→ Whole-grain flours – amaranth, spelt, etc.
→ Spices
→ Beans

### CANNED GOODS

→ Chickpeas
→ Lentils
→ Canned organic tomatoes
→ Tomato paste
→ Water-packed tuna and/or salmon
→ Corn
→ Peas
→ Low-sodium chicken and/or vegetable stock

### CONDIMENTS

→ All-natural, sugar-free tomato sauce
→ Mustard
→ Salsa
→ Unsweetened applesauce
→ Honey
→ Tahini (for making hummus)

### SUPPLEMENTS

→ Bee pollen
→ Protein powder
→ Fish oil supplements
→ Multivitamins
→ Creatine
→ MSM
→ Magnesium
→ Calcium
→ Spirulina

### MISCELLANEOUS

→ Balsamic vinegar
→ Rice vinegar
→ Lemon juice
→ Apple cider vinegar
→ Other exotic vinegars

# EAT-CLEAN SUCCESS STORY!

**PAUL LOGAN**

From an email dated August 8, 2008

*Walking into my doctor's office was supposed to be a routine affair. I didn't feel unhealthy; in fact, I thought playing racquetball twice a week meant I was in pretty good shape. I knew from previous visits that my blood pressure was getting a little high, and for that matter, my cholesterol levels weren't great. But I thought I was eating pretty well.*

*This visit to my doctor did not turn out to be routine like the others. After reviewing the recent history of my health and taking a new blood-pressure reading, my doctor informed me that I would need to start taking medication for my high blood pressure and that medication for my high cholesterol would be next. It was a shock when he informed me that I would be taking these pills for the rest of my life. As a 50-year-old man who has always been healthy, even if I was a little overweight at 183 pounds, this was quite a shock. I told him I wanted to try and make a lifestyle change instead, as I had heard that changing eating and exercise habits could affect blood pressure. He was quite insistent that I take the medication, as he didn't believe that a lifestyle change could produce the necessary results.*

*On March 19, 2008 I began a strength-training routine twice a week with a personal trainer. A friend committed to playing racquetball with me three times per week, and I started yoga once per week. Shortly after this I asked my personal trainer about nutritional guidance and he recommended* The Eat-Clean Diet *and* The Eat-Clean Diet Cookbook. *I ran out and bought these right away.* The Eat-Clean Diet *was a great book to help me get started. It gave me the insight and knowledge of how to cook and eat in healthy ways. The second book gave me a repertoire of recipes that allowed me to*

*Soon I was buying new spices and herbs, knives and cooking pots and had taken complete control of what food I was eating. I was able to eliminate salt, eat lots of blueberries and increase my intake of various grains and oats. As the weeks rolled by, I started to become comfortable in the kitchen and was able to start experimenting with my own blend of herbs and spices.*

*After about five weeks, I was looking at my reflection in my bathroom mirror when I noticed my stomach looked odd. Over the next few weeks I realized that this "odd" look was actually muscle, appearing under the fat that was melting away.*

*At the end of June I returned to my doctor's office. He was shocked by the results. I had lost 20 pounds, my blood pressure average was 124/80, and my bad cholesterol was down to two. (Two-and-a-half would have been really good for my age.) Over the next few weeks I lost another five pounds.*

*Over the summer I had to shop for an entire new wardrobe. I now wear size 30 pants and shirts that are a size small. I haven't felt so good or healthy since I was in high school, or had as much fun buying "stylish" clothes. A recent visit to my doctor showed that my blood pressure is now 110/70.*

*I don't think I could have been this successful without the guidance of* The Eat-Clean Diet *books. Tosca's insightful recipes that are easy to read and prepare allowed me to avoid being on meds for the rest of my life.*

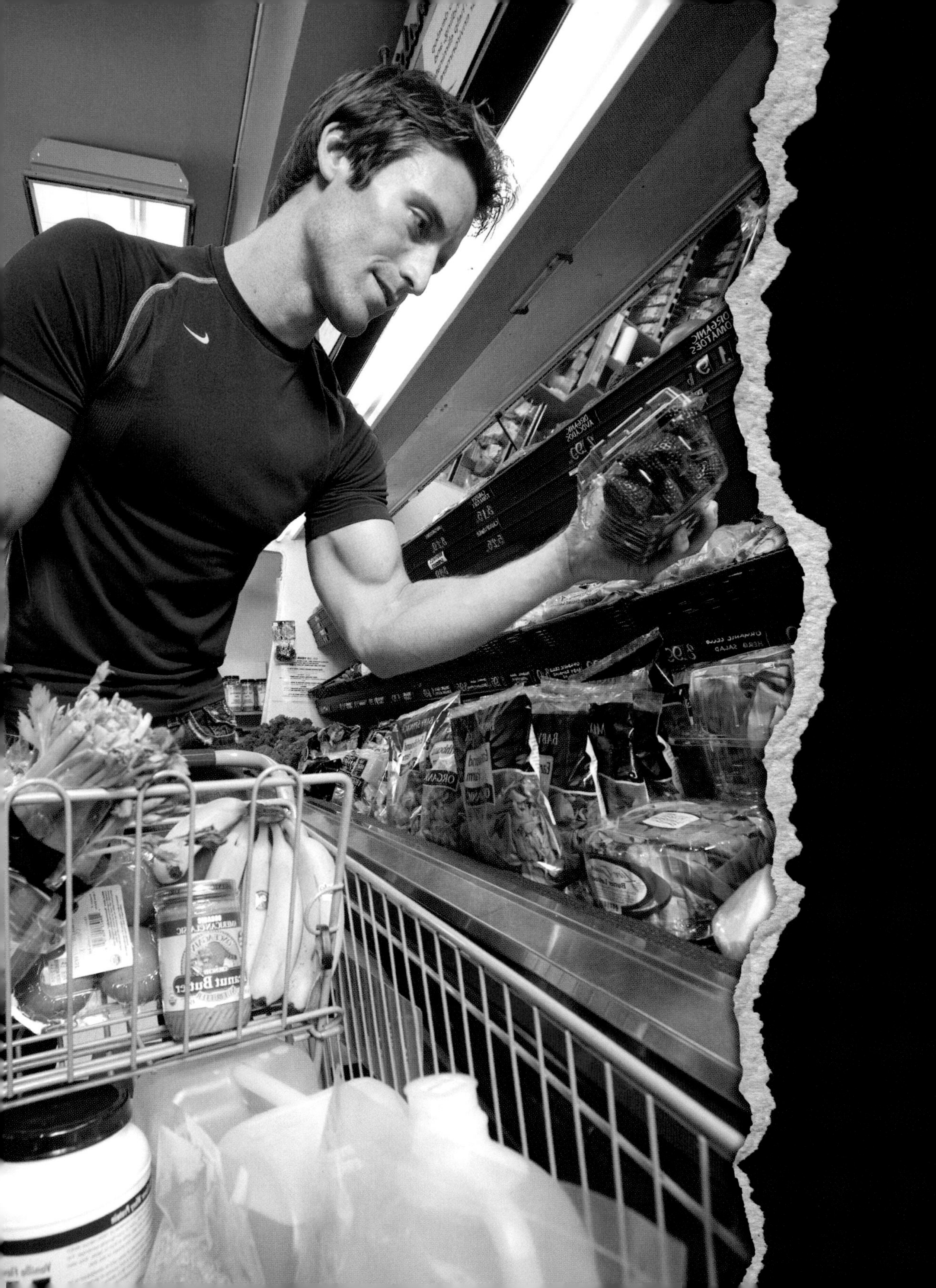
ORGANIC TOMATOES

# [CHAPTER EIGHT]

# AT THE SUPERMARKET — CLEAN SHOPPING

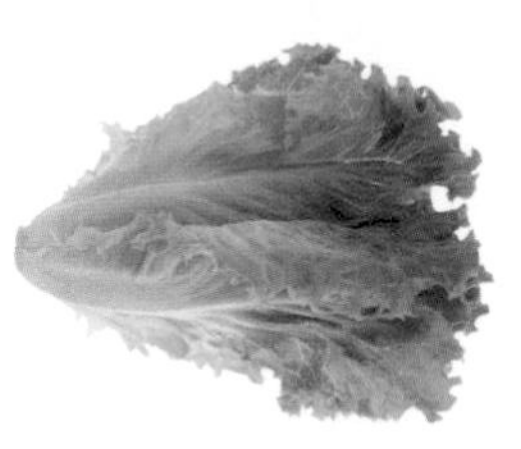

## GAME TIME

Think of it as game time. You have prepared yourself emotionally for the big day – you know where your head and heart are at. You have done your homework and studied up on the situation – you are reading this book and have assessed yourself. The playing field has been prepped – you have cleared out your cupboards, fridge and other hiding spots. Your mind is made up and now you need to fill that kitchen of yours with excellent Clean eats.

You have the details of your game plan in hand – the shopping list. Studies show that although 70 percent of us create a shopping list, most of us abandon it at the grocery store, choosing instead to select impulse buys once there. However, the exercise of creating the list has helped you review exactly what needs to be in your grocery cart in order to be successful, so whether or not you use it you are already ahead of the game. We especially believe in using a shopping list for the first big stock-up because you will need to familiarize yourself with your local supermarket and where certain previously unfamiliar foods are located. The list will also help you remember what you need. It doesn't matter if you pick up a few extra items not on your grocery list as long as they qualify as Clean-Eating foods.

## SHOPPING CLEAN – Getting your game on in the grocery store

Grocery shopping and cooking are not just for women. We have seen plenty of men doing their thing at the supermarket, although some of you may be convinced that food shopping and preparation are not your department. We want you to reconsider that notion. Stop for just a minute and think about the plethora of male celebrity chefs out there. There is one for every kind of man, from the uber-aggressive, always-shouting Gordon Ramsay to the ever-cheery naked chef, Jamie Oliver. Then there is the hugely successful Food Network, a television station devoted entirely to food. With a 44 percent (and growing) male viewing audience it is a no-brainer that the kitchen is no longer off-limits to men. Christopher Knight of Knight Productions is becoming hugely successful with numerous male-hosted, food-related TV shows, some of which are hosted by professional athletes. All the manly men we know are up to the task and just need a few skills to get it down.

## ONCE THERE

Here you are at the supermarket. Whether small, big, or just plain enormous, let the buyer beware – that means you – that grocery stores are set up in such a way to make the customer stay as long as possible, increasing the chance of pulling your money out of your pockets and dumping it into theirs. Not to belabor the point, but this is another reason a shopping list is so helpful. It keeps you from buying what you don't need. In general, supermarkets are laid out so foods requiring chilling and freezing are placed on the perimeter where the electrical outlets are located. Makes sense, right? Here is where you will find produce, meats, dairy, eggs, cheese, yogurt and anything else that needs to be kept cold.

Pay attention to labels right from the start. It is not enough to have "lean ground turkey" on your grocery list. Once you have arrived at the meat department you will now have to put your glasses on and actually read the label on your lean ground turkey package. Check to make sure the ingredient list, even in something as simple as this item, contains nothing but lean ground meat from a turkey. For it to be lean there must be no skin or other bits in the meat. You may be in for a surprise if you don't check carefully. We also like to purchase hormone- and antibiotic-free meats, which have been cut from grass-fed animals. It is slightly more difficult to find these, but the more you vote with your dollars for this kind of food the more readily available and less expensive they will be.

We are fortunate to have in our vicinity a wonderful butcher shop where all cuts of meat and fish are sourced from environmentally friendly, raised-with-a-conscience farms. Howard, from Howard the Butcher, is happy to take orders, even from picky people like us who will request venison, bison, capon and other meats. A butcher shop like this is a godsend, but it is not impossible to find similar service elsewhere. In fact, with the dawn of the Internet and the extent of its power it is possible to purchase exotic meats online and have them delivered to your door within days. Be certain that what you are purchasing is exactly what you want.

Since lean protein is the backbone of each of the six small meals you will be eating each day it makes good sense to purchase the best, leanest, healthiest cuts of meat available. Lean cuts of red meats include beef or bison tenderloin, eye of round, top round, round tip, top sirloin and bottom round. Venison and lamb with the excess fat cut off are also highly nutritious and lean cuts of red meats. Don't cut corners here. And relax! The money you are spending here is money you won't be spending on junk food or health-care bills.

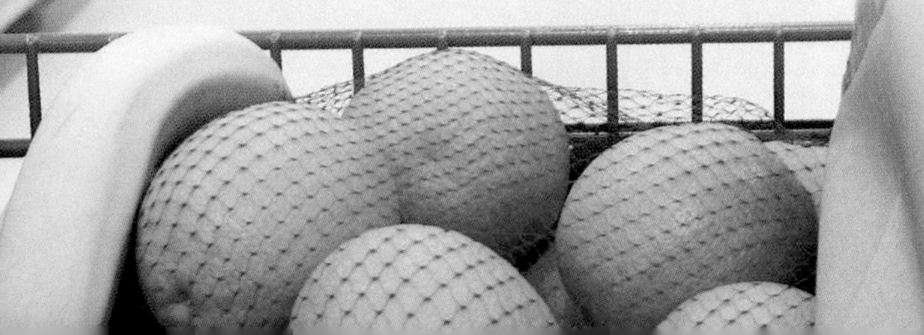

## A WORD ABOUT MONEY

If you are concerned about your food budget and wish to approach with caution, there is a way to accomplish that too. Many protein superstars are not expensive. Think eggs, egg whites, water-packed tuna, cottage cheese, quinoa, yogurt, beans, tofu and liver. If you buy these items in bulk they are even more cost effective. Wander over to the bulk-packaged items in the meat department and look for family-sized packages of chicken breasts. Although you may not have a family, buying your meat this way helps to keep the cost down, especially if you make good use of your freezer and fridge.

Here's another wallet-friendly tip. Purchase a whole chicken or turkey and roast it. Discard the skin. Remove all the meat from the carcass and place it in storage containers. You will now have plenty of cooked meat for sandwiches, stir-fries, soups and so on. Then you can toss the carcass into a big soup pot with loads of vegetables and make your own soup. Stock made from simmered bones contains a highly nutritious form of protein that is rarely seen these days. Called gelatin, this protein comes from the bones once they have been allowed to bubble away on the stove for several hours. A Dutchman who is serious about his soup stock won't touch any stock unless it is gelatinous! In our house, where Dutch heritage prevails, a concoction of chopped vegetables including celery, onions and carrots is essential to creating the best stock. These vegetables draw out the nutrients of the bones and ultimately make a thick gelatin. The gelatin forms after a long period of cooking and cooling. At this point, skimming fat off the stock is a simple matter, since it will sit on top of the gelatin in a hardened layer. Use a spoon to remove and discard the fat.* (See below.) Now you have a beautifully flavored, highly nutritious stock with which to make your own soups, sauce for stews and even as the liquid in which to cook rice. Easy!

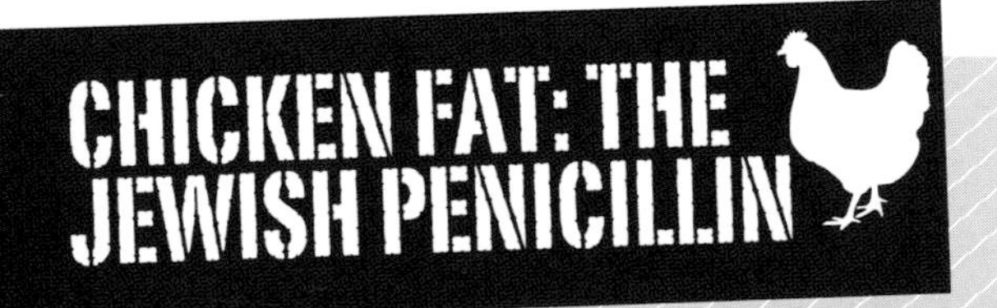


A word about chicken fat from grass-fed free-range chickens. In many Jewish households chicken fat is called "Jewish penicillin" for its immune-boosting ability. "The Jewish penicillin wasn't skinless chicken breasts; it was chicken soup, with droplets of golden fat that also makes chicken soup silky," writes Nina Planck in *Real Food.* Pulmonary medicine specialist Dr. Stephen Rennard tested his wife's grandmother's chicken soup recipe to learn what, if anything, chicken soup could do for the common cold. Rennard found that chicken soup actually has a "mild medicinal effect, inhibiting inflammation of the cells in the nasal passage, reducing the symptoms of a cold."

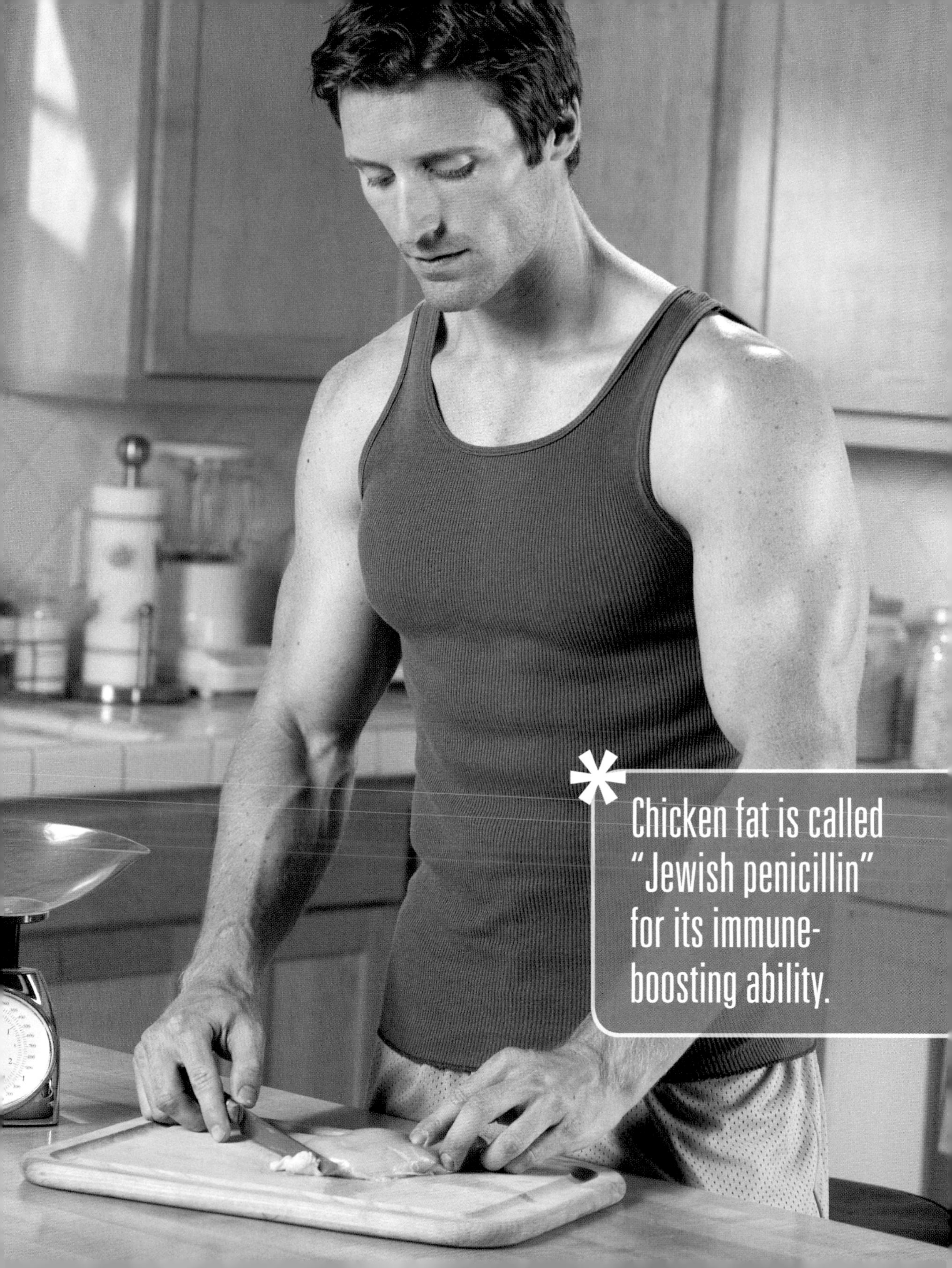

*

Chicken fat is called "Jewish penicillin" for its immune-boosting ability.

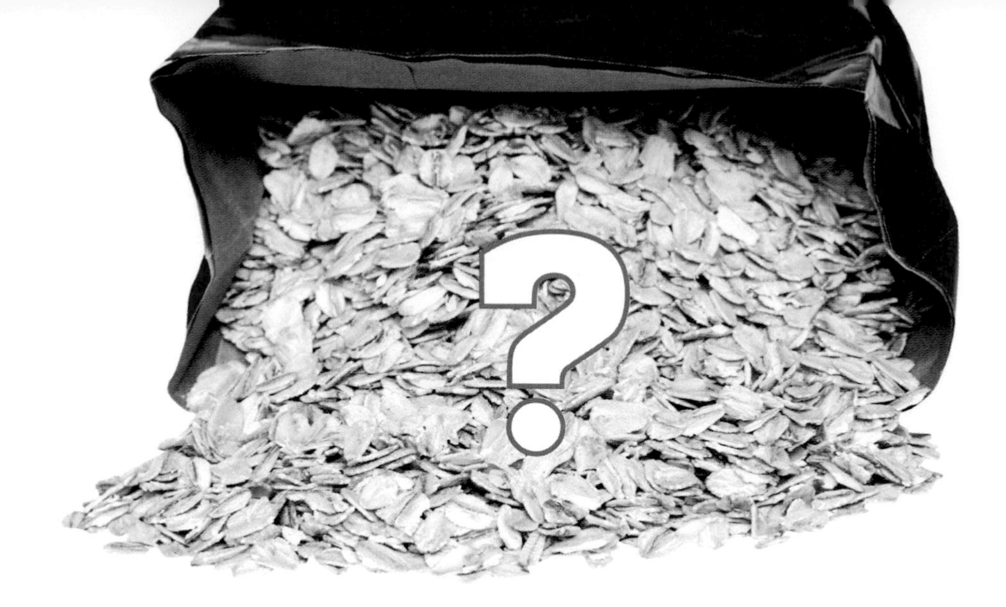

# THOROUGHLY CONFUSED ABOUT CEREAL!

We are all for simplicity in our house. We strive to keep life as simple and uncomplicated as possible, since it is already as nutty as you can imagine with two busy careers, deadlines, a house, five children, aging parents and two dogs! Food shopping and preparation needs to be simple too. Why then do we feel completely outwitted when we arrive in the cereal aisle? Is there any other aisle as big and with so many different products? We doubt it! There are literally hundreds of brands and varieties in that monstrous aisle and all are made from very simple, basic starting ingredients – whole grains, those powerful complex carbohydrates needed for perfect Clean Eating. However, this aisle is where the most subterfuge is happening.

These big food companies really want your bucks. Grains by themselves cost pennies per serving, but when you pay someone called a "food engineer" to create a so-called "new" way of eating that grain – puffing, popping, coloring, flavoring and pretty much disguising it beyond any recognition – and put it in nice packaging, then you can charge a lot more money for that lowly grain. Consider a box of Froot Loops. At our grocery store today a jumbo box weighing 925 grams cost $7.99, out of which you can get 35 three-quarter-cup servings, the recommend serving size on the box. (Although few kids, let alone men, would be satisfied with such a small serving.) Each serving costs 22.8 cents. Now consider the lowly oat. We purchased a bag of oats weighing 2.2 kilograms for $3.29. We measured 70 one-third-cup servings of dry oats. Each serving cost 4.7 cents. Need we say more? Not only is a serving of oats healthier and less expensive, we are certain that a serving of hot oatmeal will satisfy much longer than a bowl of Froot Loops.

The argument for simplicity is never more sensible than when in the cereal aisle. Our confusion ends every time when we pick up a bag of oatmeal. We feel a bit sheepish when we walk past box after box of colored fluff and bend down to the bottom shelf to pick up the lowly bag of oats. Sheepish maybe, but we are on to something with those oats.

Try to remember that the natural whole grains are already packaged perfectly, nutritionally speaking. A whole grain is one that is in its complete form and not stripped of its nutrition-giving goodness that includes fiber, minerals, healthy fats, protein, enzymes and vitamins. Without the glitz and glam of a colorful cereal box, oats, Cream of Wheat, rice, quinoa, amaranth, spelt, kamut, wheat berries, millet and wheat germ are nutritional superfoods that fly under the radar but are exactly what you need. Don't be seduced by the boxes. Eat these humble grains as nature intended. These cereals provide hardcore nutrition that help to fuel your body in the healthiest way possible. They don't strip your body of nutrients on their way through the digestive tract, they don't spike hormone levels and they don't compact waste materials in your bowels – heck, they are so good for you it's almost too simple. Eat them every day!

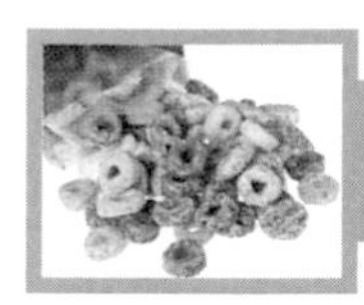

Don't be seduced by the boxes.
Eat these humble grains as nature intended.

# BOB AND TOSCA EAT BREAKFAST

## WHAT TOSCA EATS, OFF-SEASON:

- 1 cup cooked oatmeal topped with 2 Tbsp each wheat germ, ground flax-seed, bee pollen and Salba
- ½ cup mixed berries
- 4 egg whites and 1 yolk
- 250 ml water with 6 oz wheat grass
- Black coffee

## WHAT BOB EATS:

- 1 cup cooked oatmeal with ½ cup mixed berries topped with ½ cup skim milk
- 4 egg whites and 1 yolk
- 2 pieces multi-grain toast with unsweetened applesauce
- 250 ml water
- 1 cup black coffee

# STILL SHOPPING THE PERIMETER

You will also find the produce section on the perimeter, usually quite near the entrance of the supermarket. It will be very difficult for you to find a food in the produce department that carries a nutrition label. And that is what we like about this area. That and the fact that here is the place where you will find a pirate's treasure of complex carbohydrates to partner with lean protein in your Clean-Eating regimen. We always begin our food shopping in the produce department. For us, it is difficult to resist piling the cart with the colorful abundance that we know delivers our best health. Berries, bananas, apples, peppers, sprouts, sweet potatoes, celery, spinach, radishes and more – such foods spell health. Purchase plenty of these fresh foods and depend on them for the bulk of your daily Clean Eating.

Think fresh foods are expensive? Think again. Marion Nestle writes in *What to Eat* that canned foods actually cost more: "After accounting for the parts that get thrown out, the economists reported that most of the fresh fruits and vegetables they examined cost less than they did either canned or frozen ... marketing is an important barrier. American food and beverage producers spend $36 billion annually to advertise and market their products, but practically none of this goes to promote fruits and vegetables ... produce is just not profitable enough." In other words, the simplest of fruits and vegetables are the more cost-effective ones to eat. So don't worry that the whole budget will go into the red when you begin to Eat Clean; it is just not true. And if you begin to factor in long-term health-care costs, well, there is just no argument. When you're healthy you are not a burden on the health-care system.

Think fresh foods are expensive?

Think again.

Marion Nestle writes in **What to Eat** that canned foods actually cost more.

# SHOPPING LOWDOWN

✔ **Perimeter shop.** Fresh foods live here. Avoid center aisles of the grocery store unless you are stocking up on whole grains.

✔ **Shop with a grocery list.** Stick to your preplanned shopping list to help you avoid center aisles where junk foods live. This will save time, money and pounds.

✔ **Buy fresh!** Your greatest chance for Clean-Eating success is to eat fresh, unprocessed foods. Forget cans and boxes and eat closer to the ground, the way nature intended food to be.

✔ **Never shop hungry.** If you shop when hungry you will be at a far greater risk of impulse buying.

✔ **Buy organic if possible.** Conventionally grown fruits and vegetables contain harmful levels of pesticides and herbicides, and they are often produced with growth hormones, antibiotics and genetic manipulation.

✔ **Canned tomatoes are a good buy.** Cooked tomatoes found in sauces and other canned-tomato products contain higher amounts of the antioxidant lycopene. Canned tomatoes are essential in the hungry man's kitchen because they can easily become the basis of a quick meal.

✔ **Don't buy all produce at the same stage of ripeness.** You can't eat all your produce at once, so try to stagger the stage of ripeness of the various fruits and vegetables. Buy bananas green and never purchase overripe berries. They won't last.

✔ **Buy in season.** Fruits and vegetables purchased in season are often sourced from farms and suppliers that are much closer to home. That translates into saved money and higher nutrition for you, since foods in season are usually fresher and picked in a riper state.

✔ **Avoid high fructose corn syrup and other sugars.** High fructose corn syrup and other sweeteners are quite simply poisonous to your health and should be avoided at all costs.

✔ **Load up on canned beans.** Beans and lentils can be mixed with brown rice to make the perfect protein for vegetarians or even carnivores wanting to take a break from eating meat. Beans can be added to soups and stews, puréed with other ingredients to make hummus as an alternative spread for bread, or served in pastas, stews, salads and soups.

- ✔ **Look for one-item or short ingredient lists.** The fewer items on the ingredient list, the healthier the food.

- ✔ **More fiber.** Eat more fiber on a daily basis. The more you eat the less hungry you will be and the less likely you will be overweight.

- ✔ **Avoid partially hydrogenated oil** and other trans fatty acids at all costs.

- ✔ **Experiment with whole-grain alternatives.** Today you can find healthful varieties of whole-grain pastas and couscous, brown rice and quinoa that beg for a place in your Clean-Eating kitchen.

- ✔ **Cook with macadamia nut or olive oil.** These oils contain the better monounsaturated fats and have a higher smoke point, so less trans fatty acid will be formed during cooking.

- ✔ **Stick to plain yogurt.** Plain low-fat yogurt can be made to taste as sweet as commercially flavored yogurt by adding your own chopped fruits or unsweetened applesauce to it. Doing it this way saves money too.

## SHOPPING IS FOR EVERYONE!

Shopping is not usually such a page turner for you gentlemen, but we think now that you have gotten the idea you won't feel so overwhelmed when you next arrive at a supermarket. Remember to keep your dollars in your pocket as much as possible by buying Clean-Eating foods that are as close as possible to their natural state – the healthiest, most nutritious state for you. Before long you will relish the taste of fresh fruits and vegetables and realize that you feel a completely renewed sense of wellness and energy. In the next chapter you will learn all about how to supplement or enhance your Clean Eating with various additional foods.

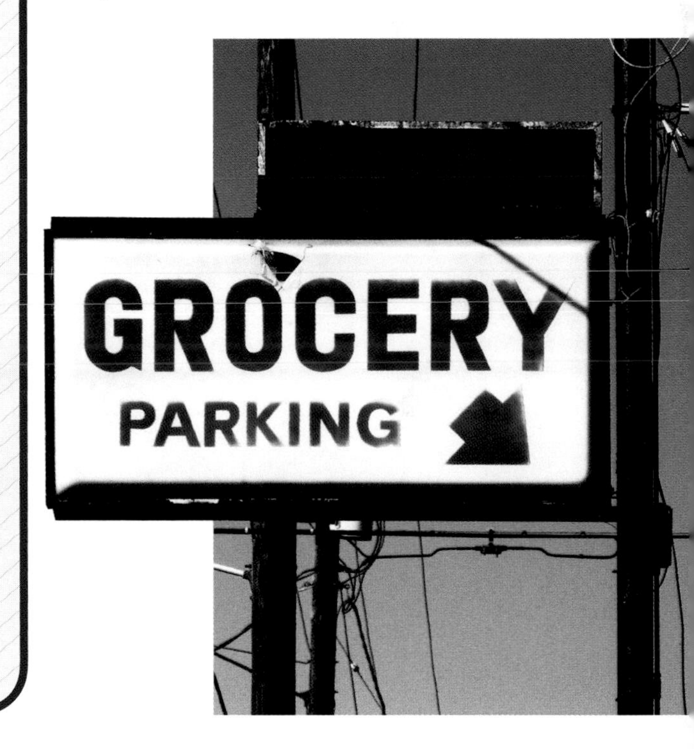

# SHOP HEALTHY AT THESE GROCERY STORES

The job of grocery shopping has changed greatly since the days of our parents. There isn't just one store around the corner from which to purchase your food needs. Today you can shop at large chain supermarkets or your local grocer; even the retail giant Walmart sells groceries. Buying healthy is the goal, so here is a list of the healthiest grocery stores in North America. Don't forget the little guy though. We can purchase all our Clean-Eating groceries at our local natural-food store, butcher, vegetable stand and bulk store with no trouble at all.

### WHOLE FOODS MARKET

Who isn't aware that Whole Foods Market is *the* place to go for healthy eats? The store builds its sales platform on natural foods, but you can find conventionally grown produce right beside the organic options. It is one of the few places we have been able to find bison meat, as well as antibiotic- and hormone-free meats. This is the place to buy quinoa – the superfood whole grain we are always kvetching about. There are 279 Whole Foods Market locations in the United States and six in Canada (hopefully with more on the way).

### SAFEWAY

This grocery chain is found both in the United States and Canada. On first glance the store looks a lot like a regular supermarket, but the owners/managers have noticed the desire for folks to Eat Clean so they have included organic foods as well as many natural foods that you will need to stock up on, including flaxseeds, bee pollen and more. There are 1,700 stores in the United States and 219 locations in western Canada.

### TRADER JOE'S

We have visited this store in Portland, Oregon, where one of our daughters is studying. It seems we can find everything there except for a lot of what we don't want – junk. This supermarket feels like you are entering a place where whatever you are about to buy will be good for you. We love it! There are 314 stores in the United States with more locations opening soon.

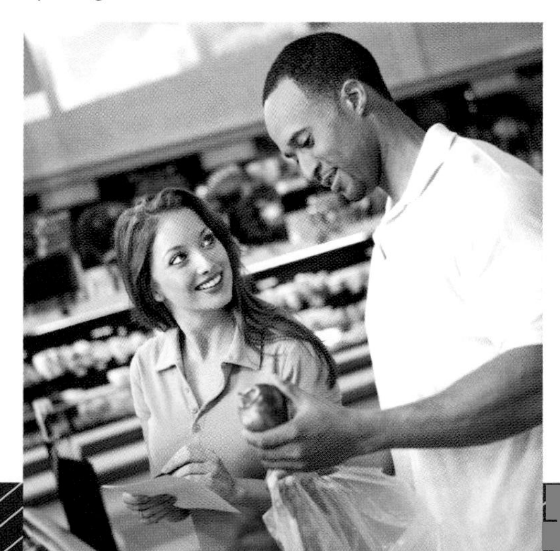

### ALBERTSONS

This is another big food chain that has added a healthy-food line. Wild Harvest foods entice organic and health-minded customers to shop here. There are 529 stores located in the United States, predominantly in the west.

### PUBLIX

With 952 stores located in the southeast, this food chain offers plenty of healthy fare. Load up on produce, both natural and organic, and pay attention to their At Season's Peak program. When produce is in season it is usually at its peak nutritionally and it costs less.

### LOBLAWS / ZEHRS

Canadians can find healthy, Clean-Eating options at the Loblaws chain, including Zehrs, where we have never seen a greater selection of fresh produce. The variety of apples, greens and other fruits and vegetables is staggering; we end up buying more than we need just because it looks so good. The chain carries lovely fresh fish and organic meats and has a well-stocked natural-foods section in most of their larger stores. Look for Ezekiel products in the freezer section. As there are over 1,000 stores across Canada you will always find healthy, Clean-Eating options just around the corner.

### SUPERTARGET

Who knew Target doubles as a healthy grocer? They offer some of the better-known organic names including Kashi, Quaker and Barbara's. Target also offers a small array of fresh produce and dairy, perfect for the customer who needs to pick something up for dinner – you'll find just enough to get the job done.

### YOUR LOCAL HEALTHY-FOODS MARKET

Don't forget to support the little guy in your neck of the woods. Some of these forward-thinking folks were spouting healthy eating long before the big chains even thought of it. We find our local Harmony Whole Foods will actually take requests if we are looking for something special that we can't already find on their shelves. They also carry local foods, particularly dairy and meat products that aren't widely available. We feel as if we often stumble on a well-kept secret when we shop there.

References:

*CNN.com* November 2008

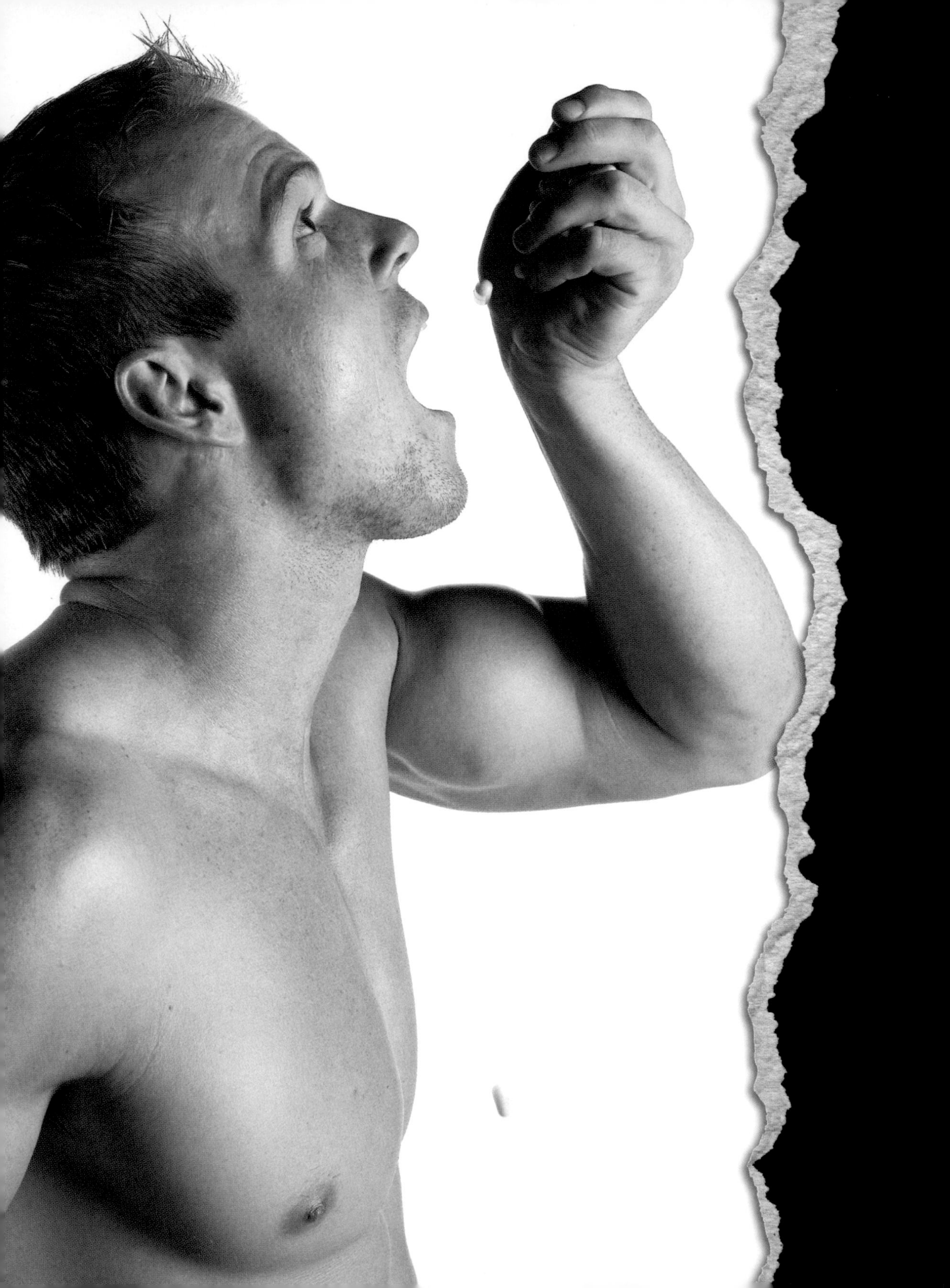

# [CHAPTER NINE]

# SUPPLEMENT ROSTER

## SUPPLEMENTS AND SUPERFOODS

The world of supplements is a multi-billion-dollar business. If you doubt this statement, have a look at the shelves in your local health food or grocery store. There are so many pills, powders and liquids proclaiming health that we all might wonder what we are missing by not taking some of these products. However, in these containers lurks plenty of snake oil! At every turn we are being warned to take this or that product to prevent a potentially damaging health condition. Who knows what is right or wrong to take? And what really works?

We urge you to carefully consider your selection of what you may or may not want to add to your nutrition in the way of supplements. While considering your choices, remember that a supplement is, by definition, something *added* to your daily food in order to boost levels of vitamins, minerals, enzymes and other nutrients. There are many supplemental ingredients you can live without, just as there are many that can improve health significantly when added to the diet on a regular basis. We would like to share in this chapter which supplements, in our collective experience, have been helpful to us or to the masses. Although supplements are no substitute for good, regular, wholesome nutrition, they can give you that extra edge.

## WHY SHOULD WE TAKE SUPPLEMENTS?

Today, the way we eat and drink is not the same as it was in the days of our parents, their parents and certainly not our primitive ancestors. Global industrialization and the population explosion have stressed every aspect of our environment. As a result our bodies have become similarly overburdened with toxins. In fact, much of the experimentation our food companies have dabbled in for the last several decades could be called chemical soup. The challenge is to sort out what will help us detoxify our bodies and strengthen our immune systems so we can forge ahead under these stressful conditions in the best health possible. Some supplements really can help us accomplish this. Knowing what works and what doesn't is a matter of educating yourself. This chapter should clarify the murky supplement waters for you.

## WHAT IS A SUPPLEMENT?

A supplement is, by definition, an ingredient added to complete a thing, make up a deficiency or extend or strengthen the whole. Vitamins, minerals, enzymes, supplements and superfoods all help to make up for nutritional deficiencies.

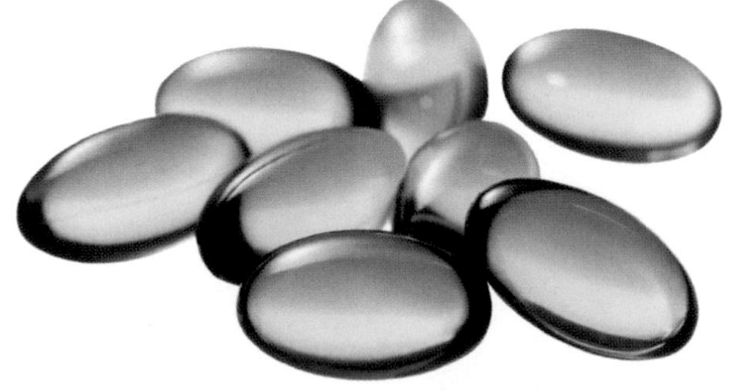

# SUPERFOODS

When people ate closer to the ground, as in the days of our forefathers, no one talked about superfoods because foods such as oats, grass-fed beef and natural milk were routinely eaten. Today, many foods have earned the title of superfood simply because the general population has eliminated eating them in favor of factory-formed quasi foods. Superfoods are not really that special; it's just that if you add them to your current roster of foods you are supplementing your diet, and yes, certain foods are densely charged with nutritional elements.

If you currently eat loads of refined carbohydrates, adding fresh fruits and vegetables will supplement the lesser ingredients. When Clean Eating becomes routine for you, you may not need to be reminded to eat tomatoes any longer. Until then, consider fresh produce, whole grains, legumes and lean meats to be your supplemental superfoods. Should kale, broccoli and sweet potatoes regularly appear on your plate, good for you, but consider adding a few more items from the Clean-Eating superfoods and supplements list.

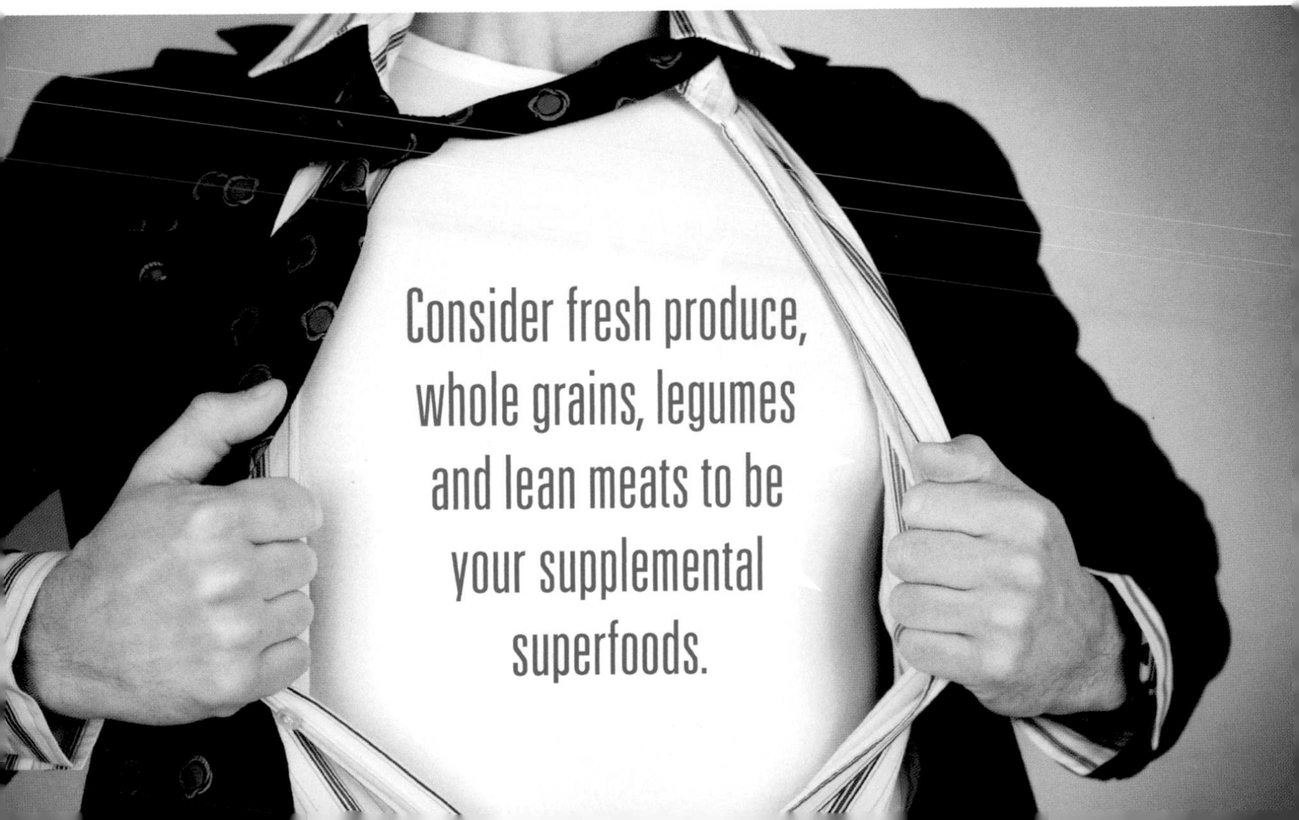

Consider fresh produce, whole grains, legumes and lean meats to be your supplemental superfoods.

# SUPERHERO SUPERFOODS

## VEGETABLES

- Artichokes
- Asparagus
- Beet greens
- Beets
- Broccoli
- Brussels sprouts
- Cabbage
- Carrots
- Cauliflower
- Celeriac
- Chervil
- Chicory
- Chinese cabbage
- Chives
- Corn
- Cucumbers
- Dandelion greens
- Eggplant
- Endive
- Garlic
- Green beans
- Kale
- Kohlrabi
- Leeks
- Lettuce
- Mushrooms
- Mustard greens
- Okra
- Onions
- Parsley
- Parsnips
- Peas
- Peppers
- Pumpkin
- Squash
- Radishes
- Red cabbage
- Rutabaga
- Turnip
- Spinach and leafy green vegetables
- Tomatoes
- Watercress

## FRUITS

- Acai and goji berries
- Apples
- Apricots
- Blackberries
- Blueberries
- Cherries
- Cranberries
- Currants
- Grapefruit
- Grapes
- Lemons
- Limes
- Mangoes
- Melons
- Nectarines
- Oranges
- Papaya
- Peaches
- Pears
- Pineapple
- Plums
- Pomegranates
- Prunes
- Raspberries
- Rhubarb
- Strawberries
- Tangerines
- Watermelon

## PROTEIN

- Beef tenderloin
- Bison
- Chicken breast
- Clams
- Cod
- Egg whites
- Mussels
- Pork tenderloin
- Salmon
- Sea bass
- Tofu
- Turkey breast
- Unsalted nuts
- Water-packed tuna
- Whitefish

## DAIRY

- Skim milk
- Low-fat yogurt
- Low-fat hard cheese
- Low-fat cottage cheese

# TOP-10 SUPERFOODS

## Tomatoes

The tomato, although American in origin, had its culinary debut in Europe, where it was widely eaten well before Americans embraced it. Considered poisonous by many until barely 100 years ago, it is now the most popular vegetable, eaten in varying forms from soups and stews to raw right off the vine. At one time regarded to be a giant berry, the tomato is an ideal Clean-Eating food. Tomatoes are dense with nutrients and complex carbohydrates. Phytochemicals in the ripe red flesh of a tomato prevent free radicals from damaging joints, muscles and brain cells. Lycopene, one of the most powerful anticancer agents (especially effective against prostate cancer) and found in good supply in the tomato, is more readily absorbed by the body after the tomato has been cooked, so load up on tomato soup, pasta and pizza sauce too – the Clean-Eating kind, of course.

**STAR NUTRIENTS:**

- Lycopene
- Carotenoids, especially the antioxidant beta-carotene

**FACT:** Only red tomatoes contain lycopene.

**HINT:** Roasting in the oven improves the flavor of mid-winter tomatoes. To roast, simply wash plum tomatoes, halve them and lay them flat on a nonstick cookie sheet. Roast them at 350°F for 25 minutes. Purée the flesh and add to soups, stews and sauces.

**STORAGE TIPS:** Don't store fresh tomatoes in the fridge or with other fruits. Ripening tomatoes emit a gas that causes other fruits in proximity to rot. Instead, place them in a bowl on your kitchen counter to ripen. This will also help to improve their flavor.

**NUTRIENTS PER ½-CUP SERVING:**

Calories: 17
Protein: 1 g
Fiber: 1 g
Potassium: 250 mg
Beta-carotene: 620 mcg
Vitamin C: 17 mg
Vitamin E: 1 mg
Folate: 17 mcg

# Skinless Turkey Breast

Don't reserve turkey for Thanksgiving and Christmas. This lean poultry is a superfood thanks to its high nutrition profile. What makes turkey supercharged is that it is loaded with lean protein, vitamins and minerals, which fits nicely in your Clean-Eating lifestyle. Use lean ground turkey breast in place of ground beef; just check that the skin has not been ground into the meat. When choosing a whole turkey, be careful to select a bird that has not been injected with oil or butter – this takes the "lean" out of lean protein.

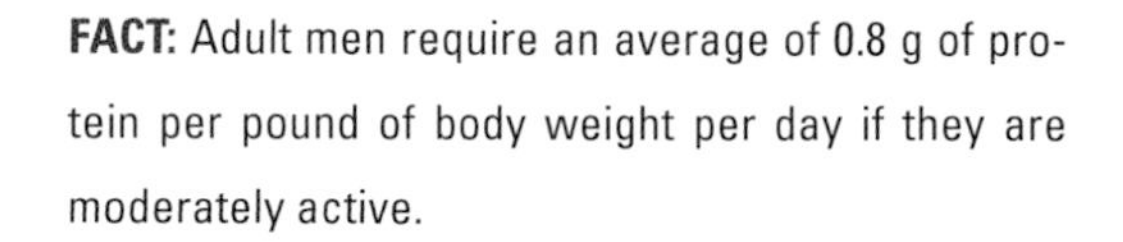

**FACT:** Adult men require an average of 0.8 g of protein per pound of body weight per day if they are moderately active.

Adult men training with weights require 1.1 to 1.4 g of protein or more per pound of body weight each day. It takes 1 g of protein per day per pound of body weight to grow muscle.

**TIP:** Turkey breast meat contains the phytochemical carnosine. This compound preserves muscle and brain tissue. Carnosine is often given to performance athletes to improve endurance and to enhance muscle formation.

**STAR NUTRIENTS:**

- Lean protein
- Minerals

**NUTRIENTS PER 6-OZ SERVING:**

| | |
|---|---|
| Calories: 230 | Niacin: 6.3 mg |
| Protein: 51 g | Vitamin B-6: 6.6 mg |
| Cholesterol: 142 mg | Vitamin B-12: 3.2mcg |
| Potassium: 699 mcg | Iron: 2.4 mg |
| Calcium: 5 mg | Selenium: 38.4 mcg |
| Sodium: 90 mg | Zinc: 2.4 mg |

## Wild Salmon

In places where indigenous peoples have access to plenty of wild salmon, modern-day diseases like heart attacks, hypertension, diabetes and strokes are unheard of. Wild salmon contains highly specialized EFAs – essential fatty acids – necessary for keeping body tissues healthy and free from inflammation. These fats play an important role in controlling metabolism, and so it is essential to add this fish to your daily diet. Wild salmon is a nutrient-dense source of quality, easily digested protein, vitamins and minerals and is low in saturated fat. Since it contains fewer hormones, toxins and chemicals than its farm-raised cousin, it is worth the extra money to include wild salmon in your diet at least once a week.

**TONING FACTOR:**

The flesh of wild salmon contains a powerful antioxidant – DMAE, or dimethylaminoethanol – which stimulates nerve function and tones muscle. Recently, it has shown up in facial creams, where it is said to "lift" sagging, wrinkled skin.

**WILD IS RED:**

The intense red flesh of wild salmon comes from carotenoids that the fish ingests in its diet of krill and other shellfish. Farmed salmon is usually much lighter in color, but if it is densely colored this is because it has had dye injected into its diet. Stay away from that kind of fish!

**STAR NUTRIENTS:**

- Protein
- Essential fatty acids

**NUTRIENTS PER 3-OZ SERVING:**

Calories: 121
Protein: 17 g
Sodium: 37 mg
Essential fatty acids: 7 g
Marine omega-3 fatty acids: 1,716 mg
Vitamin B-6: 1.6 mg
Vitamin B-12: 6.3 mcg
Selenium: 31 mcg

## Broccoli

Deeply colored green plants such as broccoli are among the most important foods to include on your superfoods list. You will want these on your menu often, since their impact on your body is not just to help create lean muscle mass. A great deal of their power lies in what you can't see, which are phytochemicals known to boost the immune system, fortifying it with the cancer-fighting agent called sulforaphane. This crunchy vegetable appears on our plates frequently, not only because its heavy fiber content keeps us full for long periods of time, but also because it's easy to steam a batch; just cook it until it turns bright green. We save the water to throw into soup stock. Oh, and let's not forget, a serving of broccoli contains more vitamin C than a glass of orange juice.

**EAT IT!**

Steamed or raw broccoli is a key vegetable for Clean-Eating nutrition.

**STAR NUTRIENTS:**

- Folate
- Vitamin C

**NUTRIENTS PER 1¼-CUP SERVING:**

Calories: 33
Beta-carotene: 575 mcg
Iron: 2 mg
Calcium: 56 mg
Folate: 90 mcg
Potassium: 370 mg
Vitamin C: 87 mg
Fiber: 3 g

# Berries

Berries of any kind should be on your Clean-Eating superfoods list. Think about it! Bears in the wild eat tons of berries, and most bears we have seen are muscular and enormous. Berries will keep you lean and healthy because they pack a load of nutritious factors in each one, including disease-fighting antioxidants and heaps of fiber. Blueberries are especially good. Berries are packed with iron, vitamins A and C, fiber, carotenoids and anthocyanins. Eating one cup of berries per day virtually guarantees good health. Try them in salads, on cold or hot cereal, in smoothies or just plain out of your hand.

**STAR NUTRIENTS:**

- Fiber
- Vitamin C

**NUTRIENTS PER 1-CUP SERVING:**

Calories: 30
Vitamin C: 17 mg
Fiber: 2 g
Carbohydrates: 57 g
Calcium: 12 mg
Folate: 6 mcg
Carotene: 30 mcg

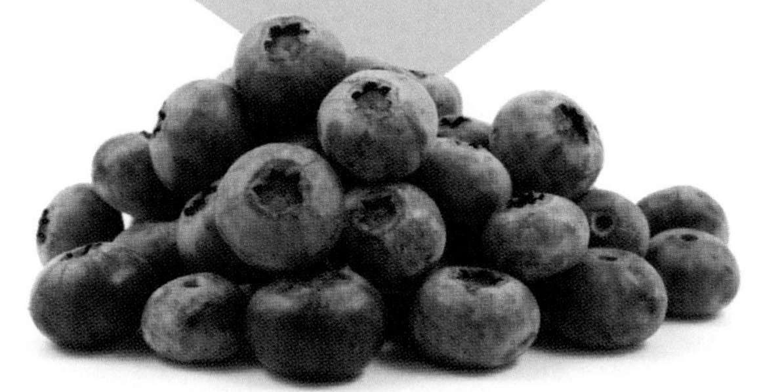

**EASY TO EAT.** Berries are at their prime right off the bush, but they are equally delicious raw, sitting atop your morning oatmeal or yogurt and as a snack to appease hunger before bed.

**AÇAI AND GOJI BERRIES.** Goji berries are a nutritional powerhouse hailing from the Himalayan mountains. Bursting with antioxidants, the tiny red berries are becoming more and more popular with savvy nutritionists and physique enthusiasts. You will never find the berries fresh because they perish much too quickly, but you can eat them dried or drink their juice. Ounce for ounce they contain more vitamin C than any other vitamin C-containing food.

Açai berries grow in the Amazon rain forest on açai palm trees and look like purple marbles. They contain high levels of anthocyanins – cancer- and disease-fighting agents. They also contain healthy omega fatty acids, amino acids, fiber and iron. For such small berries they pack a load of easily digestible plant protein along with carbohydrates – the perfect Clean-Eating meal all in one package! Oprah Winfrey and Dr. Nicolas Perricone recommend them for anti-aging and health factors.

## Beans and Legumes

Beans, sometimes called pulses, are an important and economical way to supplement your diet with protein, fiber and vitamins. Be careful to eat beans in combination with other foods (see page 63 for protein combos) because the protein from beans is incomplete. When combined with nuts, seeds or grains, they form a complete high-fiber vegetable protein. Beans are a good source of protein, calcium, iron and fiber, which make them perfect for including as part of your Clean-Eating meals. Studies show beans, which contain no cholesterol, help to reduce cholesterol levels while providing excellent nutrition, because of their high fiber content.

**STAR NUTRIENTS:**

- Fiber
- Protein

**NUTRIENTS PER 4-OZ SERVING:**

| | |
|---|---|
| Calories: 266 | Calcium: 100 mg |
| Protein: 22 g | Iron: 6 mg |
| Carbohydrates: 44 g | Zinc: 3 mg |

## WAS THAT YOU?

Soak beans overnight to eliminate some of those gassy problems.

**HUMMUS:** Instead of fatty dips made with sour cream or mayonnaise, try hummus or bean spreads. Sometimes called white peanut butter, bean dips make a great dip or spread alternative.

## Spinach

Spinach is a Clean-Eating superfood. It can be added to everything from salads, wraps and soups to omelets and other egg dishes. We are currently on a juicing trend in our house, so we purchase loads of spinach to put through our juicer. The color so identifiable with spinach is a sign that it is loaded with good-for-you nutrients, the most significant of which is chlorophyll, a potent anti-cancer agent. Spinach contains a wealth of vitamins A, B-6, C, E and K along with the minerals iron, calcium, magnesium, manganese and zinc and the phytochemicals lutein, zeaxanthin, beta-carotene, omega-3 fatty acids, glutathione, alpha-lipoic acid, coenzyme Q10, thiamine, riboflavin and folate.

**FAST FOOD IN THE KITCH!** Spinach leaves are the perfect fast-food supper fix for you gentlemen. All you have to do is place the leaves in a bowl. Pour boiling hot water over top and let sit covered for about 5 minutes. Voilà! Your veggies are ready to eat. Fresh spinach leaves can be used in salads with plenty of chopped vegetables and nuts. Toss with a little pumpkin seed oil and rice wine vinegar and serve with a grilled chicken breast or water-packed tuna for a complete, fast, Clean-Eating meal.

**STAR NUTRIENTS:**

- Vitamin K
- Vitamin C

**NUTRIENTS PER 2-CUP SERVING (RAW):**

Calories: 25
Potassium: 500 mg
Folate: 150 mcg
Fiber: 2 g
Calcium: 170 mg
Iron: 2 mg
Vitamin C: 26 mg
Vitamin E: 2 mg

## Bison – The Other Red Meat

Bison is an excellent protein alternative to conventionally raised beef. The rich red meat sometimes called buffalo tastes like beef but is sweeter and richer in flavor. Bison depend on grass and grazing as their main food sources. Farmers allow the animals to range on open land rather than tossing them into concentrated feed lots. There is no need for hormones and antibiotics thanks to this practice, so the meat is cleaner too. Grass-fed bison, or cattle for that matter, always provide a healthier, leaner meat with a far higher nutrition profile than their commercial counterparts. Nutritionists are beginning to recommend bison over beef for its superior nutrition profile.

**STAR NUTRIENTS:**

- Protein
- Calcium

**NUTRITIONAL VALUE PER 4-OZ SERVING:**

| | |
|---|---|
| Calories: 123 | Saturated fat: 1 g |
| Protein: 24 g | Cholesterol: 75 mg |
| Fat: 2 g | Calcium: 9 mg |

**ONLINE**

www.thebuffaloshop.com
www.gunpowderbison.com
www.buffalogal.com

**HEART HEALTHY!** The American Heart Association recommends eating bison due to its nutritional profile and low-fat, low-cholesterol status.

**CONJUGATED LINOLEIC ACID (CLA):** Bison meat is one of the few meats high in CLA, which has been found useful in promoting weight loss. The high concentration of CLA comes from the fact that the bison is a grass-fed animal.

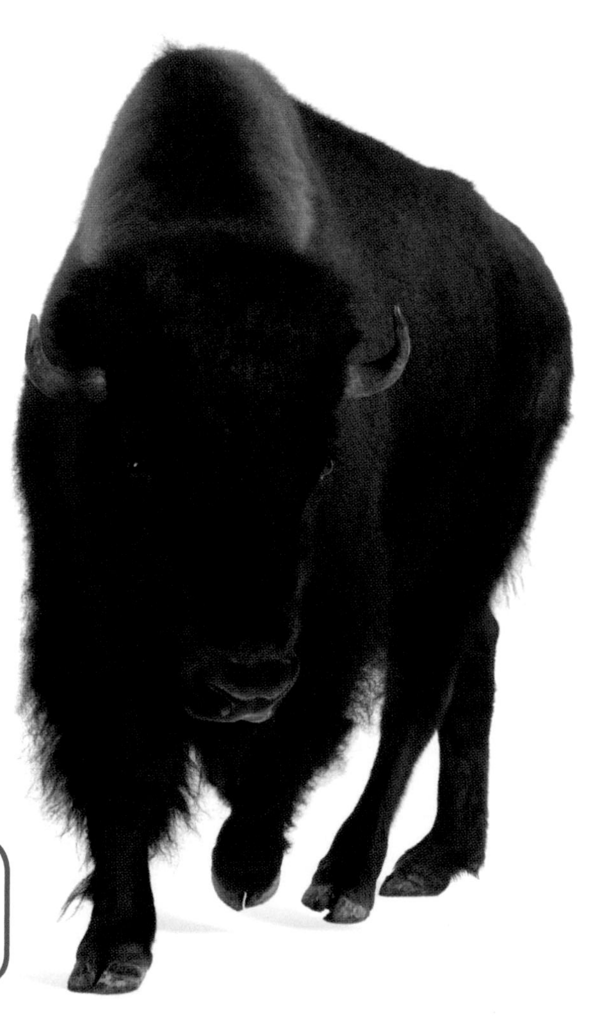

# Pumpkins

Pumpkins can be eaten sweet or savory year round. A staple food of our First Nation peoples, this inexpensive foodstuff is dense with nutrients and fiber. The bright orange flesh indicates they are loaded with the powerful antioxidant beta-carotene, also found in carrots and sweet potatoes. One cup of boiled pumpkin flesh provides 310 percent of the recommended daily allowance for vitamin A. We use pumpkin flesh as a sweet potato alternative, but one of our favorite ways to eat pumpkin is in the form of pumpkin hummus. We spread it on everything!

**DID YOU KNOW?** Pumpkins are 90 percent water and high in fiber.

**PUMPKIN-SEED VIAGRA?** Pumpkin seeds contain loads of zinc, which helps stimulate libido! They are a lot cheaper than Viagra too.

**ONLINE**

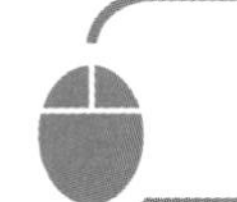

www.pumpkinnook.com
www.punkinranch.com

**STAR NUTRIENTS:**

- Carotenoids, especially beta-carotene
- Fiber

**NUTRIENTS PER 1-CUP SERVING:**

Alpha-carotene: 28 mcg
Beta-carotene: 900 mcg
Fiber: 3 g
Vitamin C: 28 mg
Vitamin E: 2 mg
Carbohydrates: 12 g
Calories: 49

# Oatmeal

One of the best ways to start your day is with a bowl of hot oatmeal. We eat this food for breakfast 90 percent of the time. The slow-burning complex carbohydrates in oatmeal prolong the feeling of fullness and stabilize blood-sugar levels. These are important factors when changing nutrition habits, since you want to feel full longer and not experience dramatic drops in blood sugar. Loaded with soluble fiber, oatmeal fills you up while lowering blood cholesterol. Oatmeal also contains plant protein and complex carbohydrates in the perfect combination, essential for building lean muscle. Oatmeal is one of the few foods rich in silicon, a mineral responsible for building beautiful skin, hair, bones and teeth.

**REV UP YOUR OATMEAL:** On its own, oatmeal is a superior food, but when you add one tablespoon each of ground flaxseed, bee pollen and wheat germ plus fresh berries, you've increased your nutrition substantially.

**OATMEAL MAKES HEALTH HISTORY:** In 1997 oatmeal made history when the FDA allowed it to be the first food labeled "heart healthy." Oats have been scientifically proven to lower blood cholesterol if eaten regularly.

**BETTER FOR YOUR BUDGET:** Check out our experiment with oatmeal and Froot Loops on page 124 to decide for yourself which is the better buy. Our money is on oatmeal every time!

**STAR NUTRIENTS:**

Soluble fiber
Plant protein
Complex carbohydrates
Silicon

**NUTRIENTS PER 1-CUP SERVING:**

Calories: 200
Fiber: 7 g
Protein: 2 g
Carbohydrates: 9 g
Iron: 1 g

# YOU COULD BE DESTROYING YOUR NUTRIENTS!

**HERE'S HOW YOU COULD BE DAMAGING THE NUTRIENTS IN YOUR FOOD.**

- Overeating
- Eating standing up
- Eating in a hurry
- Not chewing adequately or properly
- Eating after 6:00 p.m. and late into the night
- Consuming too much caffeine, alcohol, nicotine, marijuana or other drugs
- Consuming too much sugar (fake or otherwise), flour and other refined and over-processed foods
- Consuming too many chemicals found in food and water
- Over-dependence on antibiotics and other prescription drugs
- Treating symptoms of disease instead of the cause

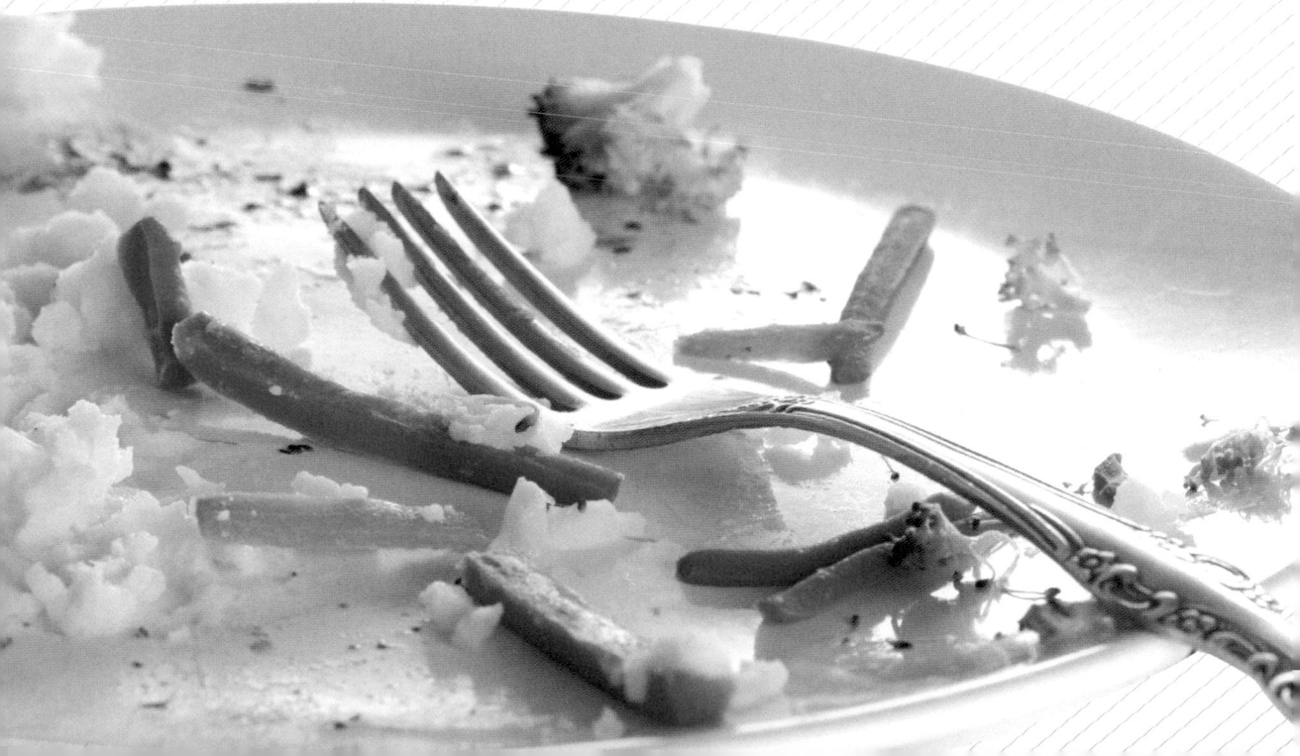

## COENZYME Q10 (CoQ10)

CoQ10 is a powerful antioxidant developed in Japan after the dropping of the Hiroshima bomb. Every cell in the body already contains this fat-soluble substance, whose main functions are to serve as a free-radical scavenger and to provide energy at the cellular level. CoQ10 was used extensively to help the people of Japan fight the devastating effects of the H-bomb to good effect. CoQ10 possesses a remarkable ability to drive metabolic reactions in the body more efficiently. Mitochondria contain the greatest amount of CoQ10, but as we age our levels of this critical antioxidant drop – a situation worsened by poor nutrition. CoQ10 also stimulates the immune system and protects the heart from damage caused by chemotherapy treatments. Lately, CoQ10 has been used to treat gum disease and Raynaud's syndrome.

**DOSAGE:** 100 to 200 mg. You may take a higher dosage, depending on your condition.

**DID YOU KNOW?** Because of the ability of CoQ10 to protect heart muscle-tissue health, its discoverer earned the Nobel Prize.

**A.K.A.** CoQ10 is also known as ubiquinone.

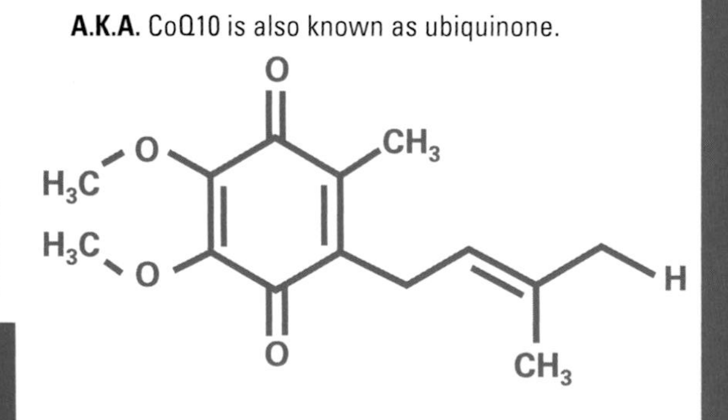


## CREATINE

Creatine exists naturally in all human muscle and to a higher degree in skeletal muscle. It is legitimately known as a supplement that can safely help you build muscle. The more lean muscle you have the higher your metabolic rate. Creatine assists the body by increasing the amount of energy readily available in muscle. The best sources of creatine include raw tuna, sushi or sashimi, but most muscle meat contains creatine. Creatine plays a critical role in lowering blood levels of homocysteine, a dangerous agent responsible for some neural diseases including Down's syndrome, Alzheimer's disease, Parkinson's disease, stroke and dementia. Creatine is also capable of lowering cholesterol levels. We are in the business of building bodies and this is one of the supplements we readily endorse.

**HOW IS IT SOLD?** Synthetic creatine is commonly used as a supplement to enhance athletic performance. It is sold as citrate, phosphate or monohydrate salts.

**DOSAGE:** 2 g to 20 g. It's best not to consume more; check with your doctor first if you have concerns or questions, although a prescription is not required.

**QUALITY:** Manufacturers like to add fillers, so be sure to check the label before you make your creatine purchase. Take special care to check for added refined or fake sugar.

## CONJUGATED LINOLEIC ACID (CLA)

CLA is a supplement used to promote fat loss and the growth of lean muscle tissue. This agent is highly effective in assisting with weight loss and seems capable of changing your body-fat composition. If you are struggling to lose stubborn fat deposits around your midsection, as many of us are, CLA seems effective at helping you do just that. If you've already lost weight and want to keep it off, studies indicate this can be achieved with CLA through its action on increasing basal metabolic rate. The action of CLA is that it prevents lipogenesis – the storage of fat after a meal. CLA is a structured lipid, or essential fatty acid, occurring naturally in beef, ground turkey, lamb, cheese and milk. It also acts as an antioxidant and enhances the immune system.

**DOSAGE:** 1-3 g per day.

**TRANS FAT:** CLA is actually a trans fat, but in this case a beneficial one.

## BEE POLLEN

In our home we like bee pollen and regularly add two tablespoons to our morning oatmeal along with ground flaxseed and wheat germ. These golden granules are valued for their complete array of proteins, vitamins, minerals and enzymes. Bee pollen supports every body system, with emphasis on the nervous and reproductive systems. The protein in bee pollen is easily digestible and readily accessible for use in the body. Also found in bee pollen are powerful antioxidants that have been proven to reduce the threat of free-radical damage from everyday toxins.

Bee pollen is known for its high rutin levels. Rutin is a quercetin found in many plants, especially buckwheat, green tea and apple skins. Rutin strengthens capillaries and therefore improves cardiovascular endurance.

Bee pollen plays an important role in weight management. Since it is so easily digested and absorbed on an empty stomach it can lessen hunger between meals. In our opinion it is delicious eaten as a snack if you can't hold out until your next meal, but to some it's an acquired taste!

**DOSAGE:** 1 teaspoon to 2 tablespoons per day.

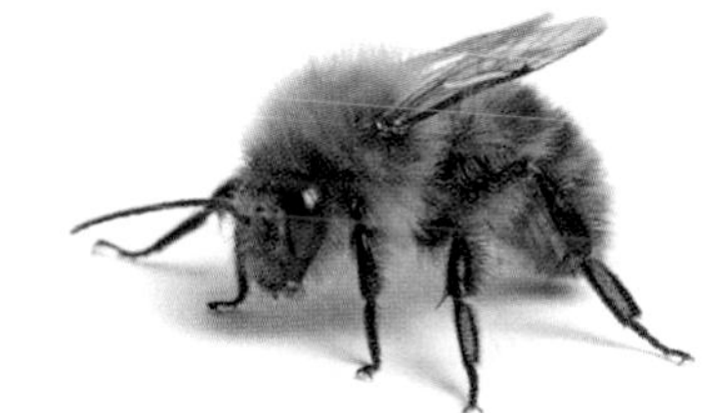

**EXCELLENT ONLINE SOURCES OF BEE POLLEN:**

**ONLINE**

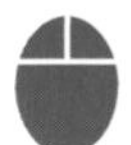

**www.honeygardens.com**
**www.gemcultures.com**

# HUMAN GROWTH HORMONE (HGH)

The body produces its own growth hormone, most of it while you are in a deep sleep and while in your youth. According to Oz Garcia, author of *Look and Feel Fabulous Forever*, "A deficiency of HGH impacts on, well . . . everything, especially by increasing the volume of fat and abdominal obesity we store, and by reducing muscle mass and strength. A drop in your natural production of HGH is a direct pathway to flab." The body produces its own HGH, particularly while you sleep, but only if the quality of your sleep is high.

Garcia further states, "In your 20s you may 'release' [HGH] about 12 times a day during a 24-hour period. After the age of 30, the number and intensity of 'releases' drop 14 percent for every decade you're alive." The other famous Oz, Dr. Mehmet Oz, claims that he regularly runs sprints because that is another time the body produces HGH. Non-prescription products are also available to stimulate the production of natural HGH. Pro-hormone products improve muscle strength and size, reduce fat and increase the ability to exercise.

**AVAILABILITY:** Actual HGH is available only by prescription and as an injectable. The cost is prohibitive at US $600 per injection, and you would need to inject yourself every day. Injected HGH is also implicated in an increased risk of prostate cancer in men. If you do choose to take HGH you must see a doctor during the course of your therapy. This is a great reason to try to get some good-quality sleep going!

# WHEY PROTEIN

In order to build and maintain lean muscle tissue you must consume adequate amounts of high-quality protein, especially if you are active and train with weights. Protein needs must be met to keep the body strong and to prevent muscle from catabolizing itself. According to Dr. Deborah Chud, author of *The Gourmet Prescription*, "Protein, fat and fiber act as brakes on the insulin-production machine because they slow the digestion of food. The slower our food is digested, the more gradually our blood-sugar levels rise and the slower the production of insulin." As an essential element of Clean Eating, protein consumed at every meal supports this mechanism. If you are not eating a high-protein food with a given meal, add some protein powder. Not only does it contain all 20 amino acids necessary for building and repairing healthy tissue, protein also contains vitamins, minerals, fatty acids and natural detoxifying agents.

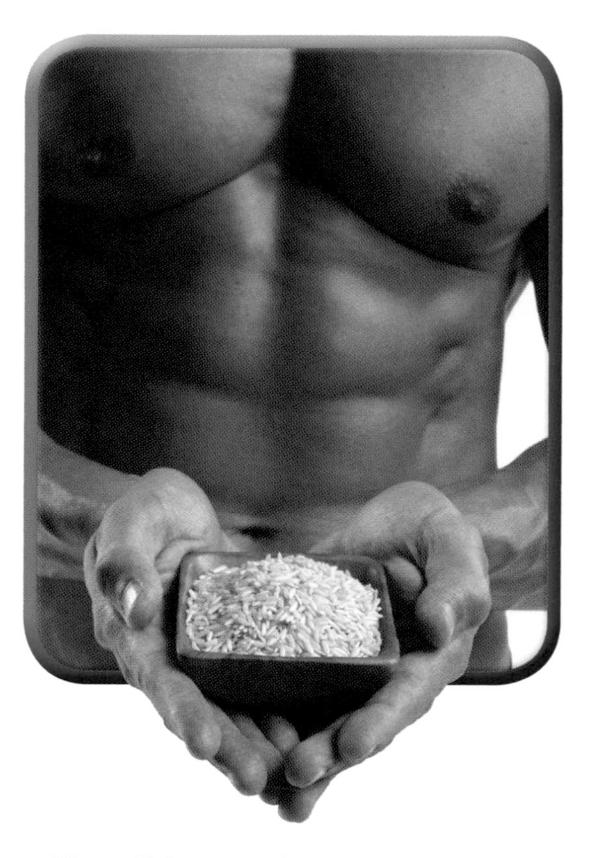

When milk is separated to make cheese, whey is the liquid left behind once the curds are removed. Whey powder is whey that has been dried. It has virtually no fat, but all the nutritional goodness of milk. Whey powders contain an array of micronutrients, antioxidants and immune globulins to sustain overall health. Look for whey powders low in carbohydrates and fats and those that don't contain high concentrations of sugar or sugar alternatives. Whey protein powder can be added to hot cereal, shakes, smoothies and yogurt or mixed with water.

**DOSAGE:** 25 g every 3 hours if not consuming other protein.

## GAMMA-ORYZANOL AND BROWN RICE

We eat only brown rice in our house, because we want the full value of this tiny grain. Unrefined brown rice is simply white rice with its exterior coating intact. We like the taste better – it is nuttier and chewier. Beyond those facts we value brown rice because it possesses the ability to balance blood-sugar levels, an important consideration in the fight against overweight and obesity. The bran coating of each grain of brown rice "is thought to be one of the most nutrient-dense substances ever studied," states Paul Pitchford, author of *Healing With Whole Foods.* "It embodies over 70 antioxidants that can protect against cellular damage and preserve youthfulness." Rice bran contains the rare form of vitamin E known as tocotrienols, which assist the body in lowering fat and cholesterol. Polysaccharides, also found in rice bran, are complex carbohydrates ideally suited for controlling high blood sugar, the implicating factor in diabetes and obesity. This is largely due to the fact that gamma-oryzanol, found in rice bran, is a potent antioxidant. This compound has the ability to strengthen muscles, reduce fat and produce lean muscle mass. Brown rice bran also contains loads of CoQ10, another supplement already discussed in this chapter.

**DOSAGE:** 1 teaspoon or 5 mg per day.

# OMEGA-3 FATTY ACIDS

Omega-3 fatty acids are one of three essential fatty acids required for overall good health. Omega-3 in particular has been proven to regulate appetite and to accelerate fat burning – beneficial when trying to lose weight. Many of the current health and weight problems we see today in North America are the result of misunderstanding fats – it is critical to consume enough healthy fats. Omega-3 is found in good supply in fish and flaxseeds. Omega-3 contains alpha-linolenic acid, which reduces fat storage – helpful in managing overweight and obesity.

**DOSAGE:** For EFAs, we have found that the answer can vary. It seems the pat answer of 1 to 3 grams per day is not really correct. There is no RDA for EFAs. Rather it is better to ensure that you are consuming at least 15% healthy fats in your daily food intake. Alternatively you can take one tablespoon of a balanced essential fatty acid supplement per 100 pounds of body weight.

**FISH:** 7 to 10 oz of fish per week.

**FLAXSEEDS:** 4 tablespoons ground flaxseed daily with meals. The oil in flaxseeds is volatile and goes off readily if not stored in a cool dry place. We store ours in the refrigerator. Grind your seeds in a coffee mill first to get their full benefit.

# MACA

Maca is a powerful adaptogenic food derived from a nutritious root vegetable originally grown in the harsh climate of the Andes mountains. It is said that Peruvian men and even their animals become more virile when they consume maca. Peruvian peoples have depended on this wrinkled root as a valuable source of nutrition for thousands of years. It is grown without pesticides or chemicals. Maca's rich nutritional content is one of the reasons it is so valuable, especially for those with weakened immune systems. It contains 31 trace minerals essential to rebuilding health.

Athletes use maca to increase energy, stamina and endurance. It is used as a safe alternative to anabolic steroids because the root is rich with sterols, natural hormone-like substances. Recently, a major US baseball team used maca as part of its nutrition program after the head coach discovered his energy was enhanced by using it. The nutrients in maca are readily digestible and therefore immediately accessible to the body. Maca is natural and completely safe to ingest.

**DOSAGE:** 1,500 to 3,000 mg per day, available over the counter as a powder, pill or tea.

# WHEAT GRASS

Wheat grass is valued as an herbal medicine for its therapeutic and nutritional properties. Whether the juice comes from wheat, kamut, barley or oat grass, it has the ability to detoxify the liver, purify the blood and cleanse the colon. It is also a food in and of itself. You could survive on the juice of wheat grass and nothing else. People who have been faced with the most destructive diseases imaginable have turned to wheat grass as an alternative to conventional medicine when there was no hope to be found elsewhere.

Nutritionally, wheat grass provides the full nutritional components for us to live. Wheat grass contains all known proteins and peptides, concentrated nutrition, all known vitamins and minerals, chlorophyll, carotenoids, antioxidants, enzymes, growth hormones and immune modulators, and is easily assimilated by the body. Wheat grass is an important step in assisting you in turning your health around.

**DOSAGE:** 6 to 10 oz each day.

Wheat grass is valued as an herbal medicine for its therapeutic and nutritional properties. Whether the juice comes from wheat, kamut, barley or oat grass, it has the ability to detoxify the liver, purify the blood and cleanse the colon.

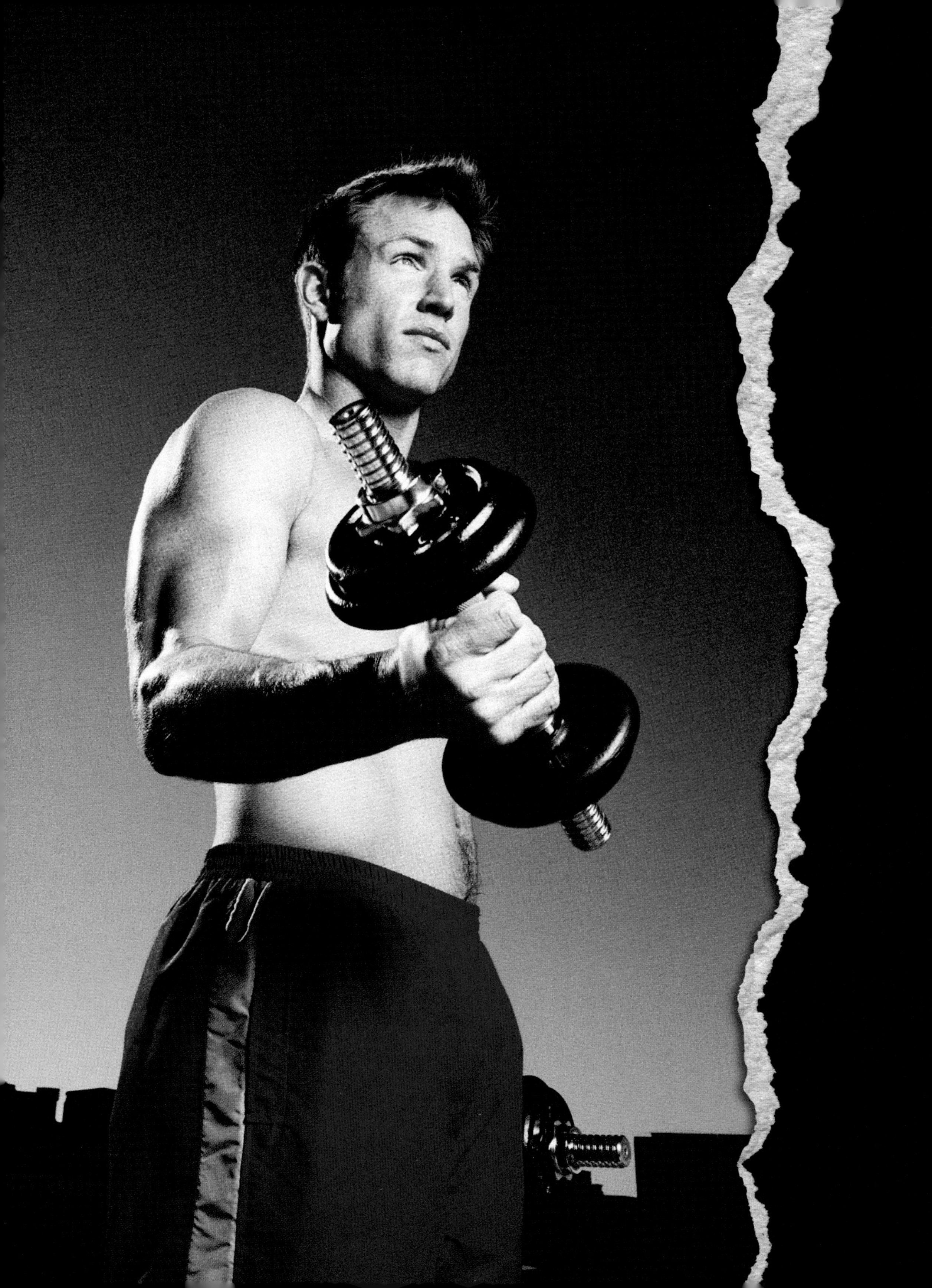

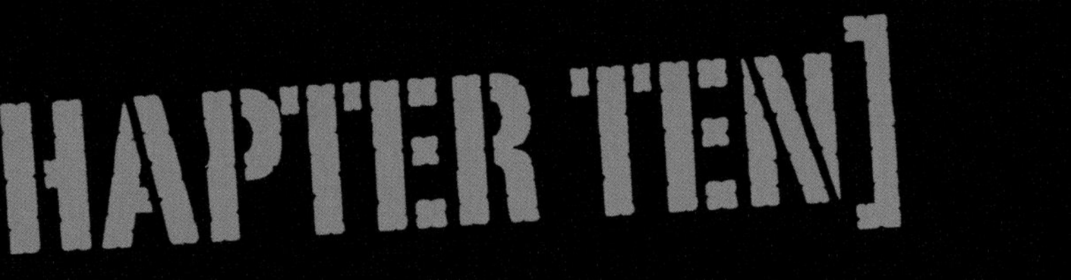
HAPTER TEN]

## EXERCISE AND OTHER FACTORS

Clean Eating really does work magic on the body. If you are too thin it will add firm flesh to your frame; should you be overweight or even obese you will burn flab like there is no tomorrow. Clean Eating works to normalize your weight. Naturally, if you are morbidly obese it will take considerably longer than if you are a mere 10 to 15 pounds overweight.

This book is principally about Eating Clean, but we'd like to touch on a couple of items that are not directly related to nutrition. Instead, they are related to your fitness level, health, energy stores, appearance and longevity.

[ Worry solves nothing. ]

## STRESS CONTROL

Worry solves nothing. Careful planning and appropriate action helps solve everything. The greatest worries come from health and relationship problems, legal concerns and financial troubles. Some men need a degree of stress in their lives to thrive while others have a low tolerance level and should avoid circumstances that can lead to high stress. Excessive worry can lead to depression, heart and stomach problems, high blood pressure, cancer and even death.

## ALCOHOL

One of the biggest questions we get at seminars is: "What about alcohol?" Alcohol is sugar and sugar is not a food. It is strongly related to obesity, heart problems and even cancer. We know that's not the answer you want to hear, but it's really hard to shed fat while drinking on a daily basis. The answer then is that if you are very serious about losing weight and getting into 100 percent shape, then drinking is not an option. Having said that, an occasional glass of wine is not exactly a cardinal sin.

Cigarettes contain over 200 poisons and cause lung cancer, leukemia, heart disease, hardening of the arteries and stroke.

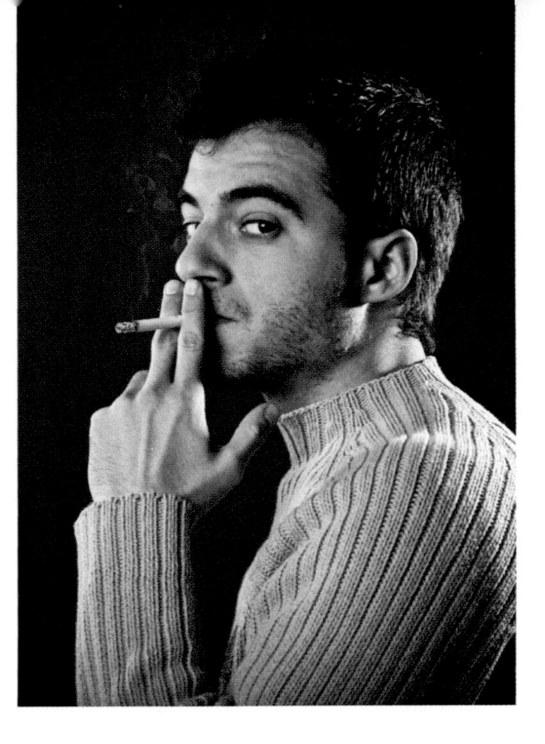

## EXERCISE

Want to make the most of your Clean Eating? Exercise is a good idea and will help you reach your goals, but it is not absolutely necessary. Naturally, before undertaking any exercise program you should consult your family doctor. Request that he or she arrange for you to have a complete physical, including a stress test. Chances are things will be perfectly normal and your physician will be delighted that you are planning a regular exercise program, but it's always best to get a checkup just to be sure. Older people may want to spend some time walking every day.

## TOBACCO

It's not our desire to come down heavy on you over your personal preferences, habits and hobbies, but when it comes to smoking we get stone-cold serious. We ask that you stop immediately. Few things a man does to himself are as devastatingly harmful as smoking. Cigarettes contain over 200 poisons and contribute to – no, cause – lung cancer, leukemia, heart disease, hardening of the arteries and stroke.

If you are a smoker and have cigarettes on you now, take them out of your pocket, crunch them up and toss them in the garbage. You will have 30 days of agony; you will be longing to "light up." Resist the temptation and you will never pine for tobacco again. In fact, when someone smokes around you, you will wave your hand in front of your face and ask that they smoke elsewhere. Oh, and did we forget to say you will feel better, have more energy, more money, have clearer eyes and skin and stand a one million percent chance of living a happier and longer life?

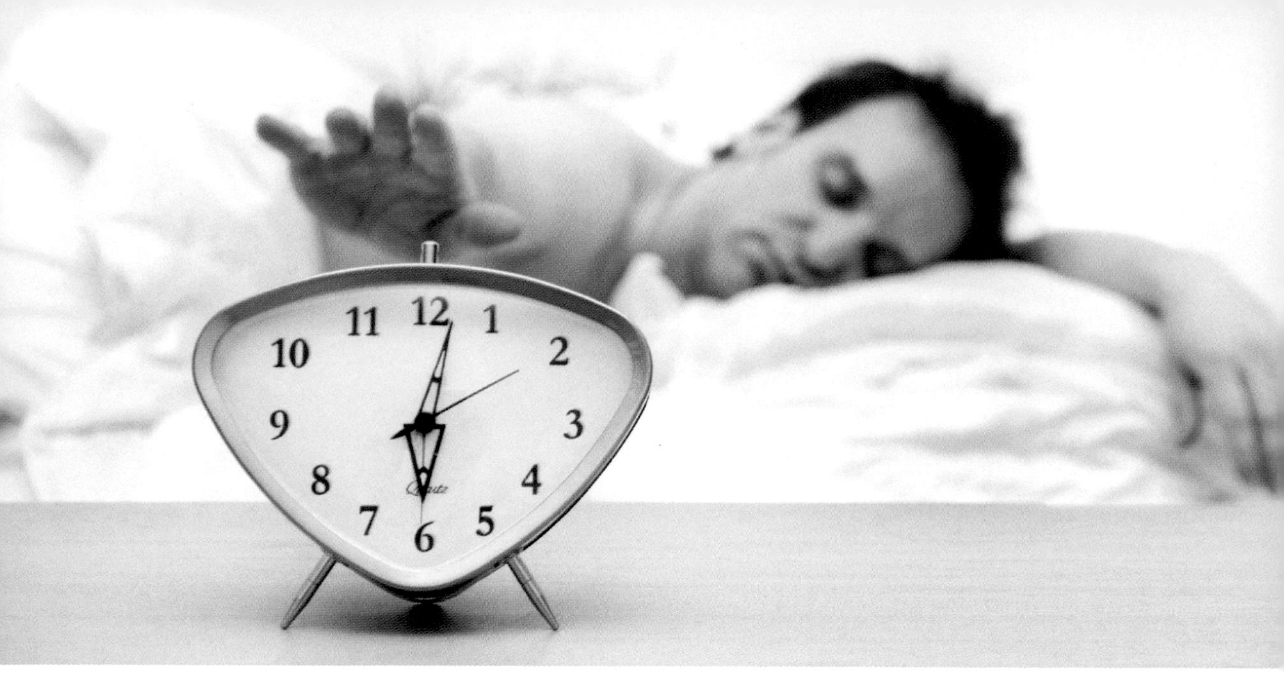


## SLEEP AND REST

Are we not all sleep deprived? One of the most frequently asked questions we get at seminars relates to tiredness. Typically, people will tell us they even wake up tired. The answer of course is to go to bed earlier, but it may not be as simple as that. Many people don't get to enjoy proper sleep. One partner might be disturbed in bed by snoring, frequent bathroom visits, sleepwalking, talking or teeth grinding. Needless to say, the other partner will have his or her sleep severely disturbed. Few people can remain energetic and alert on less than seven hours of sleep each night. And many would do better with a nightly sleep of at least eight hours.

It is a good idea to try to relax for at least half an hour after meals, although admittedly this may be hard for manual workers or those whose job it is to keep physically active.

Some men, whose lifestyles allow for it, have the luxury of an afternoon nap; this is known among athletes as muscle sleep. Many competitive athletes favor this habit, although we have never managed to find time for such repose.

## RECREATIONAL DRUGS

We have been of two minds as to whether or not to address the subject of recreational drugs, but today's statistics are staggering. Hundreds of thousands of North Americans are hooked. Some are on painkillers while others smoke pot, take ecstasy or indulge in mind-altering hard drugs such as cocaine, heroin, crystal meth or other heavy-duty concoctions. Here again we don't want to preach. Our normal philosophy is "live and let live," but this is a book about improving ourselves through lifestyle changes. Where recreational drugs are concerned, we say no, no and again no.

## YOUR REGULAR EXERCISE PROGRAM

There is no form of exercise that conditions the muscles of the body better than weight training. Why? Because barbells and dumbbells can be tailored to your age, condition and individual strength levels. An 80-year-old can start by lifting a couple of one-pound dumbbells whereas a youthful 20-year-old may begin with 30-pound dumbbells. And naturally as strength levels increase (as they always do) weights can be increased accordingly so the muscles are continuously challenged.

How effective is training with weights? Consider this: Lift a 50-pound barbell 20 times, and in less than 30 seconds you will have lifted 1,000 pounds! No other activity can tone and muscle-up your physique in such a concentrated manner. Think about it – you lift 1,000 pounds in under half a minute!

Weight training can benefit your entire body. If you take no significant rests between sets of repetitions, it will benefit your heart, lungs and circulatory system. Alternatively, if you want more direct stimulation to your cardiovascular system, you can jog, run, jump rope, swim or use the treadmill three to five times a week for 30 to 45 minutes.

We are giving you a suggested weight-training program designed to hit every body part. Perform it two or three times a week. Complete beginners to weight training should perform just one set of 12 repetitions for each exercise. Others who have some experience with weights can work up to three or four sets of each movement; resting up to a full minute between sets. Make sure you have at least one rest day (i.e., no training) between workouts. People often train on Mondays, Wednesdays and Fridays, leaving the weekend free for family and friends.

There is no form of exercise that conditions the muscles of the body better than weight training.

# HERE ARE YOUR EXERCISES

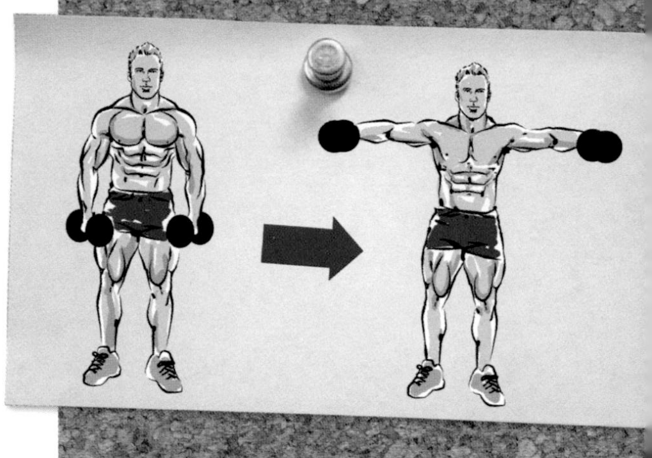

## Standing Lateral Raise (Shoulders)

Stand with your feet slightly apart. Hold two dumbbells at your sides and, keeping your arms slightly bent, raise and lower as shown. Go for 8 to 12 repetitions.

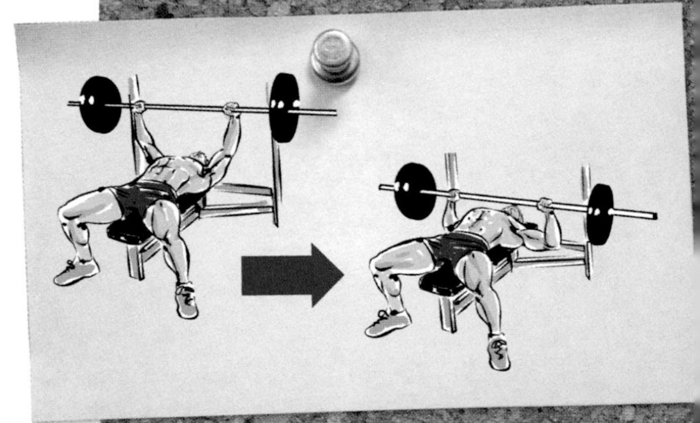

## Bench Press (Chest)

Lie on a flat bench as shown. Start by holding a loaded barbell (or pair of dumbbells) at arm's length. Lower it to your chest (no bouncing) and press to the arms-straight position. Lower and repeat. Keep your butt on the bench at all times and your feet flat on the floor. Keep your reps around 8 to 12.

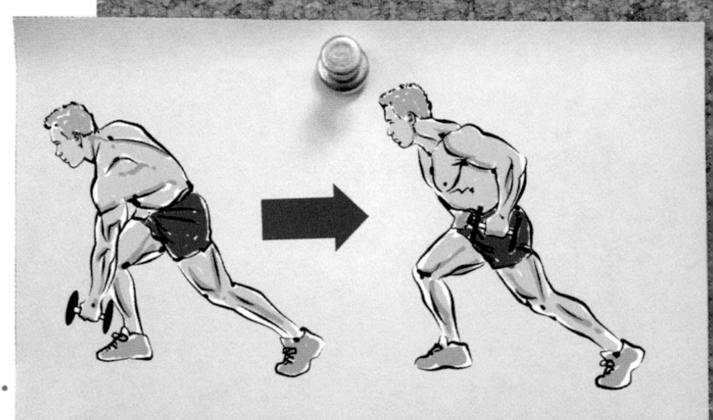

## Dumbbell Row (Upper Back)

Adopt a position as shown, holding a dumbbell in one hand. Starting from the arms-straight (hanging down) position, lift the dumbbell up as high as possible to the waist area. Lower and repeat. Work each arm for 8 to 12 repetitions.

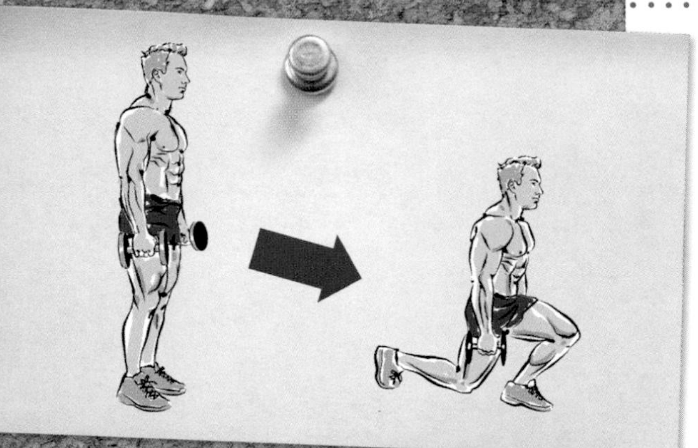

## Lunge (Thighs and Butt)

Hold a dumbbell in each hand in the start position as shown. Step forward (or backward) to the lunge position as shown. Do not allow your knee to contact the ground. Alternate your legs for 8 repetitions each leg.

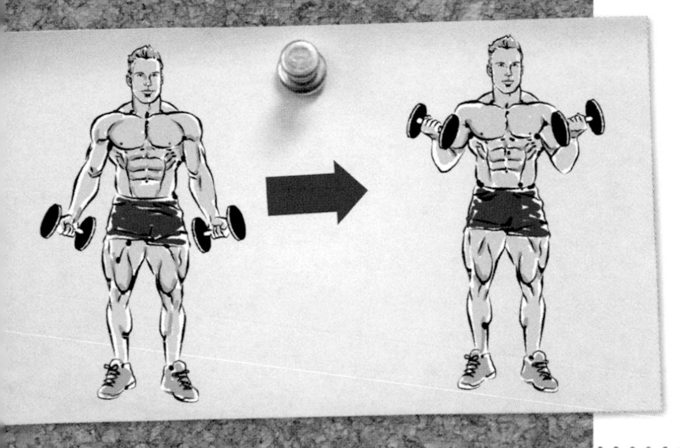

## Dumbbell Curl (Biceps)

Stand with your feet comfortably apart, your hands down and holding a pair of dumbbells. Curl the dumbbells simultaneously until the weights are at shoulder level. Lower and repeat for 8 to 12 reps.

## Calf Raise (Lower Legs)

Stand on a stair or raised area (e.g. a block of wood). Holding a dumbbell, place your feet as shown. Lift up and down so your calf muscle is fully worked over its entire range. Try 12 to 20 repetitions each leg.

## Dumbbell Shrug (Trapezius)

Hold two dumbbells at your sides as shown. Raise your shoulders up as close to your ears as possible. Lower and repeat. Try 12 repetitions.

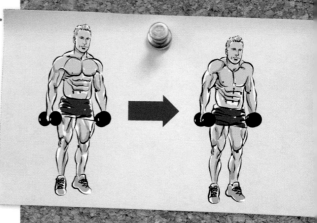

## Triceps Extension (Triceps – Rear Upper Arm)

Hold a dumbbell behind your head as shown. Try to keep your upper arm as close to the side of your head as possible. Lift the dumbbell to arm's length, keeping your upper arm still and your elbow pointed at the ceiling. Lower and repeat for 12 reps.

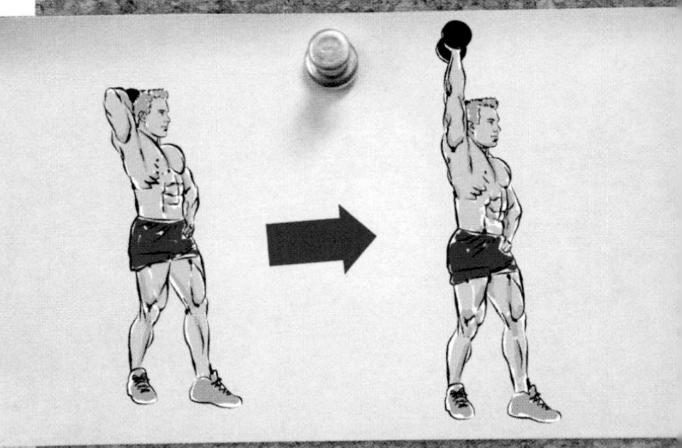

## Crunch (Abdominals)

Lie on your back as shown. Fully contract your abdominal muscles so your upper back and shoulders lift slightly off the floor. Lower and repeat for 20 repetitions.

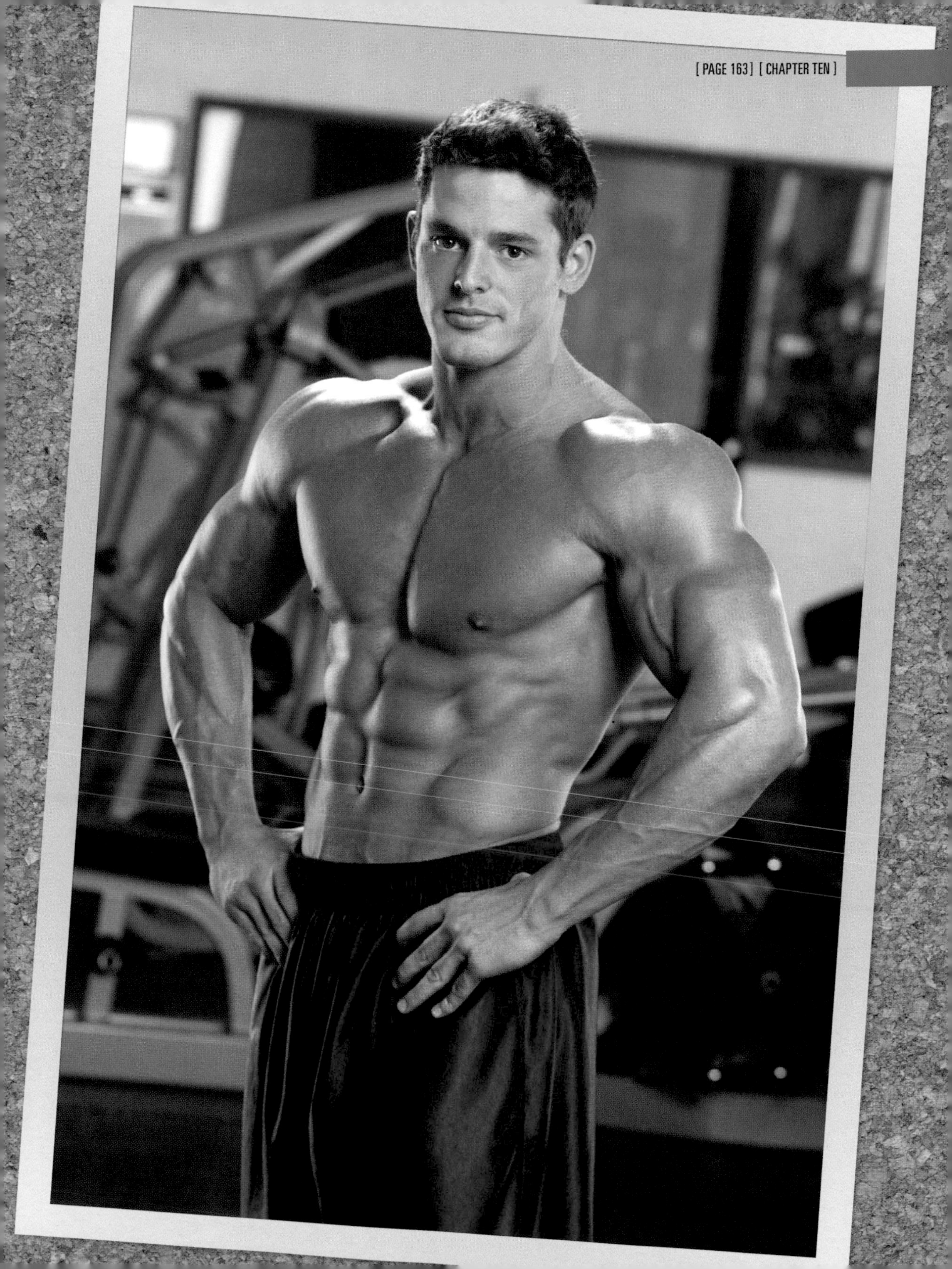

# TRAINING TIPS

### Be Progressive

After you get used to the various exercises, make sure to keep your muscles fully challenged by adding weight whenever possible. Never add too much weight, or you will compromise proper exercise form.

You should always focus on performing the repetitions. Feel your muscles reacting to the movement.

### Keep Focused

Learn to concentrate on each movement. Looking around the room (or gym) when exercising is not the way to make progress. You should always focus on performing the repetitions. Feel your muscles reacting to the movement.

### Minimal Rest Between Sets

After performing a set of an exercise (eg. 12 counts, or reps) take a rest of about one to two minutes, not more. The general rule is to go for your next set when your breathing has returned to normal. If you are aiming for a cardio effect then limit your rest periods to 30 seconds.

### Strict Form

All exercises should be done with an even cadence, and good form should be observed. Repetitions should be smooth and strict. Avoid swinging, hoisting or bouncing the weights.

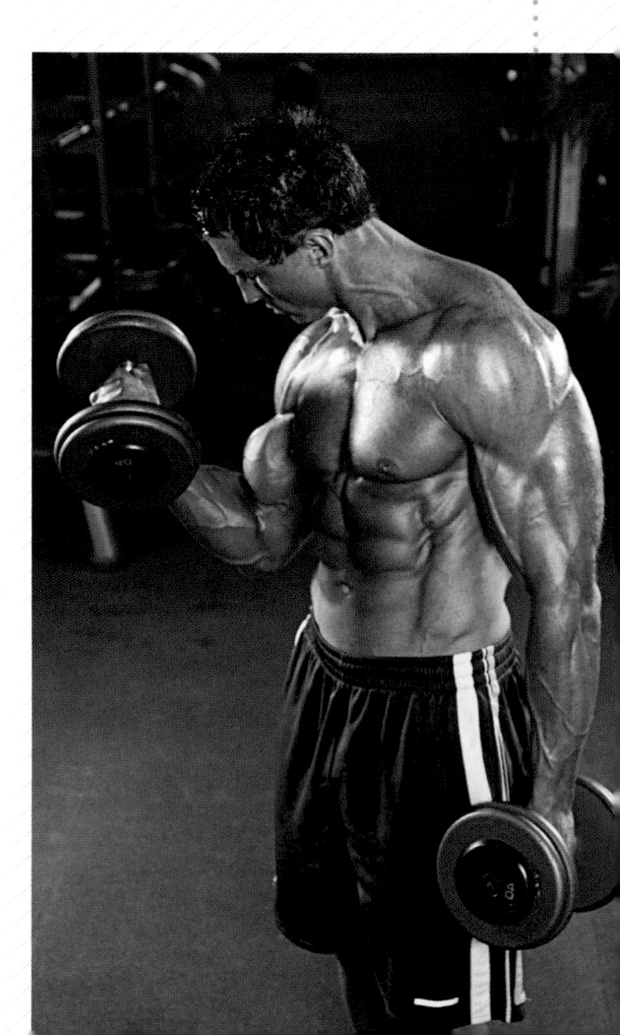

### Don't Be Casual

Do not allow yourself to get distracted while exercising. When performing an exercise, your head should be facing the same direction as your body. Do not turn your head to view another gym member. Do not talk while lifting weights. Injury can easily occur when one deviates from the standard performance of a specific exercise.

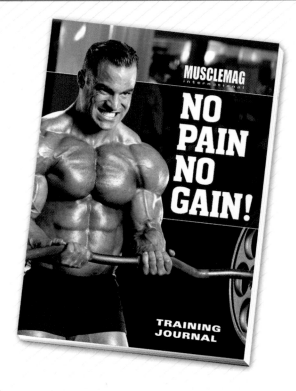


### Good Manners

Observe basic gym etiquette. Place a towel on a bench before lying down or sitting. Wipe off any sweat after using a particular piece of apparatus. Place dumbbells and barbells in racks after use. Don't shout, growl or groan while exercising.

### Write it Down

Keep a journal. It is a good practice to write down all your exercises, poundages, sets and reps. (Order the *No Pain No Gain!* workout journal by calling 1-888-254-0767.) The act of recording each workout will help you see what poundages to select for your next workout. Additionally, as the years go by it is fun to look back to see what you used to do. Have you progressed or regressed?

### Be Consistent

Regular workouts are important. Being an "on and off" exerciser won't work. Naturally, if you are sick a workout is not a good idea. In addition there are times when a few days away from training will be beneficial. Just don't make it too much of a habit – for the most part, you should work out regularly and consistently.

# COMMON TRAINING QUESTIONS AND ANSWERS

### Q Do I need to use a training belt and weightlifting gloves during my workouts?

Some people like to use a belt for heavy exercises such as squats, overhead presses or lunges because it gives additional support. A belt should never be used for all exercises from the beginning to the end of a workout. Gloves are a personal choice. If callouses are a problem then gloves are the answer.

### Q How many repetitions should I do?

The general rule is that low reps (2 to 4) build strength, medium reps (8 to 12) build muscle, and high reps (15 to 20) build endurance and definition. While the above statement is true, it should be understood that all repetitions, whether high or low, build a combination of strength, muscle and endurance.

### Q What results can I expect from weight training?

Results vary from one individual to another. There are three basic body types: endomorphs (fat, lethargic types), mesomorphs (naturally muscular types) and ectomorphs (thin, nervous types). Endomorphs have to struggle to keep fat away, mesomorphs tend to gain muscle size easily, while ectomorphs are regarded as hard gainers. Of course, few people are exactly one or another of these body types – most are a combination. All body types, however, can expect to make measurable gains within a few months, but nutrition is the big catalyst. Added food intake will lead to increased body weight. Junk food intake will lead to increased body-fat levels. Clean Eating will lead to lean muscle.

### Q Do I have to join a gym to do my workouts?

A gym is ideal. However, you can train successfully at home if you invest in an adjustable bench (with flat and incline capabilities) and several

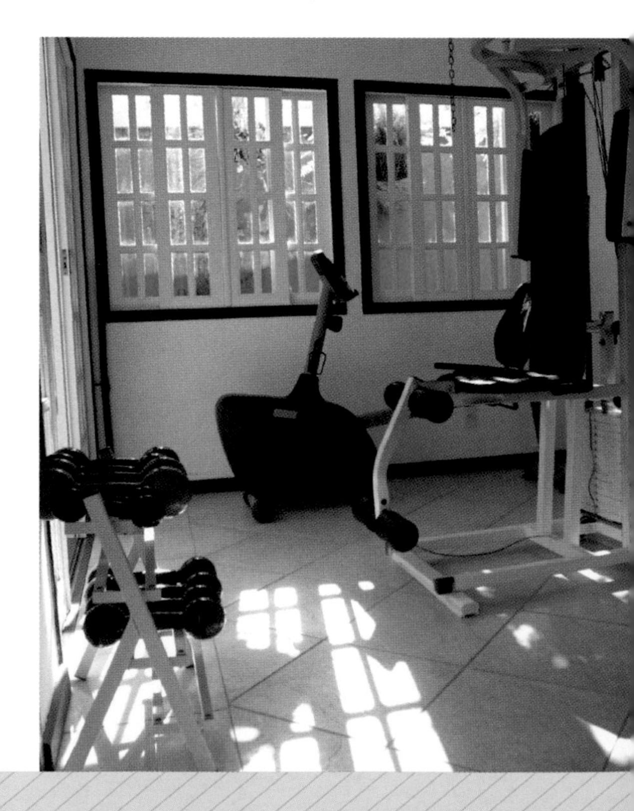

pairs of fixed dumbbells weighing 10, 20 and 30 pounds. Later, as your strength skyrockets, you might need to add pairs of 40s and 50s. A longer bar (five to six feet) on which weight discs can be added is a nice extra to have, but it is not necessary. Needless to say, a gym offers greater variety and you can vary your exercises to avoid boredom.

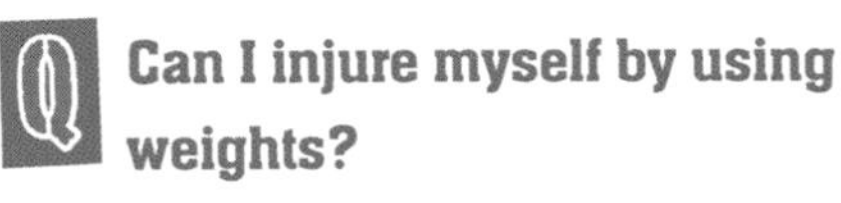

### Can I injure myself by using weights?

Yes, you can. You can also injure yourself by sneezing. Your first set of each exercise should be a warm-up set, for which you use only about 70 percent of the weight you can handle when really "going for it" in your subsequent "working sets."

### Do I have to use weights? Why can't I just run or use a treadmill?

A great amount of conditioning can be gained from running, swimming, cycling, etc., but true all-round muscle conditioning can come only from regular weight training. All Olympic athletes use weights to fully strengthen and maximize body efficiency for their individual sports.

### How can I tell if I'm overtraining?

You will feel tired all the time. Your muscles will be eternally sore and your physique will take on a stringy appearance. Cut down on your exercises and eat and sleep more.

All-round muscle conditioning can come only from regular weight training.

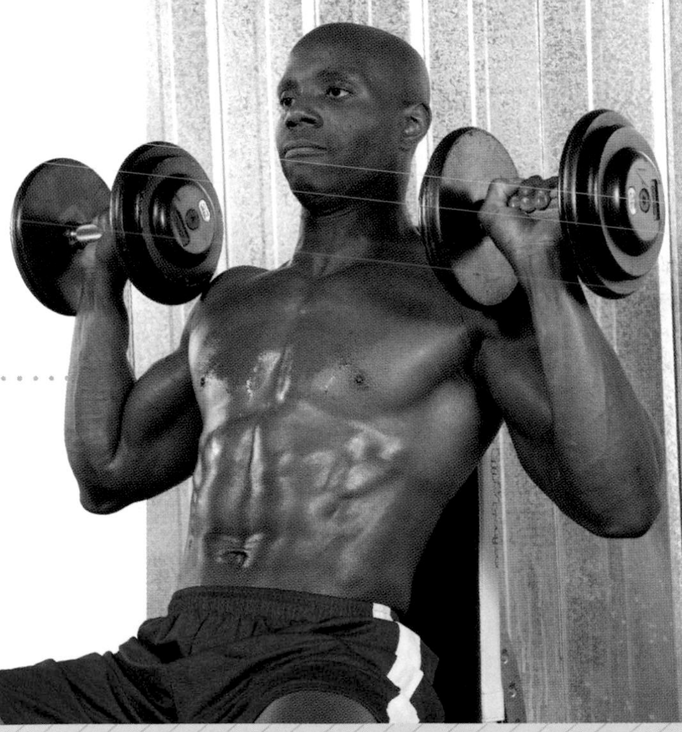

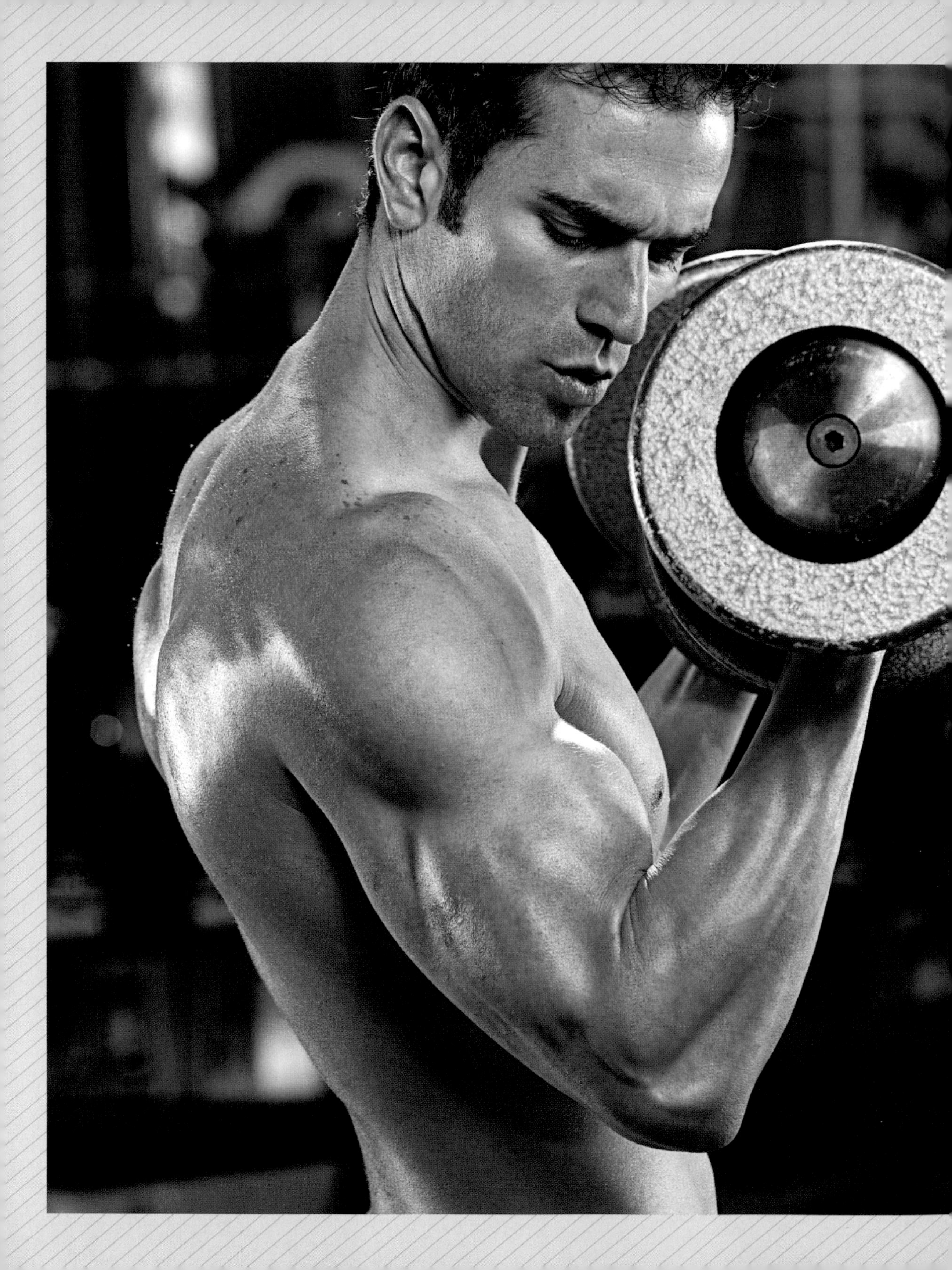

### Q How soon after eating can I work out?

It's a good practice to wait at least an hour after eating to train. The Clean-Eating program recommends eating every two-and-a-half to three hours, so your formal exercise workouts have to be carefully planned. Should you indulge in a heavy three-course meal, at least a two-hour rest is recommended.

### Q I have very skinny arms. How do I get more size in the quickest possible time?

You will need to gain weight. Eat more at each meal, but still eat five or six times a day. If you are super skinny, make an additional habit of drinking a quart of milk each day. You can perform up to five sets of dumbbell curls and five sets of triceps extensions twice a week with a two-day rest between arm workouts.

### Q My doctor says I should exercise more because, in his words, I am clinically obese and need to lose 80 pounds. When I look at myself in the mirror I cannot believe I could ever be as slim as I used to be in my college days.

Losing weight is simple, but many people fail when it doesn't happen quickly. You can't lose 80 pounds in a few weeks. Our advice is to exercise (after getting a complete physical) and to eat good wholesome (Clean) foods. Above all, stick with the plan. Look at yourself in a full-length mirror tonight, get motivated and promise yourself you will never give in. Envision yourself as you want to look, write down the weight you want to be and don't give up on your new lifestyle, even when you get to your target weight.

It's a good practice to wait at least an hour after eating to train.

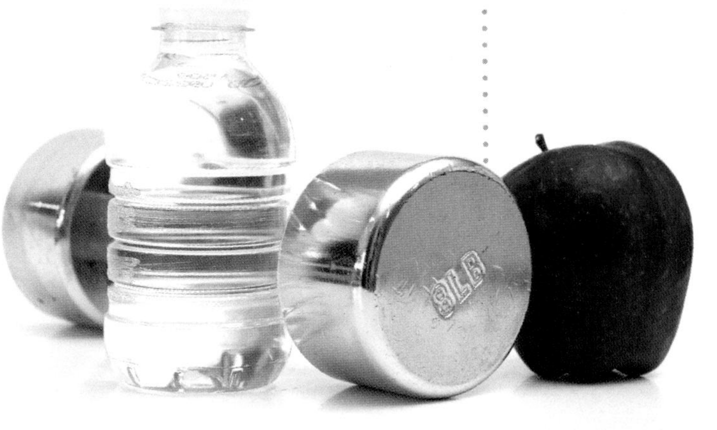

# EAT-CLEAN SUCCESS STORY!

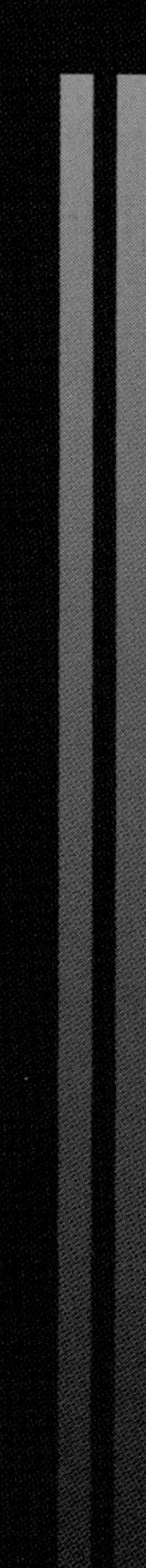

**Kevin Hennessy,**
**Age:** 44
**Height:** 5'6"
**Heaviest weight:** 312 lbs
**Current weight:** 178 lbs
From an email dated January 8, 2009

*My journey began when I realized one day that I would not see my daughter grow up. That I would not walk her down the aisle at her wedding and that I would never hold my grandchildren. That was the day my journey began. I made up my mind I was going to lose weight. No matter what it took.*

*I was very dedicated to my work and never took the time to eat properly. Breakfast consisted of a couple of coffees with two creams and two sugars. Never actual food. Lunch, if I had the time, was usually something greasy from a drive thru. Being self-employed, I worked until whenever and usually ate a huge meal late in the evening. I didn't take the time to exercise. I had no desire to.*

*Slow and steady my weight crept up until May of 2008 when some personal issues made me take a good look at my life. I realized that chasing money was meaningless. Your health and loved ones are what matter most, because without those all you have is loneliness.*

*My wife was already following the "The Eat-Clean Diet" so I started it too. I would take my cooler of food with me during the day and that's what I ate. I also joined a gym and started doing cardio, weight training, swimming and playing squash.*

*Pretty soon my weight started dropping, I had more energy and I actually liked the food I was eating. People at the gym were telling me how great I looked and were even asking me for advice! I couldn't believe it. I started working out with a personal trainer, Terry Boyd, and got hooked on bodybuilding.*

*I had weighed 312 lbs and wore size 50 jeans. Now, eight months later, I weigh 178 lbs and wear size 32 jeans! But I'm not stopping there. I still want to lose more fat and build more muscle. I feel amazing and have so many things I want to do, starting with becoming a personal trainer and opening a training studio so I can help others start their journey to a better life. Entering bodybuilding competitions, sky diving, white water rafting and scuba diving are just a few of the things on my new "to do" list of things I never dreamed of doing when I was heavy.*

*I have also established a support group within the gym. It's called "Team Hammer." We support each other in all aspects of training and one of our team members is going to make some recipes from "The Eat-Clean Diet" for everyone to try.*

*Thanks to "The Eat-Clean Diet" and exercise I am a new person and I'm loving my healthy, new life.*

*Sincerely,*
*Kevin Hennessy*
*Stay Fit.*

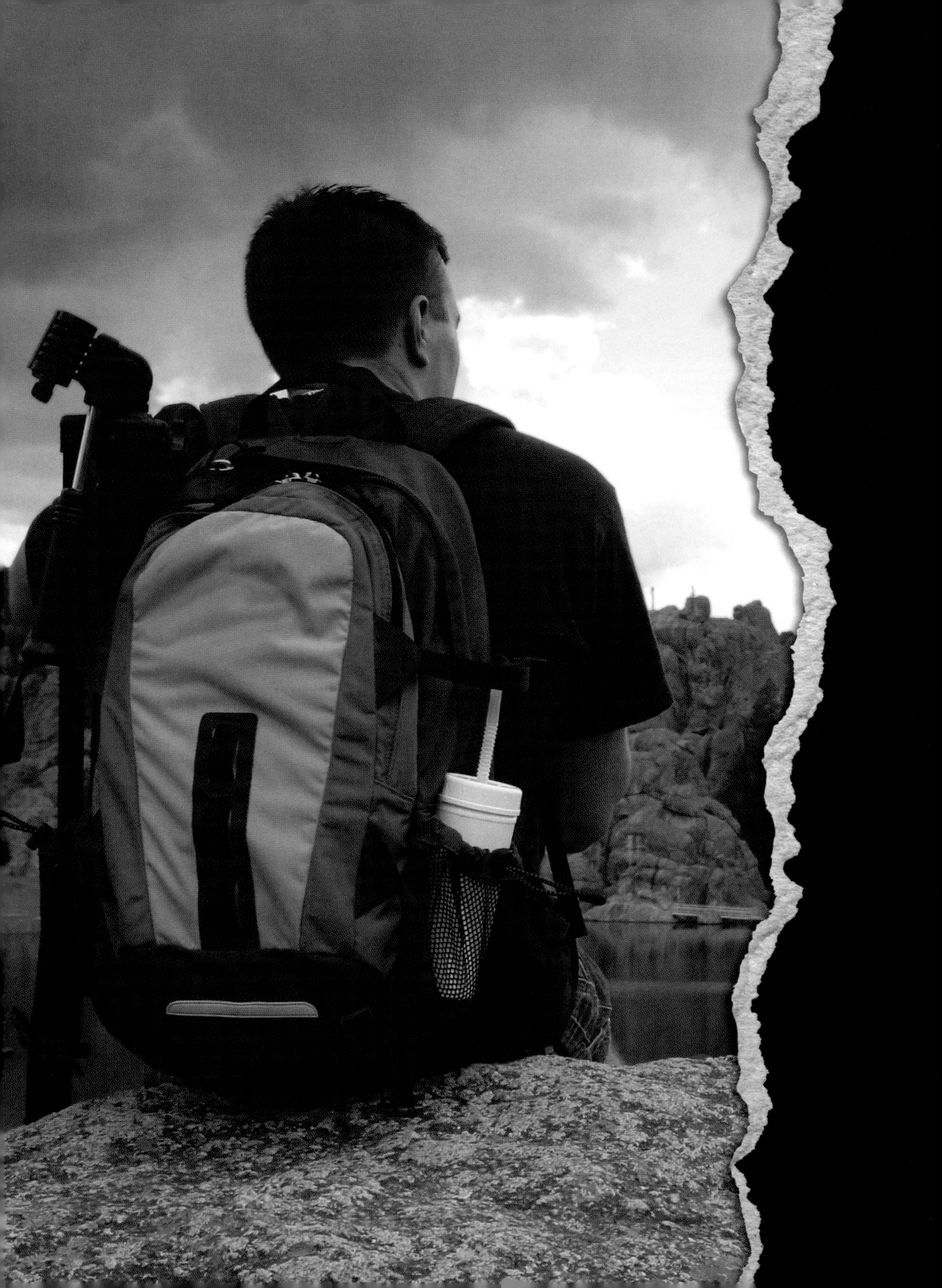

[CHAPTER ELEVEN]

# LUNCH PAILS, COOLERS AND BACKPACKS

## TAKING IT WITH YOU!

Part of the deal when you commit to Eating Clean is to eat more frequently and stick to the natural, Clean foods that make this lifestyle so successful. There is only one way to do that, and that is to take food with you and let it become your go-to tool for your physique overhaul! Doing so is your guarantee that you will eat only the foods you have prepared and not be tempted by what is offered at the drive-through of your nearest greasy spoon. We have become accustomed to carrying a cooler with us when we on the road. It is just something we do to keep us the right food track. It's a source of comfort to know that the cooler is right there with you, full of the best foods to appease a sudden hunger attack. There is just no other way to go. "When I get hungry I need to eat right away," says Tosca, "and when Robert gets hungry he will reach for a Mars bar all too quickly if the cooler isn't ready!"

## BROWN-BAG LUNCHES – WHAT'S IN YOURS?

The original purpose of a lunch break was never to satisfy a hungry workingman's stomach. Men had far more important things on their minds, such as visiting the nearest pub to down a pint and chase away the workingman's blues. Farmers traditionally ate their heaviest meal in the middle of the day at the hour we usually call "lunchtime." Most North Americans eat the heaviest meal after the workday is finished and keep lunch lighter. Until the latter 20th century men would go home in the middle of the day to be fed by their wives. Of course you know few women are at home to provide this service these days, so men have taken to carrying lunch to work.

The Brown-Bag Lunch is recognized nationwide as the way to eat the midday meal. School children carry a brown-bag lunch, as do teachers, nurses, office workers, employers and so on. You get the idea. What goes in the lunch is another question entirely, but the usual assortment is a sandwich, piece of fruit, raw vegetable crudités, cookies or a granola bar and a beverage. With the help of microwave ovens at the workplace many people also expand their lunch fare to include leftovers, which is a great idea. We often prepare our lunch for the next day while we make dinner. This saves a great deal of time and adds nutrition to our lunch.

Be sure to vary the elements in your lunch. Satisfy the desire to eat crisp, raw foods, cooked foods and thick hearty stews and soups.

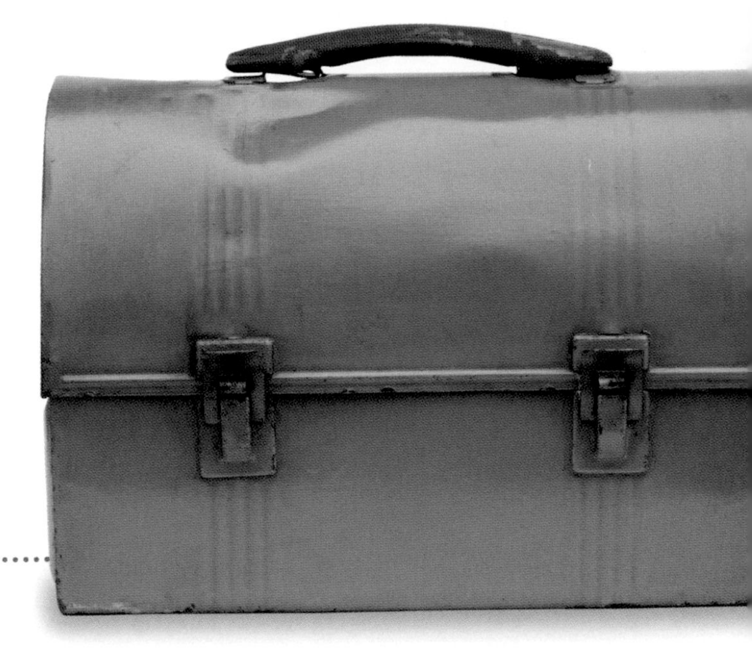

You don't have to be a chef to Eat Clean. Nor do you need much at hand to create the perfect "take it with you" lunch. We like to refer to our lunch creations as assembly cooking. If you have the right ingredients on hand it takes very little to assemble a few things into a wrap, sandwich or pita to take along to work. Preparing your own lunch has many virtues, including keeping costs down (eating out every day, even in an inexpensive restaurant, adds up!), maintains your healthy food intake and prevents you from slipping off your plan to keep your health and physique in top shape. Another bonus is that taking your lunch actually saves your precious lunch-hour time. Think how nice it is not to have to jostle the busy crowds and long lineups when you have brought your lunch with you.

Be sure to vary the elements in your lunch. Satisfy the desire to eat crisp, raw foods, cooked foods and thick hearty stews and soups. Include foods that deliver these taste experiences in every lunch and you will never get bored. Don't just throw together a smoothie. Add an apple and some raw nuts to the meal and you will enjoy it all the more.

If you can generate interest among your peers, another way to lighten the lunchtime load is to organize a lunch co-op. Invite four of your co-workers to participate in a cooperative lunch group, where each one of you takes a turn to prepare the lunch for everyone on one day of the week. Yes, it is a bit more work on your day but the other days are super easy. The more there are in your group the better.

# LUNCH IS ALL WRAPPED UP

**Fillings:**

- Homemade hummus (the white peanut butter)
- Black-bean spread
- Salsa
- An assortment of natural nut butters
- Sprouts – there are loads of varieties, so experiment with broccoli, onion, garlic or sunflower sprouts along with alfalfa
- Baby spinach or mesclun mix
- Fresh tomatoes – vine-ripened cluster tomatoes are best in the winter, field tomatoes best in late summer/early fall
- Sundried tomatoes – perfect for adding zest to a sambal
- Ground flaxseeds
- Bananas
- Apples
- Avocado
- Grilled or roasted turkey breast
- Grilled or roasted chicken breast
- Grilled salmon or other fish
- Water-packed tuna
- Hard-boiled eggs
- Skim-milk cheeses
- Yogurt cheese spreads
- Leftover brown rice
- LEFTOVERS OF ANY KIND!

**Wraps** – brown rice, whole grain, pita or any you prefer

- Ezekiel bread or wraps
- Whole-grain crackers
- Whole-grain bagels, especially traditional bagels

***NOTE:*** *A sturdy bread like rye is better for portable lunches, since it is firmer and withstands being carried around loaded with ingredients.*

**Assembly:**

- **Choose your outer wrapping** – essentially the "container" for the fillings you plan to use
- **Choose the spread you want to use** – We love almond butter sprinkled with ground flaxseeds and chopped banana, but there are endless varieties.
- **Choose the filling** – Use your imagination.
- **You can also use a pita** – spread it with hummus, stuff in some sprouts and sliced apple, sliced grilled skinless chicken breast and off you go!
- The combinations are endless – that's why it's so nice to have leftovers on hand.

## MORE ABOUT LUNCH

A Bengali luncheon often includes as many as seven courses! Shukto is the first course, consisting of lightly cooked and seasoned vegetables topped with coconut icing. Don't knock the icing. Coconuts contain important anti-viral properties helpful in fighting disease in hot climates. The next course usually involves rice, daal and a vegetable curry. Daal is a spicy stew made from split, dried beans. The third course includes rice and fish curry. The fourth is rice and meat curry. Sweet foods appear in the fifth course while payesh, a sweetened rice and milk dish, or mishti doi, a sweetened yogurt dish, are found in the sixth course. Finally, the meal is finished with a seventh course of paan. Paan is a green betel leaf, filled with various sweet or sour items, chewed to both freshen the mouth and aid digestion.

## FRENCH LUNCH

The French call their lunch *déjeuner* and make this the most substantial meal of the day. It is often a long lunch, not a rushed event, where two hours are needed to savor the food. The key here is savor. No one rushes, bolts or multi-tasks while eating lunch in France! The meal is served in courses and savored, featuring foods that are recognizable as foods. Meat and fish appear along with salads, breads and cheeses. Coffee is a common post-lunch beverage.

## THE ULTIMATE CROSS-COUNTRY WARRIORS

We have learned a lot from our truck-driving friends, who tell us how they have managed to improve their health and waistlines by packing an Eat-Clean cooler in preparation for a long drive. Contrary to what you may think, those who make their living hauling goods across the continent want good health, trim waistlines and more food choices than just the local Subway. In an effort to create their own solutions to these problems, OTR (on the road) drivers have come up with strategies to ensure healthier eating while away from home. Here are some of their tricks for portable good eats.

# SOLUTIONS FOR EATING ON THE ROAD:

**Many truck drivers eat out of a cooler throughout the week.**

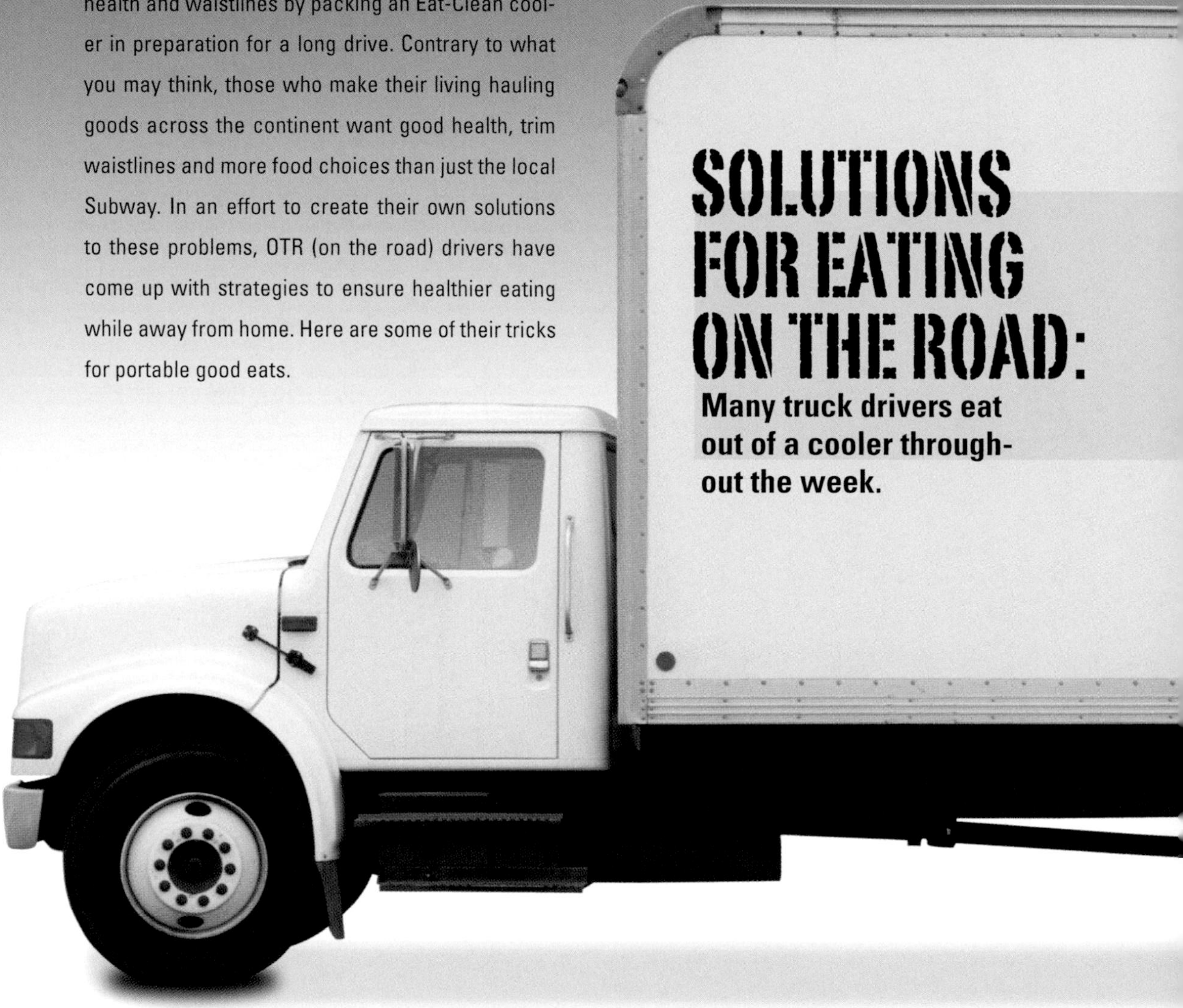

## HOW TO KEEP YOUR FOOD COLD

Some drivers use plug-in coolers and inverters to power them, while others have resorted to packaging dry ice in plastic bags and packing food around it. An inverter is a piece of equipment that facilitates the use of 110-amp appliances in a truck. Some small 12-volt coolers are very inexpensive but do not seem to last long. This is because their fans can lose steam. However, some of these products work fine. Check out www.roadtrucker.com for more information. Some drivers use a more expensive 12-volt refrigerator, which seems to do the trick. The cost is probably worth it if you spend serious hours on the road, especially considering the money you'll save on fast food.

## HOW TO KEEP YOUR FOOD HOT

Drivers also use a small microwave oven if their rig space permits. There's nothing like a hot meal. You can even get a 12-volt portable oven to heat up or toast food. It plugs into the cigarette lighter. If the truck has an inverter, then a Foreman grill is handy too. Some types of electric kettles and coffee makers can also be plugged into the cigarette lighter. Another handy heating tool is a lunch-box cooker, which again plugs into the cigarette lighter and is useful for heating leftovers and soups.

## PORTABLE FOODS

Any time you jump in the car with family or friends for a hike or day trip it is good thinking to pack a cooler. Many outdoor lovers already know the value of having trail mix, water, energy bars and oranges tucked away in their backpack. These foods have always gone along in our backpacks when downhill or cross-country skiing, since they are high in complex carbohydrates, protein and healthy fats, satisfying, highly portable, and require no preparation. In our house if we are not fed and watered regularly, we get cranky.

## PACK YOUR COOLER EVERY DAY

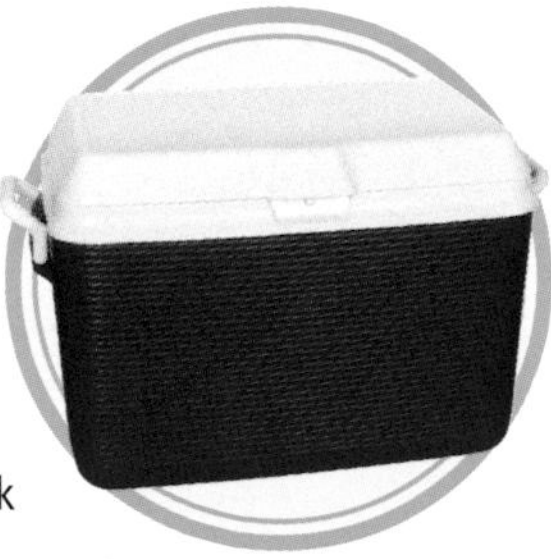

Success with Clean Eating demands that you pack a cooler every day. Eating as frequently as Clean Eating requires means that you will have to somehow carry your food to wherever it is you work or play. Doing so also reinforces your plan to overhaul your lifestyle – remember the deal you made with yourself to get leaner, fitter and healthier? The cooler will keep you from overeating or munching on nutrient-poor treats.

It isn't fun to be hungry, so we depend on that loaded cooler to keep us full. If you are ravenous you want food fast, and that is usually the time you are vulnerable to eating just about anything. If your cooler is handy you will always have the luxury of Clean foods at your finger tips. No more Twinkies and doughnuts!

## GET THE GOODS

Getting started with your Clean-Eating cooler means you may need to make a few purchases. Visit your local big-box department store, hardware store or outdoor goods store, where you will find coolers of all sizes. Look for a soft-sided cooler measuring just large enough to handle three or four small meals. We like the collapsible ones with a plastic insert, which slips out easily for washing. The collapsible part is perfect for traveling. When the cooler is empty you can fold it up and tuck it away till next time. Smaller coolers such as these usually have an adjustable carrying strap.

Don't forget to pick up some freezable ice packs for keeping cooler contents chilled. Purchase a few small ones so you can distribute them around foods. We buy extras because for some reason they go missing, just like socks in the dryer.

You will also need an array of re-sealable containers in which to pack your food. We like containers with see-through lids so you know at a glance what's inside. Stock up on incidentals such as napkins, travel wipes, cutlery and re-sealable bags in a number of sizes. The next step will be packing your cooler.

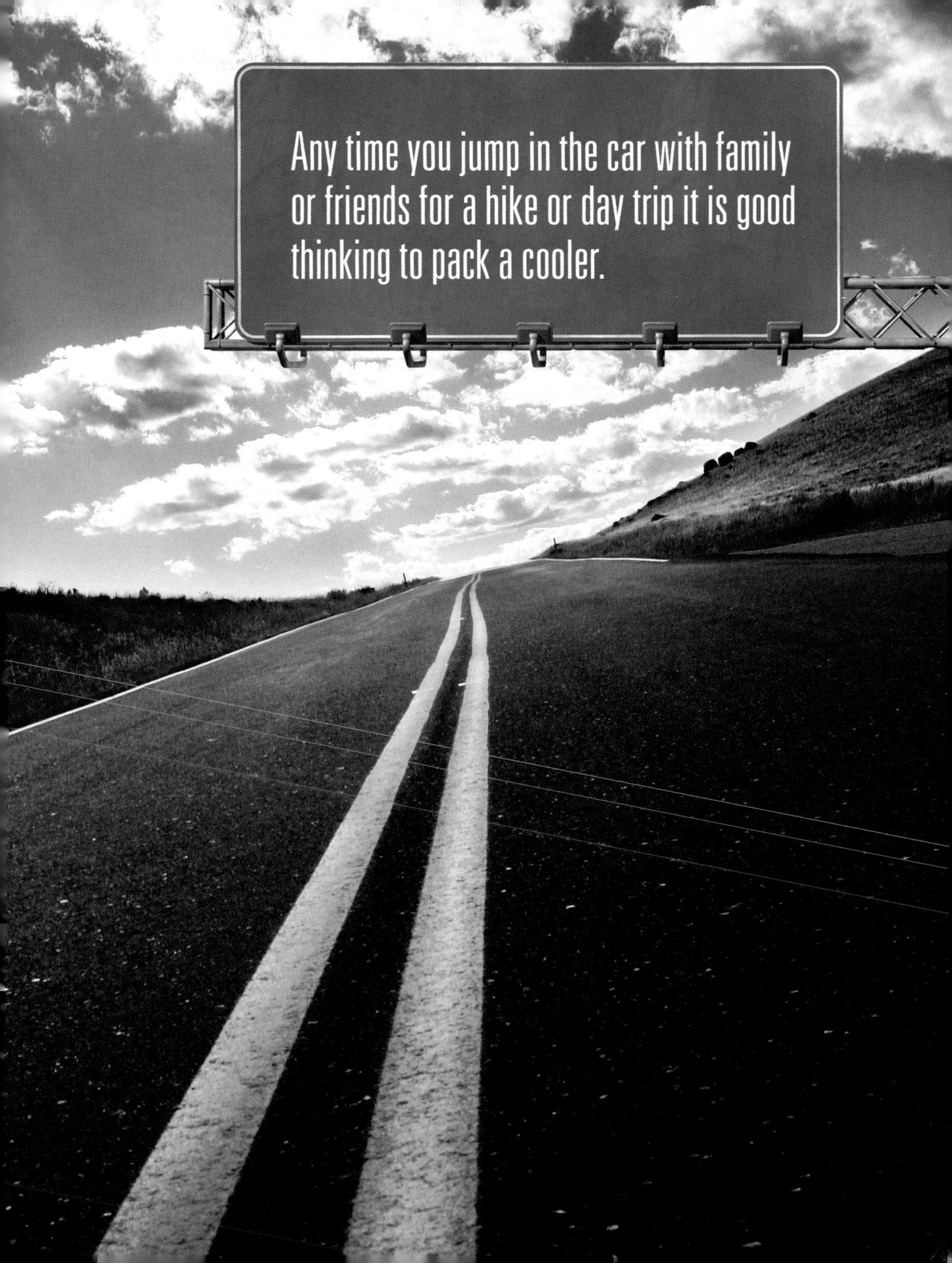

Any time you jump in the car with family or friends for a hike or day trip it is good thinking to pack a cooler.

## COOLER PLANS

The kinds of foods you pack in your cooler determine how tight your nutrition will be and also your rate of weight loss, if that is part of your plan. We have worked out three plan to get you Eating Clean with your cooler or lunch pail in hand. Each plan is different from the others in that they contain different foods that are either an introduction to Eating Clean or extremely lean, Clean foods. You may want to begin with Cooler Plan #3 to get an idea of how to start. Then you can move on to the other cooler plans to really tighten up.

## THREE PLANS

The first thing to remember is that all three plans contain Clean foods. The foods that go in each different cooler are chosen to give you a specific result. We have found this is necessary because some people need time to get into the habit of Clean Eating while others don't. Cooler Plan #1 is the tightest, and by most people's standards not the easiest way to eat. There is a good chance you will be hungry, but at the same time if weight loss is your goal you will definitely get the desired result. Cooler Plan #3 is less strict and eases a newcomer into Clean Eating.

## CHOOSE A PLAN

Having a choice of plans allows you to control how tight you want to keep your nutrition and the rate at which you would like to lose weight. Clean Eating should help you lose a healthy amount of weight each week – an average of three pounds. This is standard until you get to your set point. If you have more weight to lose at the beginning, you may find that you end up losing more each week. Bonus!

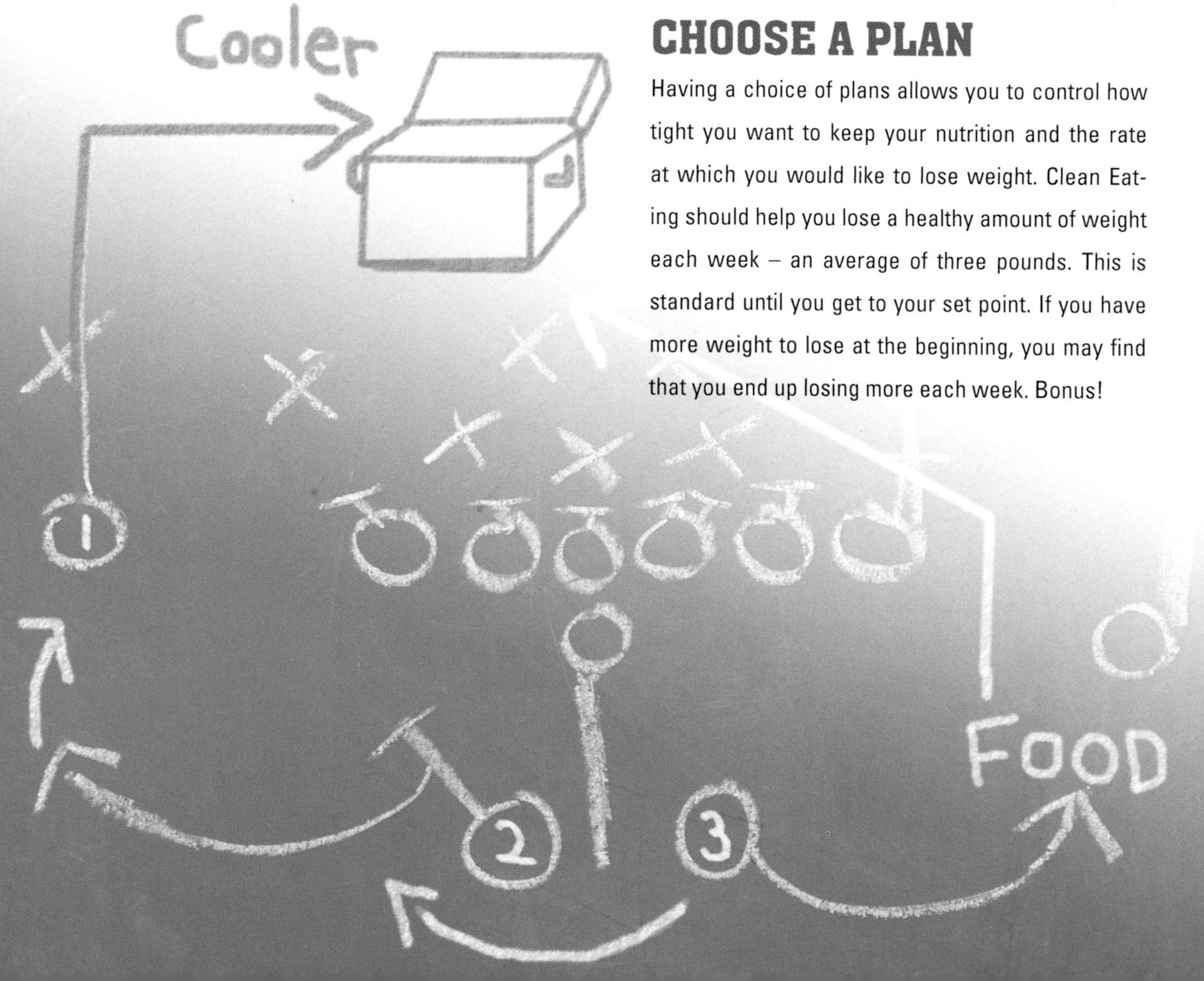

# COOLER PLAN #1

## HARDCORE EATING FOR HARDCORE EFFECT

Please note that this is the strictest of the cooler plans and will not be easy for some of you. There is little room for indulgence and you may initially experience lightheadedness due to a lack of carbs. If the feeling is too much, simply add more complex carbohydrates in the form of whole grains and fresh fruits and vegetables to one of your earlier meals. Keep in mind that this plan suggests results and that is what you will get. Lean, chiseled definition is just around the corner.

**HOW?** Eat six meals per day with the last meal at 6:00 p.m.

**WHEN?** Meals should be spread out every two to three hours.

**WHAT TO EAT FOR THE ENTIRE DAY:**

→ **PROTEIN:** 6–7, 5-oz servings of chicken, tuna, egg whites, turkey, bison, elk, fish (primarily whitefish and salmon)

→ **VEGGIES:** 5, 1½–2-cup servings cucumbers, radishes, tomatoes, leafy greens, asparagus, green beans, sprouts, celery

→ **STARCHY COMPLEX CARBOHYDRATES AND FRUITS:** Yams and/or sweet potatoes – 1 sweet potato or equivalent over the course of the day or 1½ cups brown rice throughout the day, 1 apple, 1 banana

→ **FATS:** 1 handful unsalted, raw nuts or seeds of your choice.

→ **WATER:** 1 gallon distilled water or fresh water with no sodium.

★ **NOTE:** An ideal breakfest would be 1 cup cooked oatmeal with 2–4 Tbsp each flaxseeds, wheat germ, bee pollen (optional) and scrambled egg whites.

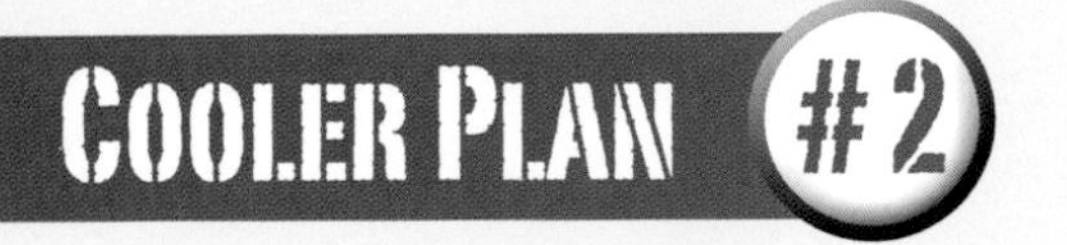


## STRICT EATING FOR BEST RESULTS AND MAINTENANCE

This plan can be considered the way to eat once you have achieved your physique goals. Begin to reintroduce some Clean foods, especially complex carbohydrates, once you have arrived at your goal weight. You will be able to eat as you ate in **Cooler Plan #1**, plus extra foods.

### COOLER PLAN #1 PLUS THE FOLLOWING:

- 2–3, 1-cup servings berries, grapefruit, apples, banana or mango
- All vegetables, but limited amounts of corn, carrots and squash
- Hot cooked cereals, muesli, Kashi Go Lean
- 2 pieces multi-grain toast, dry
- 1 cup unsweetened applesauce as sweetener on cereal or toast
- 2 whole-grain wraps
- 1 cup low-fat soy, almond, hemp or brown-rice milk, or skim milk
- Unlimited clear green tea, coffee and regular water
- 1 handful or ½ cup unsalted nuts
- 2 Tbsp nut butter

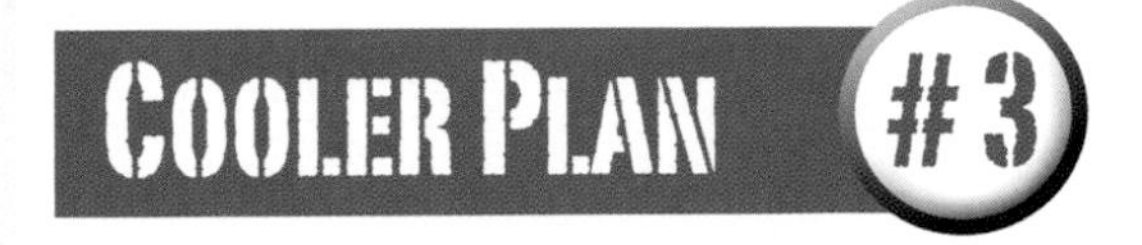


## GETTING THE IDEA OF EATING FOR HEALTH AND LIFE

We understand that you might be new to Clean Eating, and you may feel hesitant about how to go forward with it. You may wish to make simple changes fast so you can begin to understand and experience the way Clean Eating can positively affect your health and your body. Although these are simple changes, they are nonetheless powerful enough that you will soon see results. What may be the biggest surprise is how good natural foods will taste once you forego the junk.

### WHAT TO EAT

Include all the wholesome and body-building foods outlined in **Cooler Plans #1 and #2,** but avoid all refined foods including sugar, white flour, cookies, pastries, candies, snack foods and fast foods. Steer clear of unhealthy saturated and trans fats, especially cream, ice cream, fatty dressings, fatty cheeses and fatty meats.

### HAVE IN MODERATION

- Egg yolks: Have one yolk for every three or four whites
- 1 glass juice per day
- 1 handful unsalted nuts per day
- Low-fat, plain yogurt
- Low-fat cottage cheese
- Limited low-fat cheese

## LUNCH IS GOOD AGAIN

Most nights we cook our own meals rather than eat out. This provides the perfect opportunity to prepare a little extra food for our coolers the next day. We call it making "Planned Leftovers." The theory is that since you are in the kitchen anyway you should make the most of your time there. The oven is already on, you have the ingredients on hand, and making double of a particular recipe takes little extra time. We never cook just one of anything; we aim for better efficiency. This way, filling a cooler becomes a simple matter of selecting from foods you have already prepared and then you are on your way.

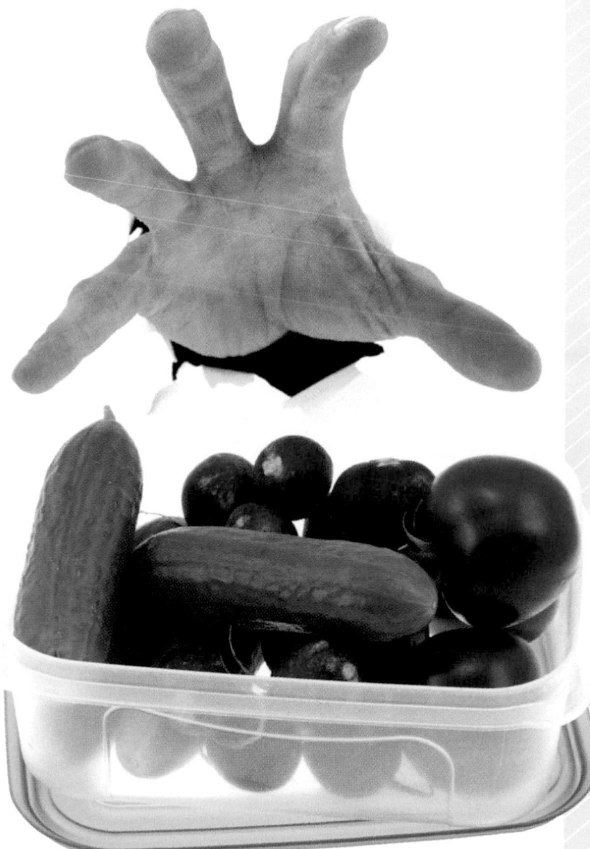

### Here are some of our favorite ways to simplify cooking time in the kitchen:

- Roast two pork tenderloins, let cool and slice into medallions, which can then be used in wraps or stir-fries.
- Roast one whole lean turkey breast without the bone and let cool. Cut into thin slices for sandwiches and wraps.
- Grill two salmon steaks for each person. Eat one for dinner and let the other cool. Use it to top a leafy green salad for lunch.
- Grill or bake a few chicken breasts at a time. Have one for dinner and the rest can be sliced for use in sandwiches or stir-fries.
- Boil a dozen eggs until they are hard-boiled. Eggs keep well for a few days and are a simple, reliable and complete protein source. Eat three or four at a time (whites only) for 21 grams of lean protein.
- Purchase water-packed tuna, either in cans or in small pouches that don't require a can opener. Either way, tuna is an inexpensive and versatile source of lean, portable protein.

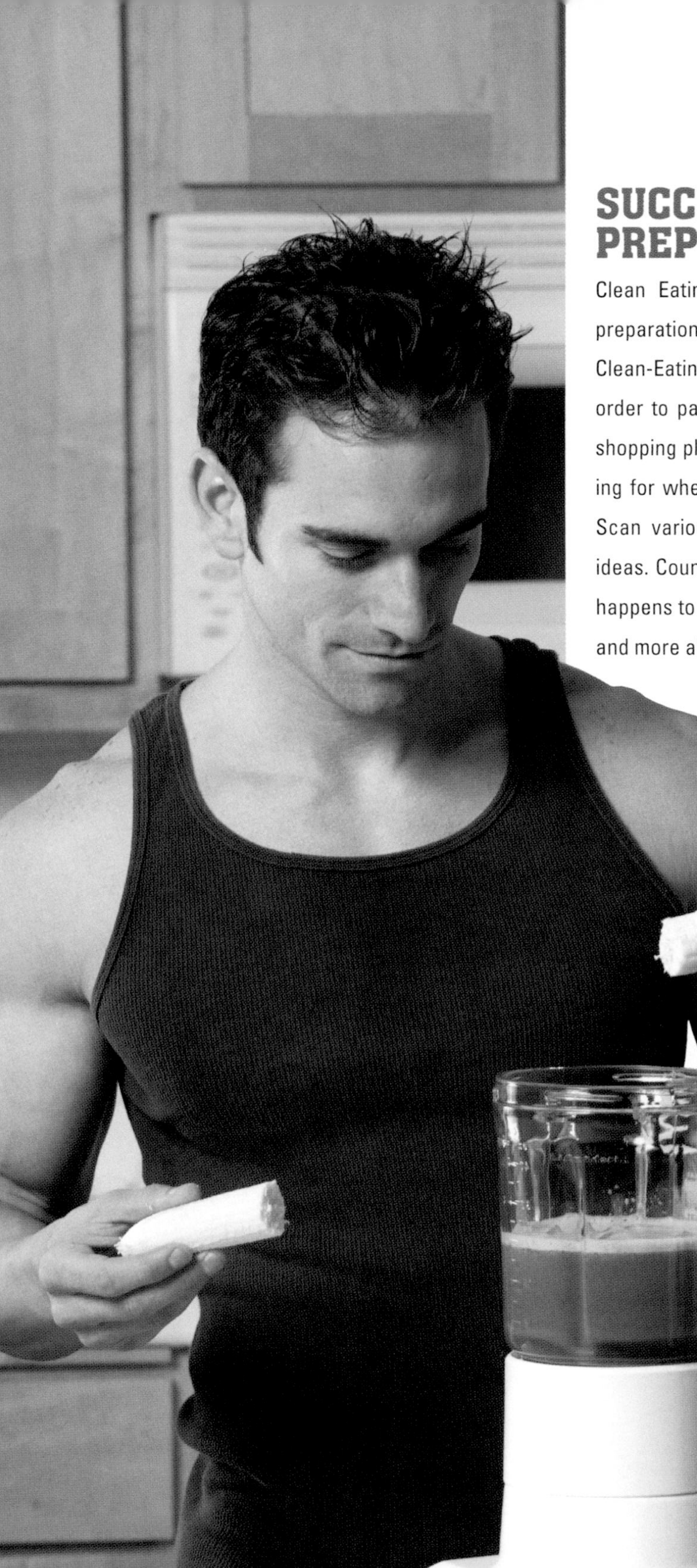

## SUCCESS IS PREPARATION

Clean Eating is simplified with organization and preparation. You need to have a good supply of Clean-Eating foods in your fridge and cupboards in order to pack a healthful lunch. Doing a little pre-shopping planning helps you get what you are looking for when you finally arrive at the supermarket. Scan various magazines and websites for recipe ideas. Count on local produce, especially whatever happens to be in season, since it is usually cheaper and more abundant.

## CRITICAL QUESTION

**Dave**

*There is one issue I have – it's about gas. If I start this diet (and I do have about 100 pounds to lose) should I buy stock in Beano or is there something I can do to offset the gas by-product?*

## ANSWER

Beano might seem like a reasonable solution, but the truth is your body just needs to adjust to eating more fiber and protein. There are several things you can do to offset this smelly problem. First, you must chew your food thoroughly – and we mean thoroughly. The more you liquefy the food the less work your digestive system will have to do, and the less it will bloat you on the way out. Next, drink plenty of water, which again helps flush out the system. You may also want to consider taking a pro-biotic or a pre-biotic, either of which helps to break down foods in a friendly way down there. Some foods that are excellent for this purpose include yogurt and kefir. Digestive enzymes are helpful, too. Other than that, perhaps your excessive gassiness is due to food intolerance. This is most often due to lactose or gluten sensitivity. Avoid the foods that trouble you the most.

# A NOT-SO-CLEAN EATING STORY!

**Sharon Johnston**

From an email dated August 3, 2008

*I must share with you my latest experience and the problem with American health care. My father (my reason for being so health conscious) is currently in ICU as a result of a blood clot. He is diabetic and has severe coronary disease. After "roto-rooting" the vessel to clear out the clot and installing four stents to keep it open because it is in such bad condition, they fed him a grilled ham and cheese sandwich. Can you believe it??? When I walked by the trays in the ICU I saw that the other patients were eating deli turkey on a white hamburger roll!! I am no dietician and certainly no health care provider, but my guess is that the majority of the patients in ICUs have a heart condition and/or diabetes. They are lying flat on their backs with absolutely no fiber in their diet and we are feeding them white bread. Today's breakfast for my father was oatmeal (OK, that was good) and scrambled eggs, bacon and pork sausage, a sugary muffin and orange juice!! Can you imagine feeding a diabetic heart patient with a blood clot this diet?? The American diet stinks, particularly in a hospital. The cafeteria there is just as bad if not worse. Trying to eat healthy there has been*

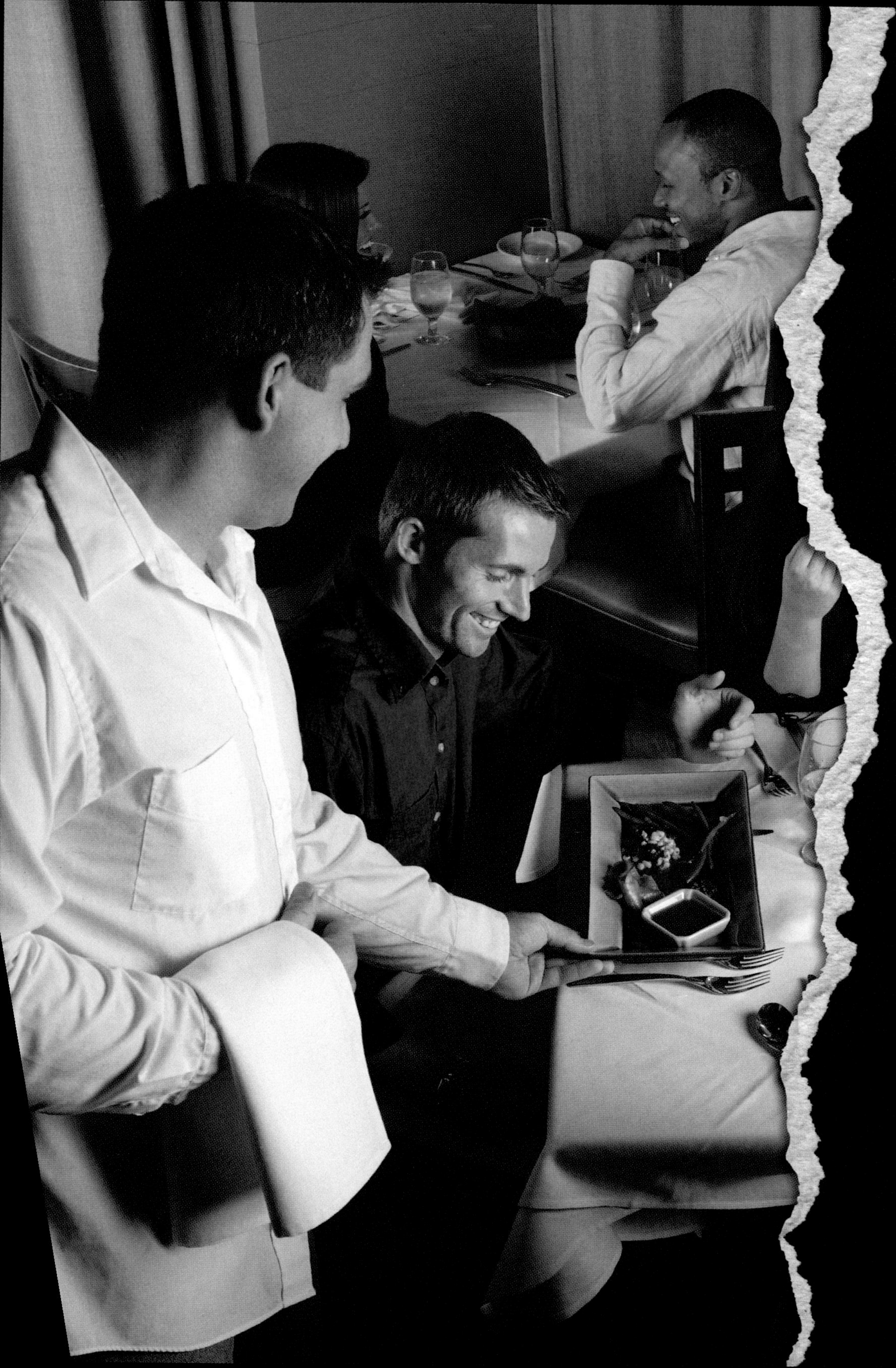

# [CHAPTER TWELVE]

# EATING OUT

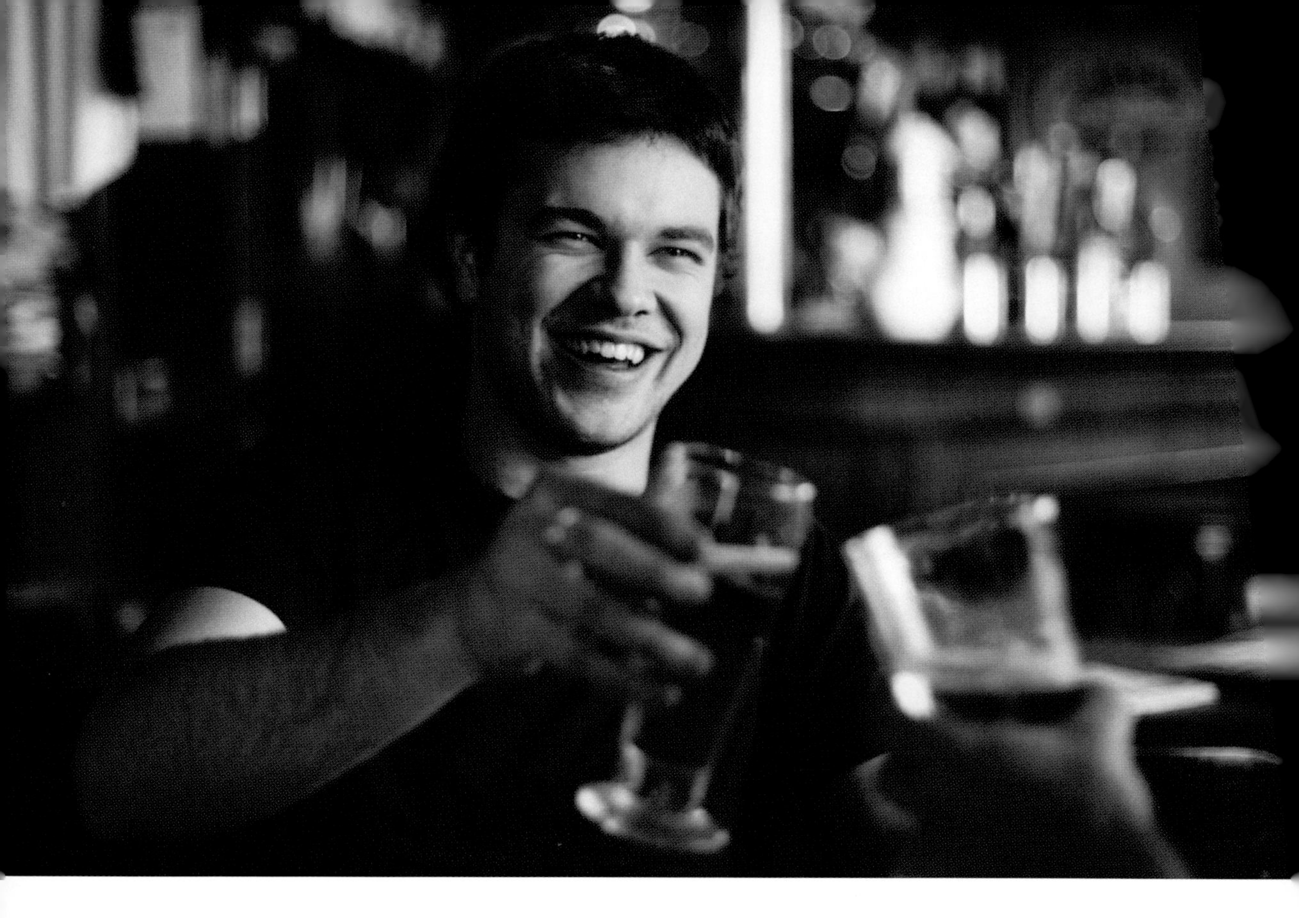

# A WAY OF LIFE

Each year North Americans spend an estimated $400 billion either in restaurants or for other foods prepared and eaten outside the home. Most of us spend so much money on foods not prepared or eaten in the home that it has become a way of life for us, so it isn't difficult to perceive that eating out has contributed to the ever-expanding waistline and health problems this nation is facing. The way food is prepared today represents an enormous departure from the way food was prepared hundreds or thousands of years ago, and in general this does not represent a trend for the better.

This may surprise you, but restaurants don't have your health in mind the way you would when preparing foods. Their priorities are elsewhere. That is fine if you are a restaurant owner, but if you are a consumer with either a weight or a health problem, you need to know more. You need to develop a strategy for navigating menus and other offerings at various restaurants. You need the translation guide for what certain terms mean when you see them on the menu. Furthermore, you need to know how to order a meal that fits with an Eat-Clean lifestyle. You may also need help figuring out what a serving is versus a portion size. Do you know the difference?

You will learn to figure out all these matters in this chapter. Trust us, we have traveled to enough cities big and small on this continent and elsewhere in the world that we are quite certain we know what we are doing when it comes to ordering Clean food in practically any restaurant.

Dining out has proven to be the most dramatic change in North American eating habits, thanks to busy schedules and the prevalence of food establishments. The problem with this trend is that most foods consumed away from home contain more questionable nutrients, including trans and saturated fats, than those prepared at home. Author Sally Fallon notes in her book *Nourishing Traditions*, "... father technology has not brought us freedom from disease. Chronic illness in industrialized nations has reached epic proportions because we have been dazzled by his stepchildren – fast foods, fractionated foods, convenience foods, packaged foods, fake foods, embalmed foods, ersatz foods." She makes an excellent point. Food is not to be trusted simply because it's called food. Additionally, restaurant foods may contain less of the more desirable components in foods including vitamins, minerals and fiber. This of course does not apply to all restaurants, but to be certain there are no standards across the board.

Restaurants don't have your health in mind the way you would when preparing foods. Their priorities are elsewhere.

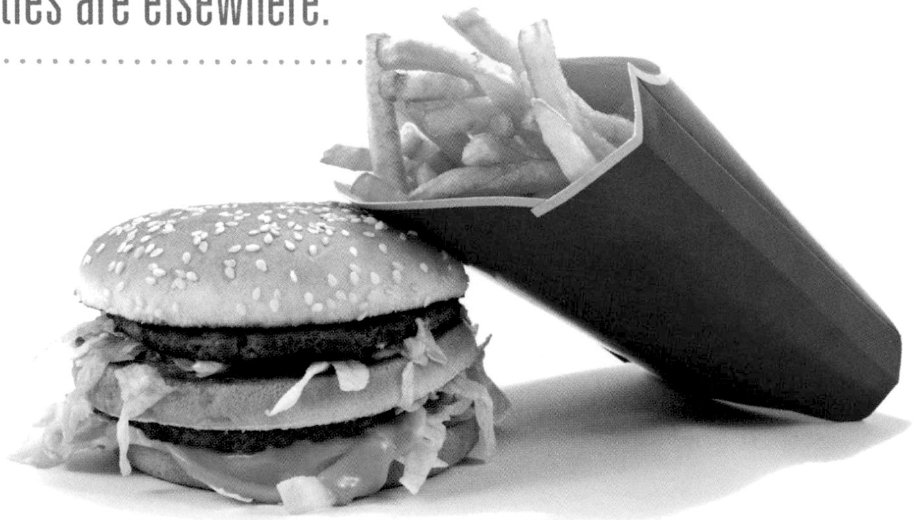

## WHAT IS YOUR MINDSET?

Eating out can be an occasion for celebration, relaxation or reward, and is more often than not a convenience factor for the harried cook. If you make your living on the road, eating out is an occupational hazard. You have to do it. As a consumer the decisions about what you eat are driven by what is offered at the particular restaurant you are visiting. If you are sitting in a McDonald's you will very likely soon be eating a burger. If you are at the International House of Pancakes you will probably order a plate of pancakes, and so on. Some of your decision making about what you will eat is therefore guided by your choice of restaurant. This is where we suggest you begin to rethink the dining-out experience at the point when you are choosing the restaurant.

Before you even leave the house you can use the Internet to search for potential restaurants. We recommend looking for those that offer some Clean-Eating choices. Restaurants often post a menu online so you can see if they serve Clean-Eating fare. Remember you are looking for lean protein – grilled salmon, chicken, beef tenderloin, bison and so on – complex carbohydrates in the form of vegetables and fruits, and slower-burning complex carbs in the form of whole grains. On one website called Healthy Dining Finder (www.healthydiningfinder.com), registered dieticians and nutrition professionals work together to help restaurants develop healthy menus or tweak existing offerings. In order for a restaurant to be considered worthy of Healthy Dining status it must meet several criteria, including serving entrées with lean protein, fruits and/or vegetables and whole grains. The restaurant must also offer entrées with calorie counts of 750 or fewer, fat content of 25 grams or less and saturated fat of less than 8 grams. They also monitor sodium and cholesterol. The Internet can be a valuable tool for determining where you will dine. Use listings like these to your advantage to help you narrow down the choice of restaurant before your final decision.

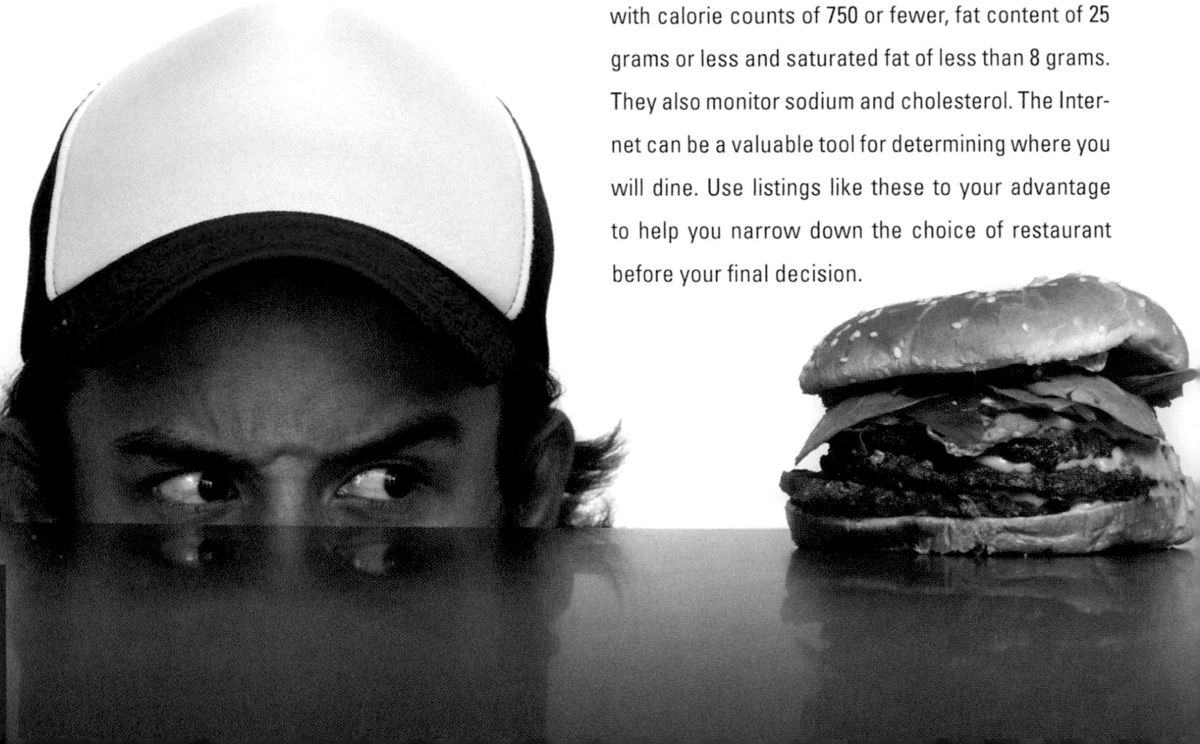

## YOUR EATING-OUT STRATEGY

Some dining-out occasions are really meant to be occasions – special events that celebrate special times. This may not be the time to avoid your favorite cocktail or rich dessert. Go ahead and celebrate; just don't do it every night. This is part of your whole dining-out strategy. Know when to party and when to keep it tight.

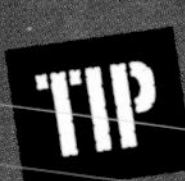


**Have a plan: You have a pretty good idea what you'll encounter during your evening out. If you are prepared in advance, then you'll be much more likely to handle it Cleanly!**

If it happens to be party time tonight, you will find it a challenge to stick to Eating Clean religiously. The question presents itself: Will you cave in when you see the menu, or will you stick to your guns and make healthier food choices? If you are celebrating a special occasion, then we feel it's best to stick to making Clean food choices for the most part, and make the decision to enjoy a glass of wine, cocktail or beer, and dessert too. You don't have to completely let go, but allow yourself a treat. Don't feel bad about it, just keep in mind ahead of time what you are getting into, and what your solution is. And a celebration is a special time – when it is over, the good-time eating needs to be over too.

## ORDER CLEAN AND EAT CLEAN

We have found with the extensive traveling we do that you can find Clean foods no matter which restaurant you plan to visit, from a five-star resort to a diner. We always approach our dining experiences with an eye to our physique goals. If we are preparing for an event where we want to look our best we stick strictly to Clean Eating. We don't touch the bread from the breadbasket, and won't order any alcohol or dessert. That way whatever progress we have made will stay with us.

You may feel the same way, particularly if you've recently lost a few pounds. You want to keep on losing weight, so you will want to keep your food choices tight. Some of you may just have started Eating Clean and there are others of you who are maintaining a Clean-Eating lifestyle. Ultimately you will have to determine both your goals and where you are in the process, and order accordingly.

[ Make friends with the waiter if you hope to get your food the way you want it. ]

## MAKE FRIENDS WITH THE SERVER

We would like to offer our best piece of advice yet. Make friends with the server if you hope to get your food the way you want it. If the server is on your side you stand a far better chance of getting the Clean food you want. We always tell our server the way we would like our food cooked, and explain that we don't want it prepared with sauces, gravy, cheese or excess fats and oils. You will have to be charming and polite, not crusty and cranky. Be clear about how you want your food but don't be rude. Once you have charmed him into your corner, tell him politely but meaningfully that you will return the food if it comes covered in ingredients you don't want.

With all the eating out we have done over the years, we notice chefs seem to really dislike leaving cheese out of food. For some reason you have to specify very clearly that you don't want melted cheese on anything, especially egg-white omelets. What is the point of ordering an egg-white omelet if it's oozing with melted cheese?

## ORDERING

Now it's time to order. Have a quick look at the menu. You might notice the chef is offering beef tenderloin as a special tonight. We love beef tenderloin or filet mignon. But you may have noticed the beef comes dressed in bacon and sauce. This is where we politely ask if the chef would prepare the filet without the bacon and sauce. Go ahead and order the filet, but don't forget to ask for it to be served grilled and without the extra ingredients. If the food in the restaurant you choose is not pre-made, then getting your dish prepared the way you want it should not be difficult.

Now for the vegetables. Vegetables often come coated in heavy sauces, butter or melted cheese. You definitely don't want these extras if you are Eating Clean. Request plain steamed vegetables instead. If the chef can't do the vegetables this way, request a salad without dressing instead.

You will be lucky if your entrée comes with brown rice. Go ahead and try to order it, but it's a rare find unless you're in a healthy-food restaurant. Ask to switch the accompanying starch, whether it's some form of potato, rice or noodle, to an extra helping of vegetables if you are keeping your food intake tight. If we are dining out late, we often omit starchy carbohydrates and request a salad or sliced tomato instead.

If you are interested in soup as an appetizer make sure to check with the server if it is broth or cream based. Puréed vegetable soups and clear broths are a delicious source of complex carbohydrates and nutrients, but if the soup is made with cream you are getting way too much fat – and the fat is saturated. You will need to check with the waiter to be sure. If there are no Clean-Eating appetizer choices, ask for a salad instead. Remember, bacon bits and croutons are not on your Clean-Eating menu, so make sure they are not on your salad. Dress the salad with lemon juice or balsamic vinegar and a splash of olive oil. Chilled shrimp cocktail with a squeeze of lemon is a good choice too.

We often ask the server not to bring the breadbasket to the table. The breadbasket is put on the table to keep the diners happy while their order is being prepared. Avoid it if you can. If the basket sits in front of you long enough you will end up eating out of it despite your best intentions.

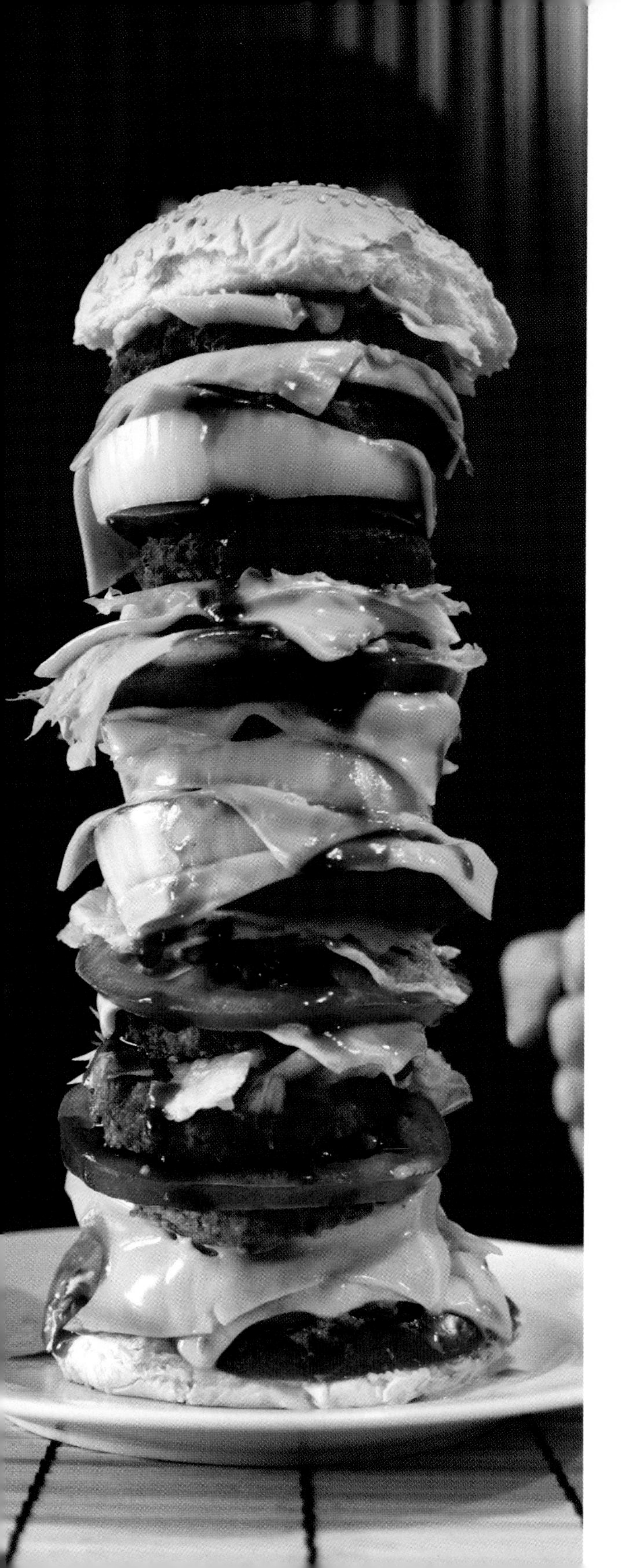

## THAT COULD FEED FOUR OF US!

Findings from a recent study show the average daily caloric intake in 1987-88 was 1,807, but that rose to 2,043 calories per day in 1995. Today that number is higher still. We already know that one in three North American adults is overweight. According to Biing-Hwan Lin, Joanne Guthrie and Elizabeth Frazao, authors of a report entitled *Nutrient Contribution of Food Away from Home*, "... when eating out, people either eat more or eat higher-calorie foods – or both." Regardless, it is up to you to control your food intake. Keep the Clean Eating recommended portion sizes in your mind (see page 66) and consider whether the entrée you just ordered should feed you or the four of you.

Remember, the protein serving should approximate the size of the palm of your hand, complex carbohydrates from fresh vegetables should be the size of two hands cupped together, and whole grains and other starches should be the size of one cupped hand. Consider ordering a starter as a main course if the restaurant you are in has a reputation for serving large portions. Also consider that at home you may not order an appetizer but in a restaurant situation you might. That means you will be eating more and taking in more calories, so you'll have to adjust your food intake accordingly if you want to stick to Clean Eating.

## GET IT TO GO

Just because you have received an enormous portion of food on your plate doesn't mean you must finish it. You can ask for a take-home container right away and put half of the food away before you even begin if it really is too much. Regardless, you are not obligated to finish the food on your plate. You bought the food, and you have the right to take the excess home. What difference does it make if you only eat half now and the rest for another meal?

## WHAT ABOUT DESSERT?

The dessert section is the trickiest part of the menu to navigate. Everything looks so delicious! To make it worse, dessert options are often posted on tables so you end up staring at a piece of yummy-looking pie throughout the entire meal. It's a form of silent torture. We normally reserve dessert eating to a few limited occasions including birthdays, holidays such as Christmas or Thanksgiving, and the odd special celebration. Even then that's about 20 desserts per year and that's more than enough for us. In fact, we usually share.

If we are hosting festive Christmas and Thanksgiving meals – and we usually do, because we have the biggest dining-room table – we always prepare Clean-Eating dessert choices. The best of these include fruit salads, fresh berry combinations, fruit platters and unsweetened applesauce. Biscotti is also an excellent dessert alternative, since this dry Italian cookie is naturally low in fat and calories. When it comes to birthday cake, we will take a very small piece but won't eat the icing and skip the ice cream.

When dining out we ask the server if it is possible to have fresh berries or a selection of fresh fruits for dessert – not that we always order dessert, but when we do fresh fruit or berries is what we order. It may seem bold to ask, especially when what we are asking for is not on the menu, but we do it anyway!

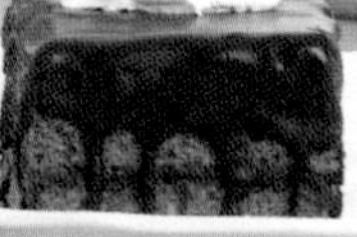

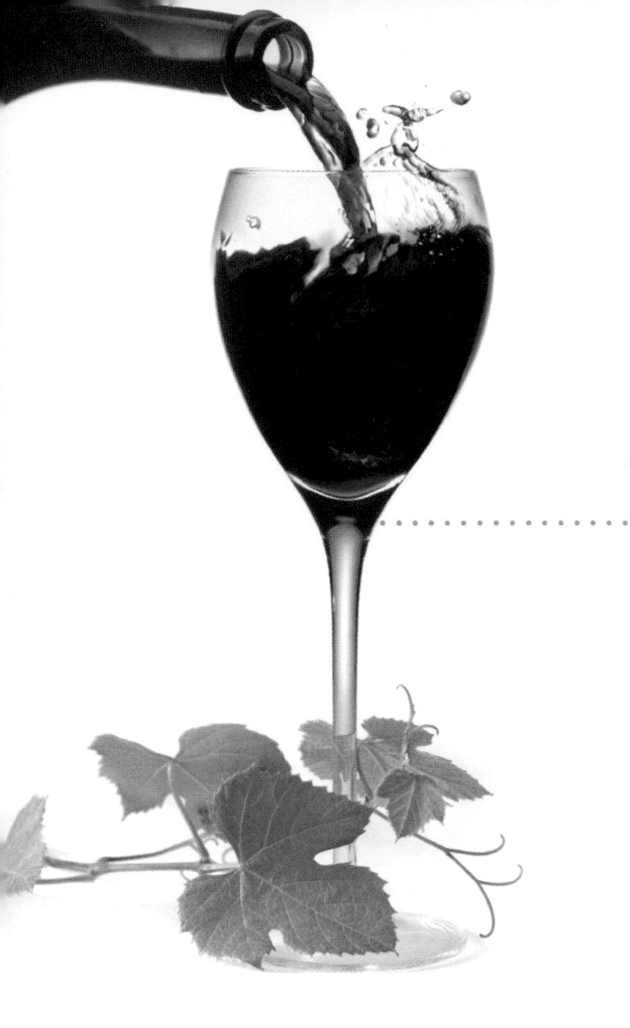

If you feel you have to drink, limit it to one glass of dry red wine or a spritzer.

## ALCOHOL – MODERATION PLEASE

Alcohol is simply another form of sugar, with as many unnecessary calories from sugar as dessert, and it helps to think of it this way. Specialty liqueurs such as Bailey's Irish Cream or Kahlua are delicious but swimming in sugar. Such beverages don't come with nutrition labels, but the ingredient list includes hefty doses of sugar – which doesn't appear on the Clean-Eating list of recommend foods.

We know this next statement will cause a groan, but ultimately it is best to limit alcohol intake. Even a couple of beers every other night will add up to the dreaded beer belly. And no matter how light that beer might be, it is still added sugar and added pounds. "Our physical nature is such that we need foods that are whole, not refined and denatured, to grow, prosper and reproduce. As the consumption of sugar has increased, so have all the 'civilized' diseases. In 1821 the average sugar intake in America was 10 pounds per person per year; today it is 170 pounds per person ..." states Sally Fallon in her astounding book, *Nourishing Traditions*.

If you feel you have to have a drink, limit it to one glass of dry red wine or a spritzer – that's white wine mixed with soda water and a few wedges of lemon. Unless people are going to join us in having a glass of wine with dinner we usually order by the glass. That way we don't feel obliged to finish the whole bottle.

# GET YOUR FOOD THE WAY YOU ORDERED IT

When you eat out, at times your food will not come to you the way you ordered it. If your Clean-Eating requests were forgotten and your entrée comes to you swimming in gravy while the accompanying potato is crowned with a blob of sour cream, you have a problem. How do you handle this situation?

Don't wimp out now! We find it is best to casually point out that the food arrived differently than we ordered it. Stick with your resolve to Eat Clean. It does not make sense to throw out your hard-earned results now when you are confronted with a pile of sour cream. Remind the waiter that you ordered your meal without accoutrement and would like it that way. Be gracious but firm. Usually the serving staff will be happy to oblige you by going back to the kitchen and cleaning up your order.

Some restaurants are better able or more willing to handle special requests and you will get to know which they are. Jack LaLanne, old-time fitness and health enthusiast, eats out with his wife Elaine every night. They know a handful of restaurants where they get Clean food with no trouble. So frequent are their visits that they even have dishes named after them, including The Jack LaLanne Special. Invariably the dish is a white fish with steamed vegetables and rice. Clean food all the way for Jack!

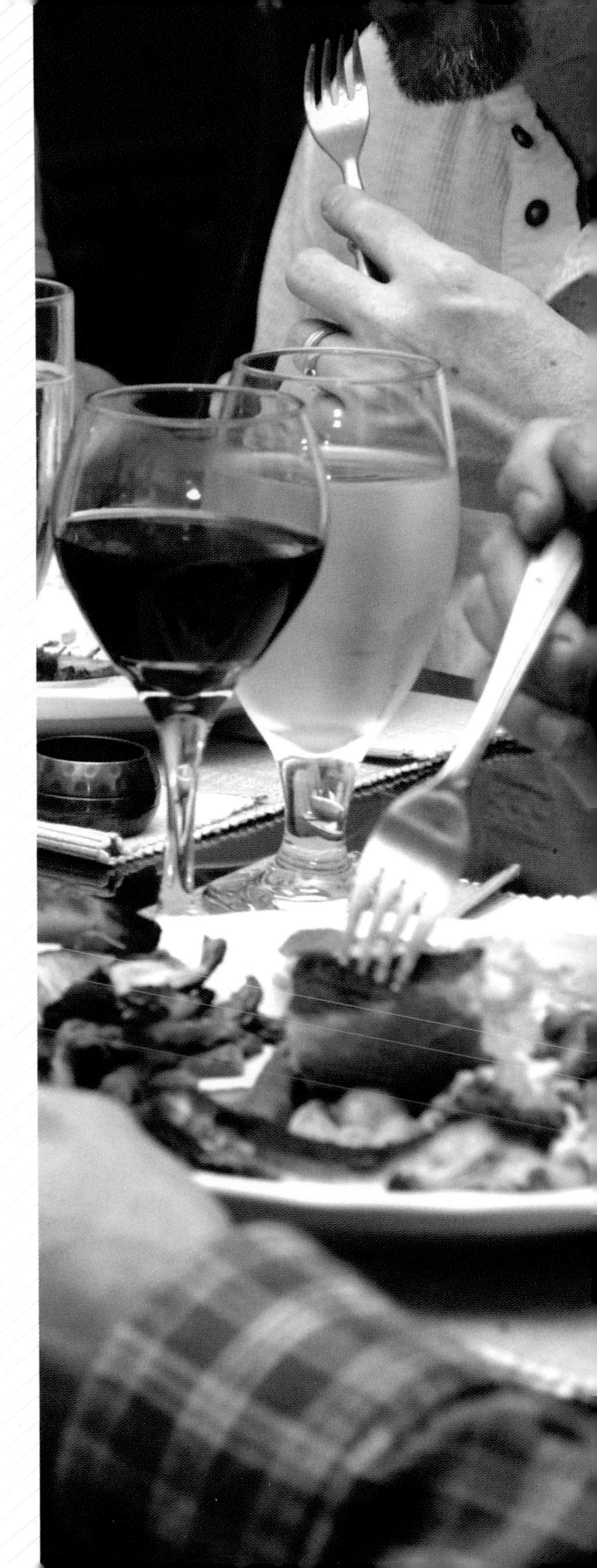

# MAKING A COMMITMENT TO YOURSELF

Your current physique reflects exactly what you are putting into it. The body doesn't lie. If you are neglecting both nutrition and exercise you'll look soft and squishy, a lot like the processed foods you love to eat. If you enjoy eating so much that you can't locate the OFF button to your mouth and on top of that have no inclination to exercise, then you'll look like the couch you're lying on – only a lot softer and squishier.

If you show respect for both nutrition and exercise your body becomes a reflection of that. Your skin, hair, eyes and nails glow with health. Muscles ripple under tight skin with not a hint of excess flesh anywhere. Your waist is trim and your heart beats at a steady, moderate pace. The blood running in your veins is no longer a chemical-soup time bomb waiting to go off at any moment. Life has a very different, positive feel when you live this way. You feel invigorated and powerful – the way you were always meant to feel.

We often hear from folks who claim they are doing everything right but are still fat. However, we know the basic truth of nature: the body doesn't lie. When we hear these stories we know they are getting something wrong, and 95 percent of the time that thing is food. Your physique paints an accurate picture of your approach to taking care of it. Eating Clean is the best and only way to achieve the physique you truly desire. If we had our way we would ask that all restaurants offer at least one broth-based soup and that there would always be a fruit option for dessert. It would make Eating Clean so much easier!

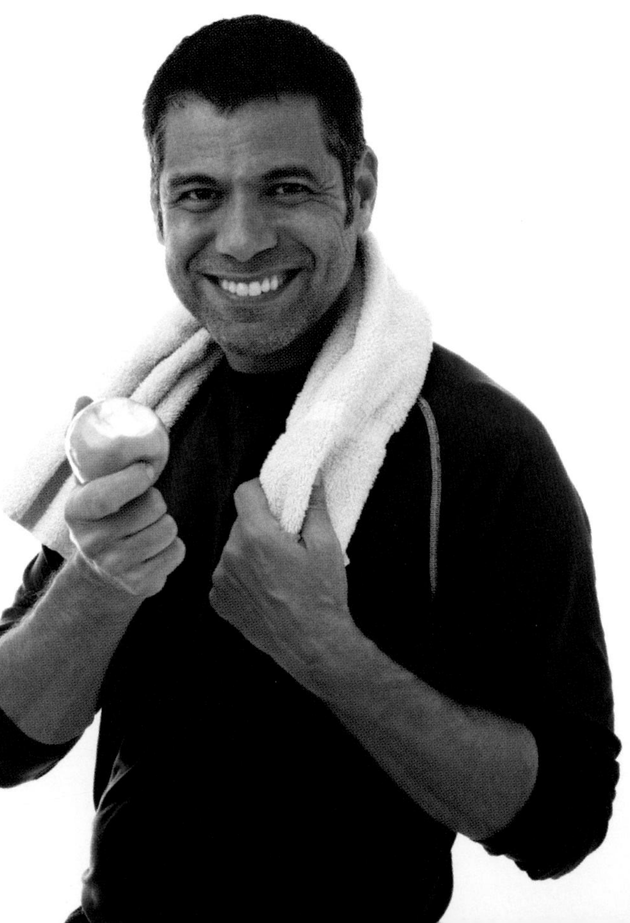

# CLEAN-EATING ORDERING

Here are several techniques to help you with your Clean-Eating ordering. Stay committed to your plan not only to improve your nutrition, but also your health. Weight loss will be the ultimate result.

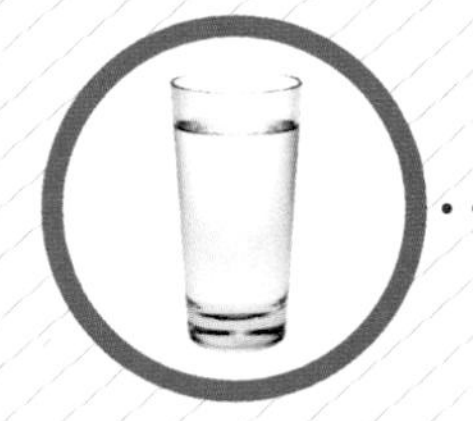

- Take the breadbasket away. The bread is on the table to keep you busy while your meal is being prepared. Occupy yourself with your companion and a glass of water.

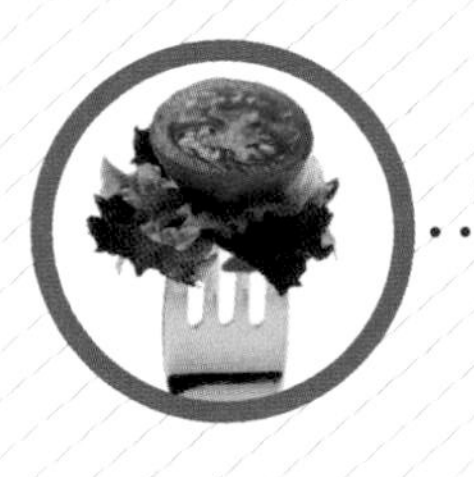

- Substitute vegetables for fries. Even salad greens and sliced tomatoes are okay.

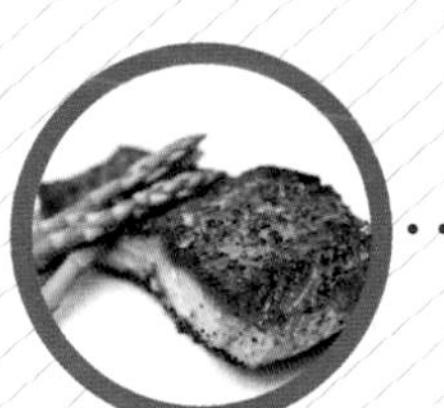

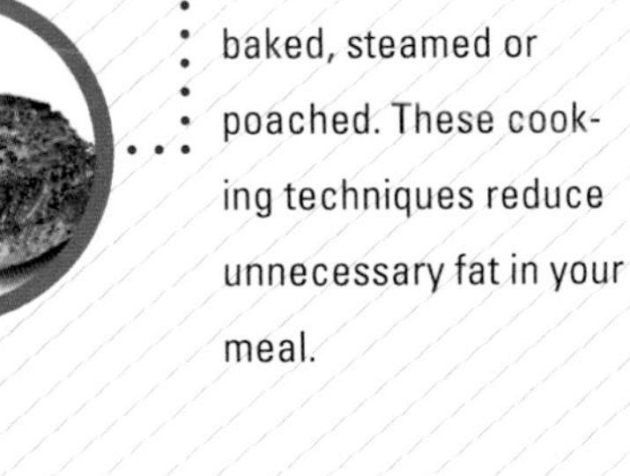

- Have your protein grilled, baked, steamed or poached. These cooking techniques reduce unnecessary fat in your meal.

- Try sushi or sashimi from a reputable source as a great Clean-Eating protein alternative.

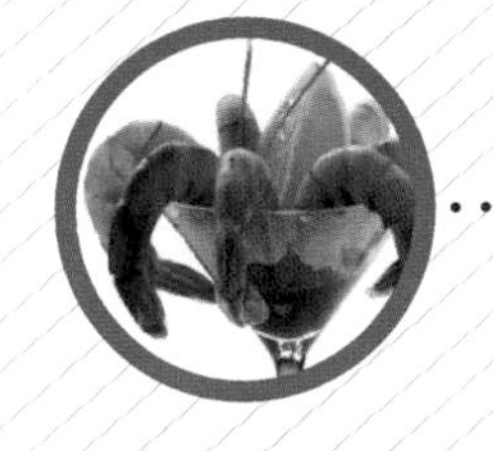

- Order an appetizer as an entrée if you aren't overly hungry or if the portions are huge.

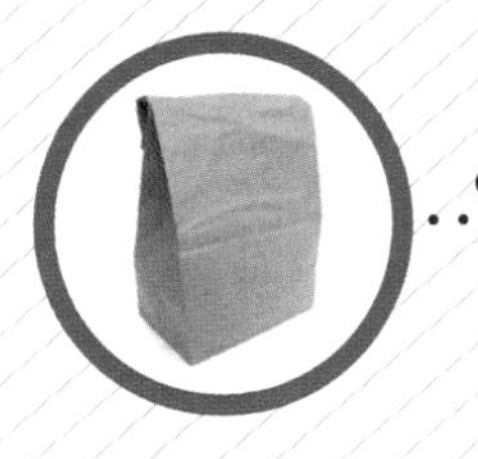

- Ask for a doggie bag right away if the portion is too large.

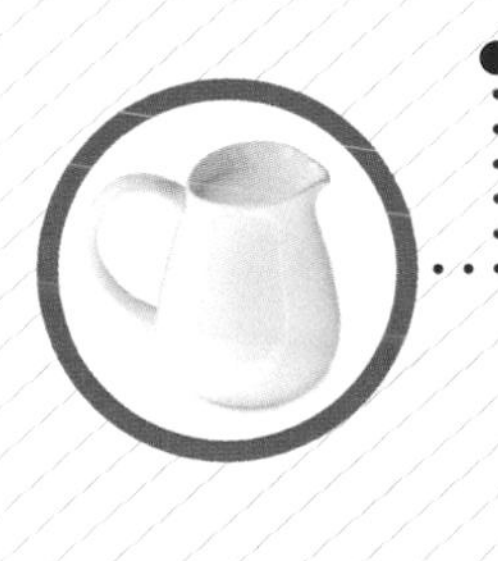

- Ask the waiter if a food item is prepared with cream, butter or other non-Clean ingredients. Don't order the entrée if you aren't sure.

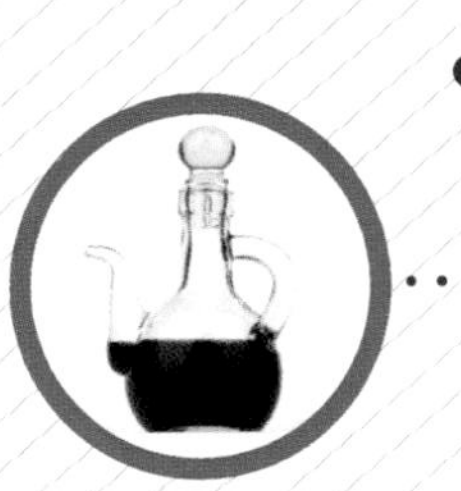

- Ask for dressings and sauces to be served on the side. Balsamic vinegar and mustard rule!

# MENU TRANSLATIONS

Take a few minutes to study the menu before placing your order. Ordering too hastily could result in a disappointing meal loaded with unnecessary fats, sodium and sugar.

| HIGH-CALORIE TRAP | TRANSLATION |
|---|---|
| **Au gratin** | with cheese |
| **Basted** | to moisten meat with fat or drippings |
| **Battered** | a fat, flour and water mixture to coat meat |
| **Béarnaise sauce** | cream sauce made of egg yolks, vinegar and butter |
| **Béchamel** | cream sauce made of milk, butter and flour |
| **Bisque** | shellfish purée made of wine, Cognac and fresh cream |
| **Breaded** | coated with mixture of breadcrumbs, egg and butter – normally fried |
| **Buttered** | butter added to the dish |
| **Creamed/creamy** | cream added to the dish |
| **Crisp (savory)** | fried in butter or oil |
| **Crisp (sweet)** | topping of butter and sugar |

| HIGH-CALORIE TRAP | TRANSLATION |
| --- | --- |
| Croquette | mixture of meat or grains bound with heavy sauce and deep fried |
| Croute | encased in pastry and fried in butter |
| Custard | sweet sauce of eggs, cream, milk, butter and sugar |
| Foie gras | duck or goose liver |
| Fried, fritters, frite | anything fried in oil |
| Hollandaise | heated sauce made of egg yolks and butter |
| Parmesan | with Parmesan cheese |
| Scalloped | layered dish of vegetables and sauce made of milk, butter and flour |
| Tempura | batter coating of ice water, flour and eggs, fried |

| CLEAN-EATING TERM | TRANSLATION |
| --- | --- |
| **Au jus** | in its own juice |
| **Baked** | oven cooked, no added oils, fats or sauce |
| **Braised** | slow cooked in own juice |
| **Broiled** | cooked under high heat |
| **Ceviche** | raw fish, citrus juice, limes, onion and tomato |
| **Gazpacho** | Spanish uncooked soup made with cucumber, onion, red pepper, olive oil, corn and spices |
| **Grilled** | cooked over high heat to seal in natural juices |
| **Lean** | without added fat |
| **Poached** | simmered in liquid |
| **Purée** | blended foods |
| **Roasted** | cooked in radiant heat of oven or over open flame |
| **Salsa** | spicy sauce of uncooked vegetables or fruit, usually tomatoes, onions, peppers and herbs |
| **Sauté** | cook meat, vegetables or fish in small amount of fat in frying pan until brown |
| **Steamed** | foods cooked over but not in boiling water |

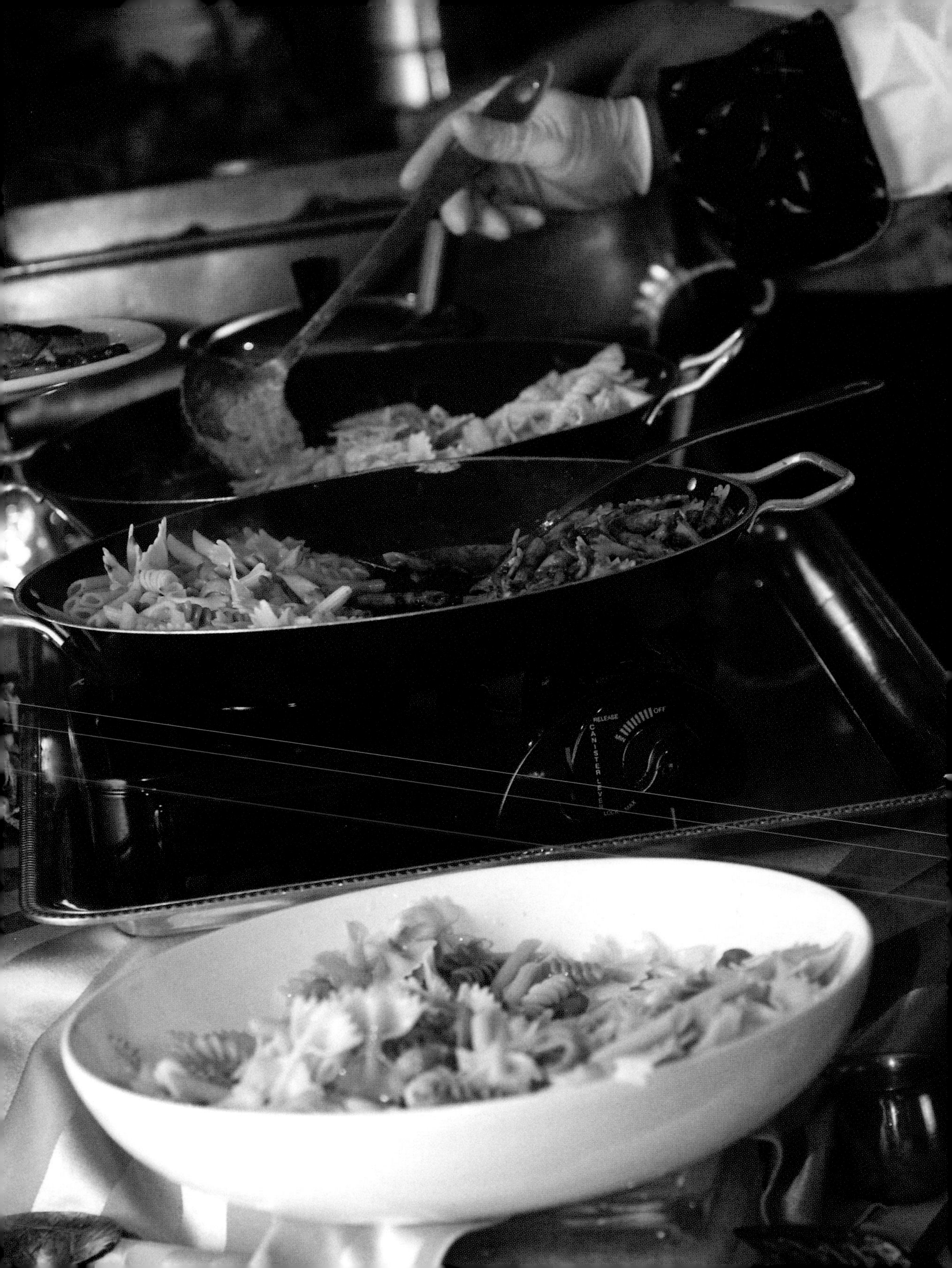
RELEASE
OFF
CANISTER LEVER

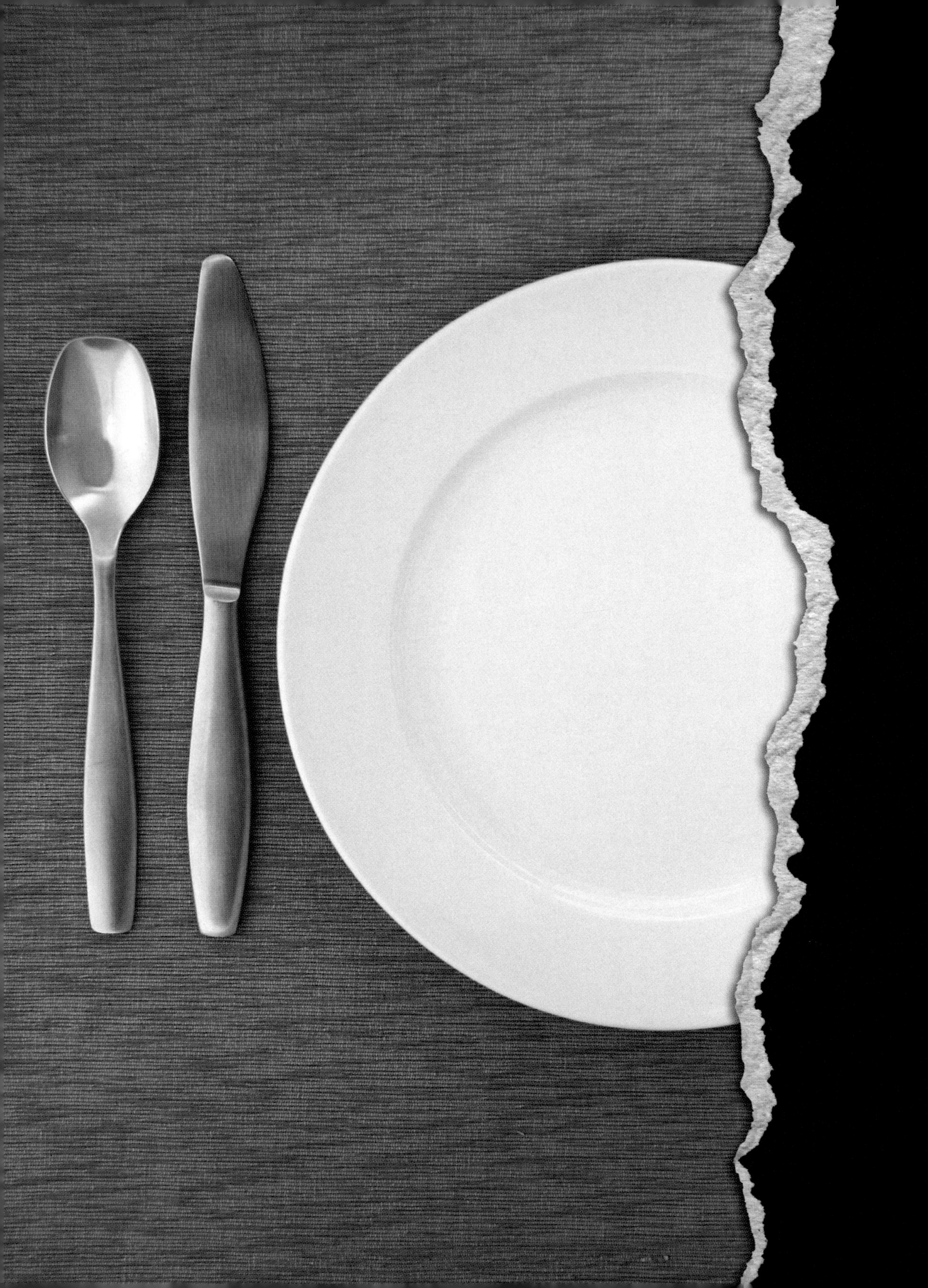

# [CHAPTER THIRTEEN]

## CLEAN-EATING RECIPES

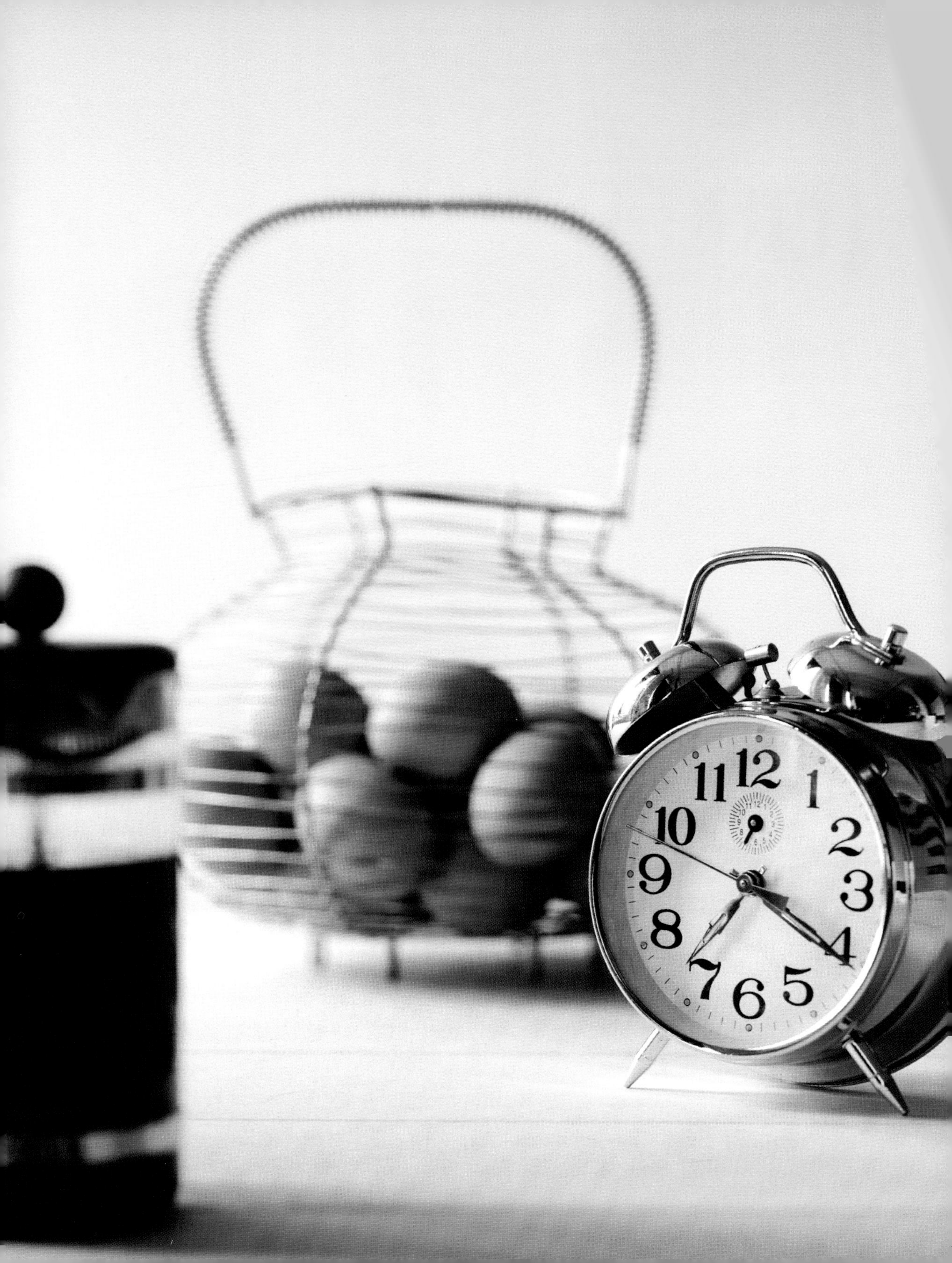

# BREAKFAST

You've heard that breakfast is the most important meal of the day, and we could not agree more. A Clean breakfast made of lean protein and good-quality complex carbs gets your metabolism revved up and your engine humming. The Power Breakfast will help you build muscle, the NYC Bagel Breakfast is perfect with the paper, and the Sweet Potato Pancakes will make you feel like you're sitting on a veranda in the deep south. Enjoy!

# POWER BREAKFAST

When you want some real stick-to-your-ribs food that will help you build muscle, burn fat and give you lots of energy to get through your morning, this is the breakfast for you! As a bonus, this breakfast takes practically no time to prepare. **WARNING: not for dainty eaters.**

### WHAT YOU'LL NEED »

Boiling water
⅓ cup / 80 ml large-flake oats
¼ cup / 60 ml sliced almonds
1 Tbsp / 15 ml ground flaxseed
1 Tbsp / 15 ml chia seed, or Salba
½ tsp / 2½ ml pure vanilla extract
1 tsp / 5 ml agave nectar
2 Tbsp / 30 ml hemp protein powder
1 Tbsp / 15 ml bee pollen
½ cup / 120 ml blueberries
¼ cup / 60 ml plain nonfat yogurt

### HOW TO MAKE IT »

1. Place first seven ingredients in a large cereal bowl. Pour boiling water over top to cover. Stir to combine. Let sit for five to ten minutes, while you shave or make coffee.
2. Add bee pollen, blueberries and yogurt. Mix together, and then sit with your morning paper and eat!

**NUTRITIONAL VALUE FOR ONE SERVING:**
Calories: 623 | Calories from Fat: 220 | Total Fat: 25 g | Saturated Fat: 2 g | Total Carbs: 77 g | Fiber: 16 g | Protein: 23 g | Sodium: 156 mg | Cholesterol: 1 mg

**Preparation time:** 1 minute
**Sitting time:** 5-10 minutes
**Yield:** 1 serving

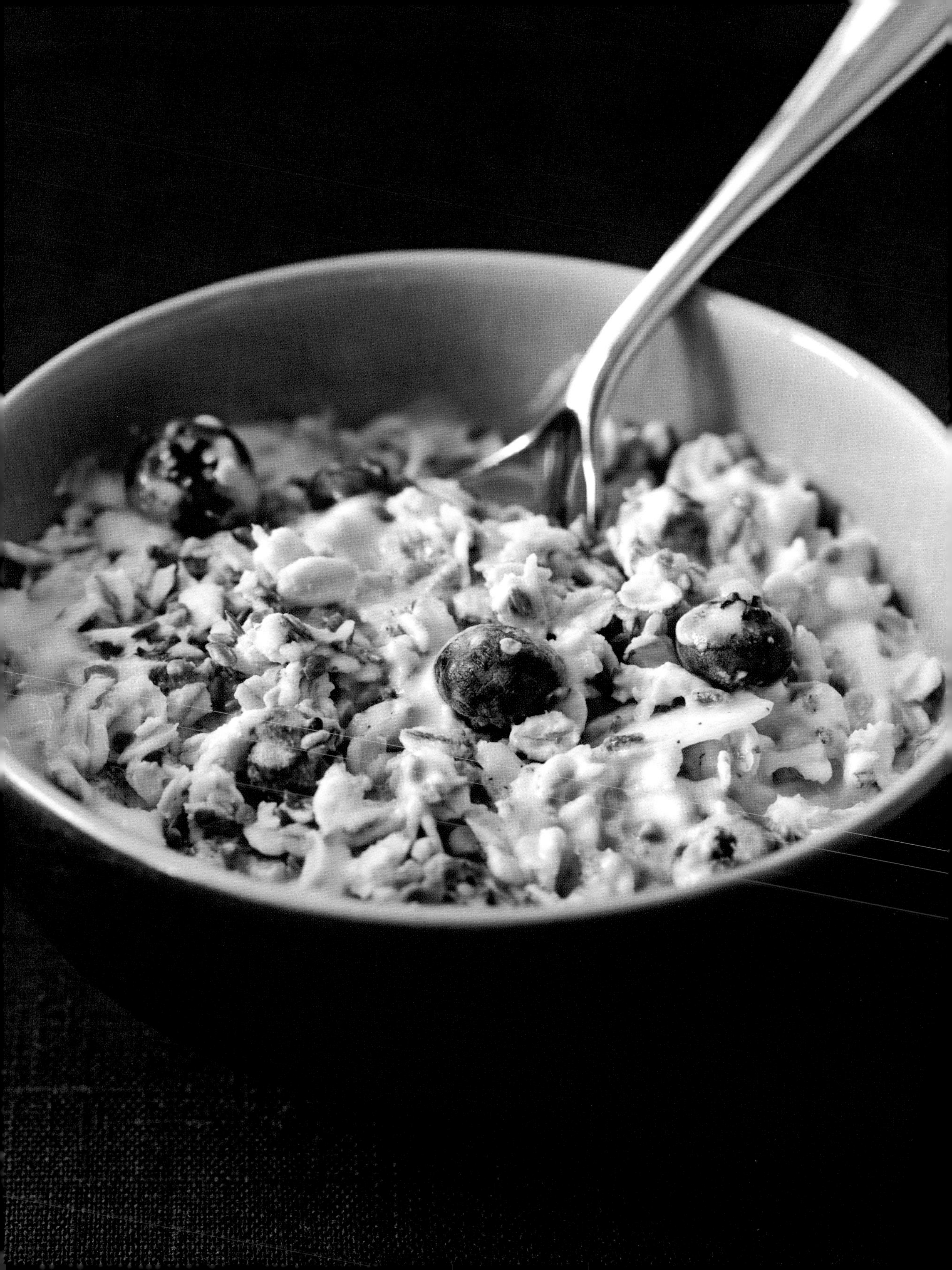

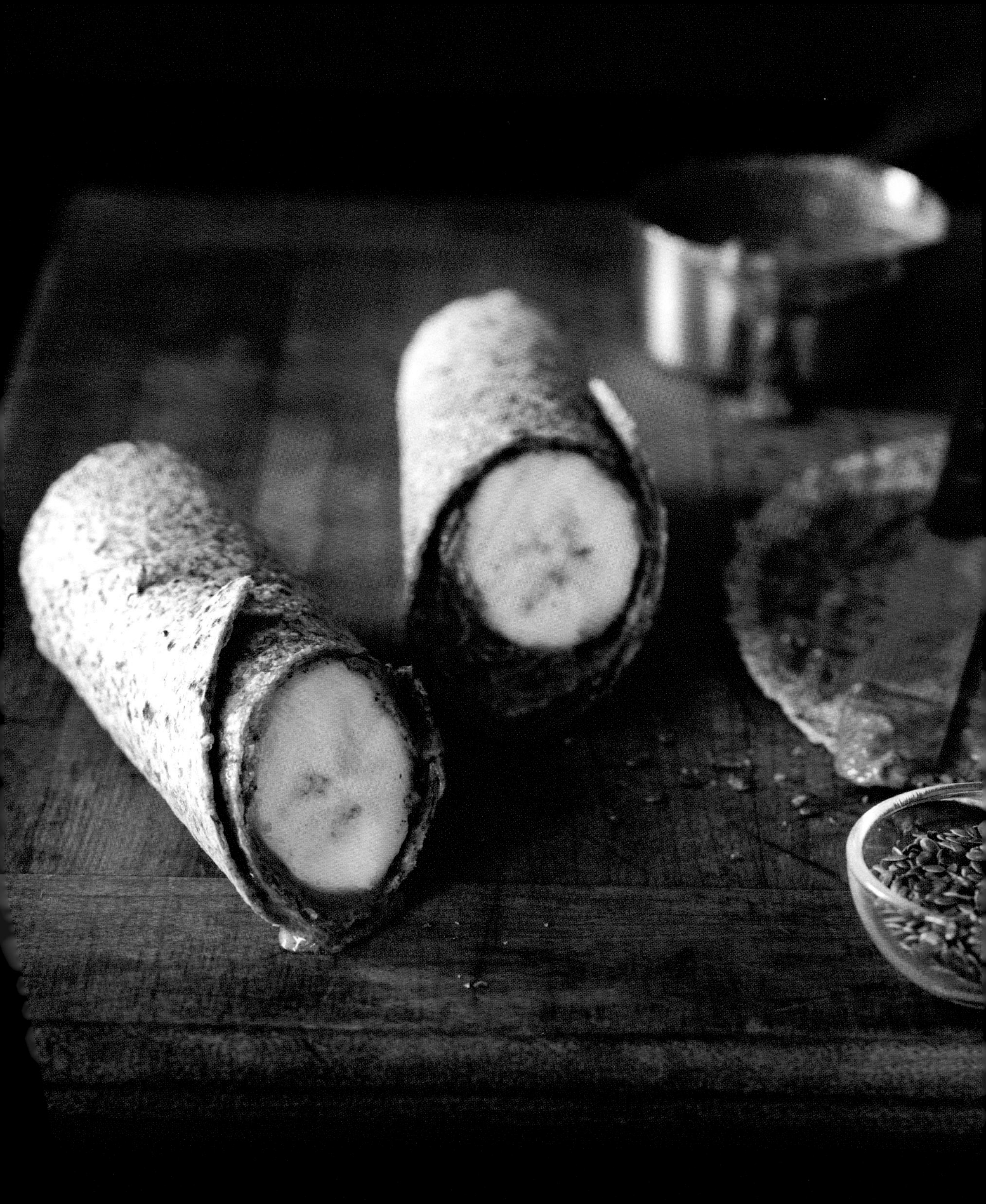

# BANANA ROLL-UP

This one's so easy we hesitate to call it a recipe, but there's no better solution when you're running late and need something faster than quick!

### WHAT YOU'LL NEED »

1 banana

1 x 7-inch / 18 cm whole-grain wrap

2 Tbsp / 30 ml natural nut butter

### HOW TO MAKE IT »

1. Spread wrap with nut butter.
2. Lay peeled banana on one end of wrap.
3. Roll up and eat!

**TIP You can sprinkle some ground flaxseed over the nut butter before adding the banana to increase the nutritional content even more!**

**NUTRITIONAL VALUE FOR ONE ROLL-UP:**
Calories: 422 | Calories from Fat: 235 | Total Fat: 26 g | Saturated Fat: 2 g | Total Carbohydrates: 52 g | Fiber: 9 g | Protein: 11 g | Sodium: 300 mg | Cholesterol: 0 mg

**Preparation time:** 1 minutes
**Cooking time:** 0 minutes
**Yield:** 1 serving

# TROPICAL SMOOTHIE

Don't like eating breakfast? Why not drink it instead? If you've read this far you know skipping breakfast is a very bad idea, but lots of people don't like to chew in the morning. Blend up this tropical treat and you'll samba your way to work.

### WHAT YOU'LL NEED »

1 cup / 240 ml pineapple chunks

1 mango, peeled – flesh only

1 banana

2 servings vanilla protein powder

4 Tbsp / 60 ml chia seed, or Salba

1 cup / 240 ml skim milk

### HOW TO MAKE IT »

1. Blend all ingredients together. Add skim milk a little at a time to thin for blending if necessary.
2. Pour into two glasses, and drink!

**NUTRITIONAL VALUE FOR ONE SERVING:**
Total Calories: 289 | Calories from Fat: 86 | Total Fat: 9.5 g | Saturated Fat: 1 g | Trans Fat: 0 g | Total Carbs: 46 g | Fiber: 13.5 g | Protein: 10 g | Sodium: 73 mg | Cholesterol: 2.5 mg

**Preparation time:** 5 minutes
**Cooking time:** 0 minutes
**Yield:** 2 servings

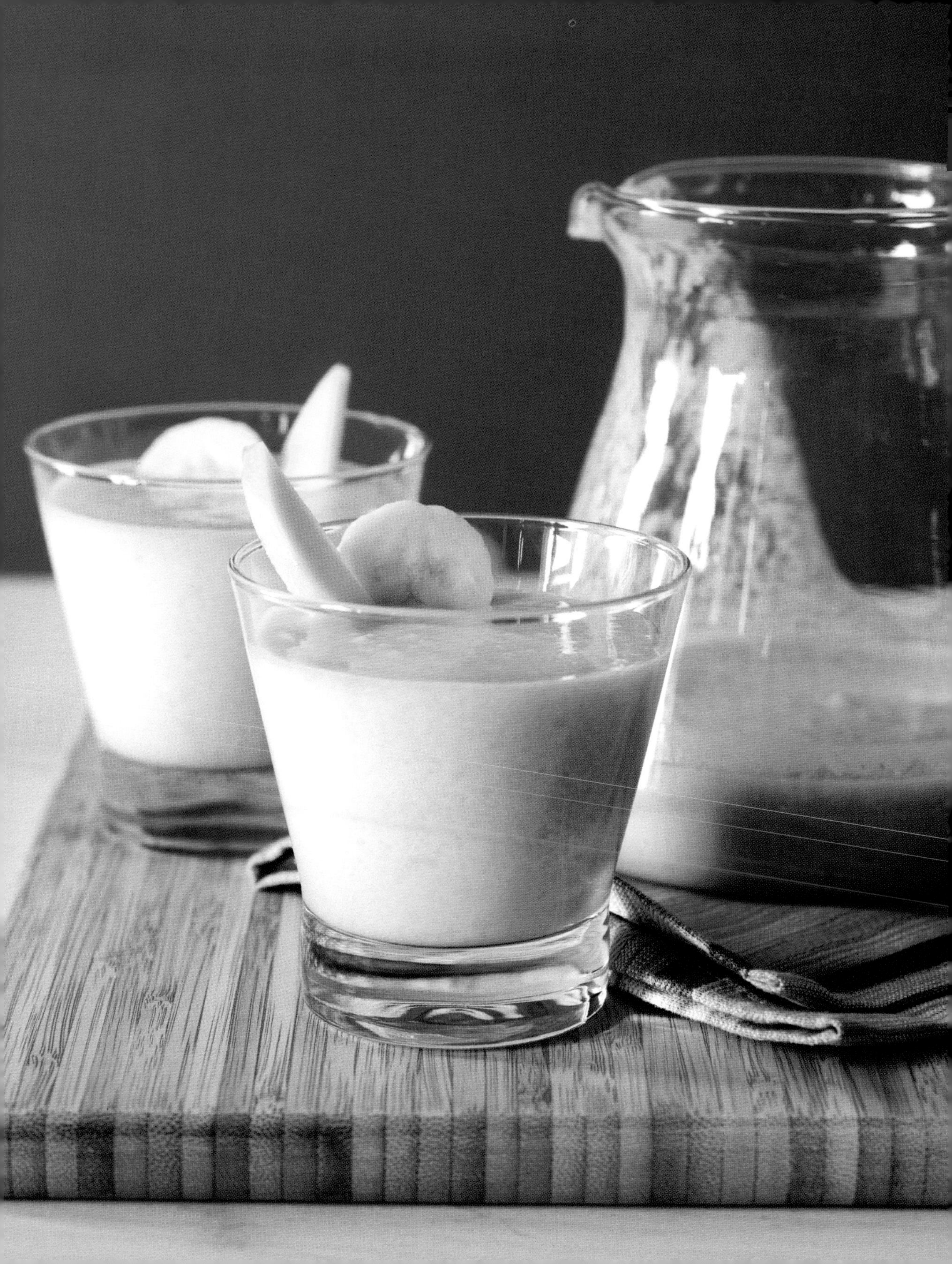

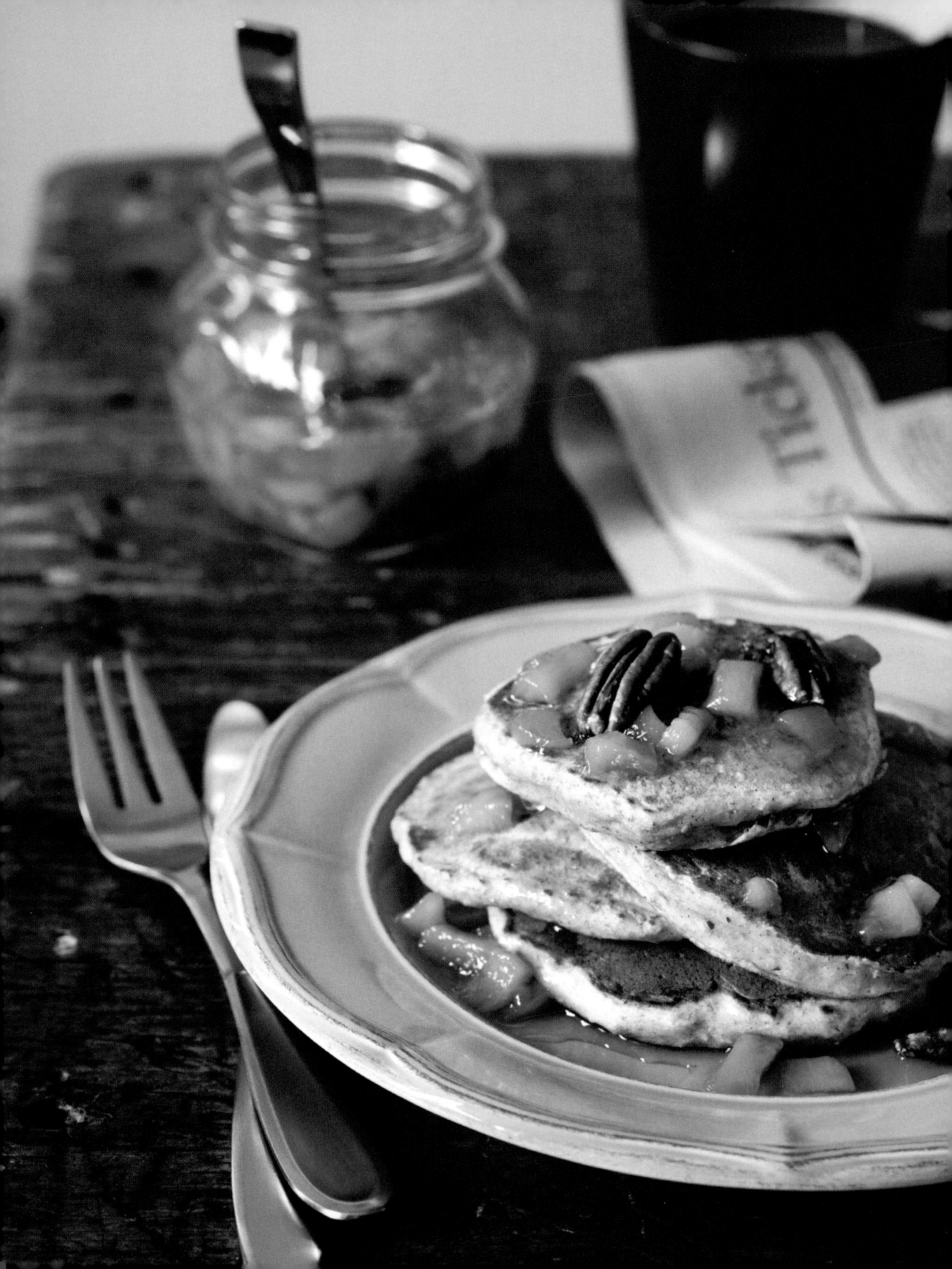

# SOUTHERN SWEET POTATO PANCAKES

**WHAT YOU'LL NEED »**

2 cups / 480 ml whole-wheat flour
4 tsp / 20 ml baking powder
1 tsp / 5 ml cinnamon
¼ tsp / 1¼ ml nutmeg
2 cups / 480 ml skim milk
2 egg whites, beaten
1 leftover cooked sweet potato, peeled and mashed
1 cup / 240 ml pecan halves
2 cups / 480 ml peach compote (recipe follows)

**HOW TO MAKE IT »**

1. Sift dry ingredients into a mixing bowl and mix thoroughly.
2. Whip together milk, beaten eggs and sweet potato. Add to flour mixture, stirring just until dry ingredients are moistened.
3. Spray a griddle or frying pan with Eat-Clean Cooking Spray (see page 262) and heat on medium-high.
4. Drop mixture by heaping tablespoons onto hot griddle. Let cook until edges are lightly browned and bubbles start to appear on the top of the pancake. Flip and continue to cook until both sides are golden brown.
5. As pancakes cook, set on ovenproof plate in 225°F / 107°C oven.
6. Meanwhile, in another hot pan, toast pecans till brown.
7. Place four mini pancakes on each plate. Ladle ½ cup / 120 ml peach compote on top of your hot pancakes, and sprinkle ¼ cup / 60 ml toasted pecans on top.

**NUTRITIONAL VALUE FOR FOUR MINI PANCAKES:**
Calories: 463 | Calories from Fat: 175 | Total Fat: 19 g | Saturated Fat: 2 g | Total Carbs: 62.5 g | Fiber: 11 g | Protein: 17.2 g | Sodium: 118 mg | Cholesterol: 2.5 mg

**Preparation time:** 10 minutes
**Cooking time:** 20 minutes
**Yield:** 4 servings – 16 mini pancakes

## PEACH COMPOTE

**THE COMPOTE CAN BE CANNED, OR IT WILL KEEP IN THE FRIDGE FOR ABOUT A WEEK.**

**WHAT YOU'LL NEED »**

6 to 7 very ripe **peaches**, peeled, pitted & chopped
2 cups / 480 ml **apple cider**
1 cup / 240 ml frozen concentrated **white grape juice**
1 Tbsp / 15 ml **lemon zest**
1 Tbsp / 15 ml **lemon juice**

**HOW TO MAKE IT »**

**1.** Simmer together in a non-aluminum pot, allowing the compote to thicken for about 1 to 1½ hours.

**NUTRITIONAL VALUE FOR ½ CUP OF PEACH COMPOTE:**
Calories: 91 | Calories from Fat: 2 | Total Fat: 0.2 g | Saturated Fat: 0.1 g | Total Carbs: 25 g | Fiber: 1.1 g | Protein: 0.6 g | Sodium: 10 mg | Cholesterol: 0 mg

**Preparation time:** 10 minutes
**Cooking time:** 60 – 90 minutes
**Yield:** 5 cups

# HOME FRIES

We all love home fries, but they do not exactly fit into the Clean-Eating lifestyle. Here's a way to get the satisfaction of home fries without excess fat. Serve alongside scrambled egg whites for a complete breakfast.

### WHAT YOU'LL NEED »

3 potatoes (1 lb / 454 g), boiled till soft but firm, and sliced
1 green bell pepper, sliced
1 cooking onion, sliced thinly
2 Tbsp / 30 ml best-quality olive oil, separated
2 tsp / 10 ml mustard seeds
Sea salt and freshly gound black pepper, to taste

### HOW TO MAKE IT »

1. Heat 1 Tbsp / 15 ml oil over medium-heat in a large skillet.
2. Cook onions for 1 to 2 minutes. Add green pepper and continue to cook, stirring, for about 4 minutes. Set aside in a bowl.
3. Add the rest of the oil to the skillet. Allow to heat. Set potato slices in single layer. Let brown, then flip. Brown the potatoes for 2 minutes, then add onions and peppers. Stir together. Add mustard seeds, salt and pepper, and serve.

**NUTRITIONAL VALUE FOR ONE SERVING:**
Calories: 134 | Calories from Fat: 42 | Total Fat: 4.5 g | Saturated Fat: 0.66 mg | Total Carbs: 21 g | Fiber: 3 g | Protein: 2.5 g | Sodium: 73 mg | Cholesterol: 0 mg

**Preparation time:** 25 minutes
**Cooking time:** 35 minutes
**Yield:** 6 servings

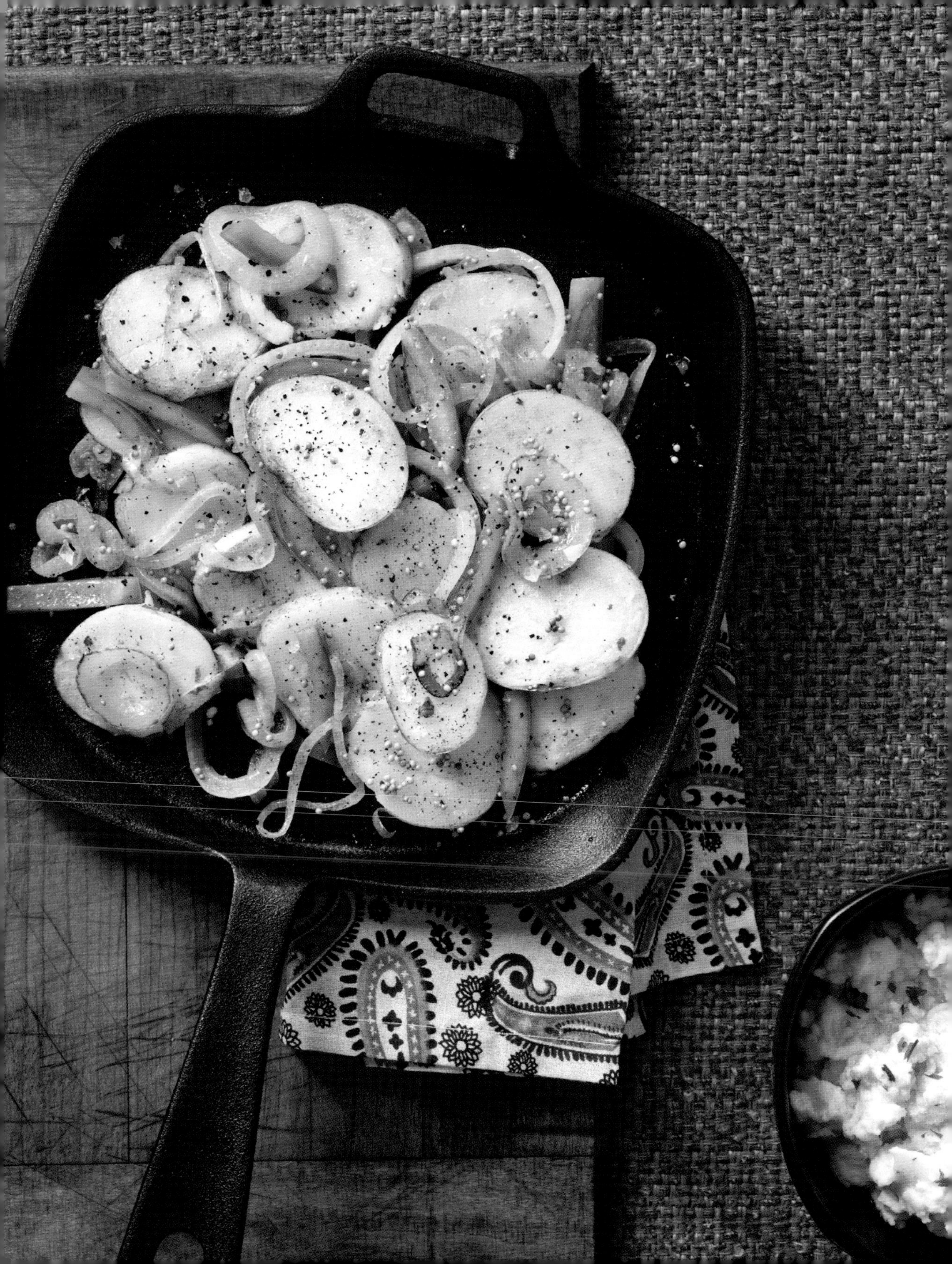

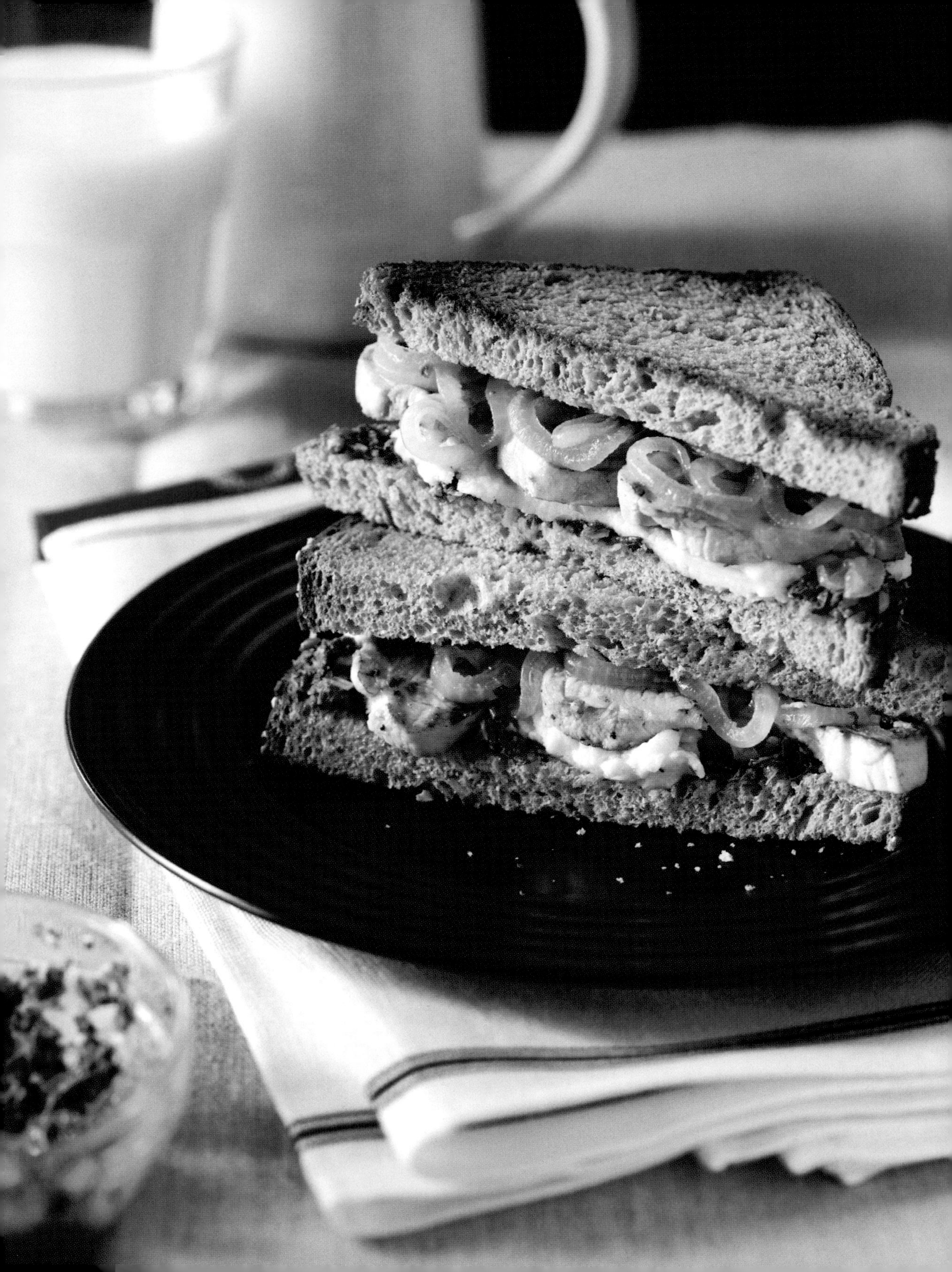

# WEEKEND EGG SANDWICH

This egg breakfast takes a little while to prepare but is both hearty and tasty. Perfect after a morning workout.

### WHAT YOU'LL NEED »

4 slices whole-grain bread

8 egg whites

1 boneless, skinless chicken breast, cooked

½ sweet Vidalia onion

1 Tbsp / 15 ml best-quality olive oil

2 Tbsp / 30 ml coriander chutney, see below

**NUTRITIONAL VALUE FOR ONE SANDWICH:**
Calories: 384 | Calories from Fat: 103 | Total Fat: 11.5 g | Saturated Fat: 2 g | Total Carbs: 30 g | Fiber: 4 g | Protein: 36 g | Sodium: 845 mg | Cholesterol: 0 mg

### HOW TO MAKE IT »

1. Preheat oven to 250°F / 120°C.
2. Slice chicken breast thinly – slices should be about ¼ inch thick.
3. Slice onion into thin rings.
4. Heat olive oil in heavy pan. Sauté onions till they just start to brown. Set in ovenproof dish and place inside oven to keep warm.
5. In the same pan on medium-high, lay chicken slices. Brown one side, then flip and brown the other. Set on ovenproof plate in oven.
6. Crack egg whites into a medium-sized bowl, then whip with a fork. Pour into the same pan. Scramble a bit until the eggs start to set, then cover and turn heat to low.
7. Meanwhile, toast the bread. Once toasted, spread one side of each piece with the coriander chutney.
8. Once eggs are cooked almost through, flip over to cook the other side till finished.
9. Cut a toast-sized piece of egg out of the pan and lay on one piece of toast, on top of the chutney. Lay chicken slices on top of the egg, and then spoon onion on top of the chicken. Top with another piece of chutney-spread toast. Repeat with other toast, egg, chicken and onions. Serve on nice heated stoneware plates.

**Preparation time:** 5 minutes
**Cooking time:** 20 minutes
**Yield:** 2 servings

## CORIANDER CHUTNEY

### WHAT YOU'LL NEED »

1 cup / 240 ml chopped **fresh coriander (cilantro)**
Juice of 1 medium **lemon**
Few sprigs **fresh mint**
1 hot **Thai chili pepper**
1 Tbsp / 15 ml best-quality **olive oil**
**Sea salt** to taste

### HOW TO MAKE IT »

1. Clean cilantro and mint well. Chop coarsely.
2. Chop chili pepper.
3. Blend all ingredients together in high-speed blender, stopping the blender every now and again to scrape sides and push unblended material toward blades.

**NUTRITIONAL VALUE FOR TWO TBSP:**
Calories: 19 | Calories from Fat: 15 | Total Fat: 2 g | Saturated Fat: 0.2 g | Total Carbs: 1 g | Fiber: 0.2 g | Protein: 0.2 g | Sodium: 50 mg | Cholesterol: 0 mg

**Preparation time:** 10 minutes
**Cooking time:** 0 minutes
**Yield:** 1 cup

# NYC BAGEL BREAKFAST
## CLEAN STYLE

The morning sun is streaming through your window, a steaming pot of fresh coffee is brewing and you've just stepped out the door in your dressing gown to pick up the Sunday paper. Now all you have to do is settle in with this NYC-style bagel breakfast to complete the scene.

### WHAT YOU'LL NEED »

1 whole-grain bagel

4 Tbsp / 60 ml dilled yogurt cheese*

6 oz / 170 g lox or smoked salmon

2 Tbsp / 30 ml capers

**NUTRITIONAL VALUE FOR ONE SERVING:**
Calories: 295 | Calories from Fat: 48 | Total Fat: 5 g | Saturated Fat: 1 g| Total Carbs: 36.5 g | Fiber: 3 g | Protein: 23.5 g | Sodium: 2.5 g | Cholesterol: 20 mg

### YOGURT CHEESE

**WHAT YOU'LL NEED »**

2 quarts / 1.9 L **low-fat plain yogurt,** dairy or soy based

**HOW TO MAKE IT »**

**1.** Place 4 layers of damp cheesecloth in a fine mesh sieve or colander. Place the colander over a bowl.
**2.** Add yogurt and let it drain overnight in the refrigerator.
**3.** Discard the water from the bowl.

### HOW TO MAKE IT »

1. Slice the bagel in two, and toast so it's crispy on the outside but still moist on the inside.
2. Spread dilled yogurt cheese evenly between two halves.
3. Lay lox, or break up smoked salmon, atop the yogurt cheese.
4. Set on two plates and garnish with capers.

### *METHOD FOR DILLED YOGURT CHEESE »

1. Make yogurt cheese following directions on left.
2. Chop ½ to 1 bunch of fresh dill very fine. Mix into yogurt cheese.
3. Add sea salt and freshly ground black pepper to taste.

**Yield:** 2 servings

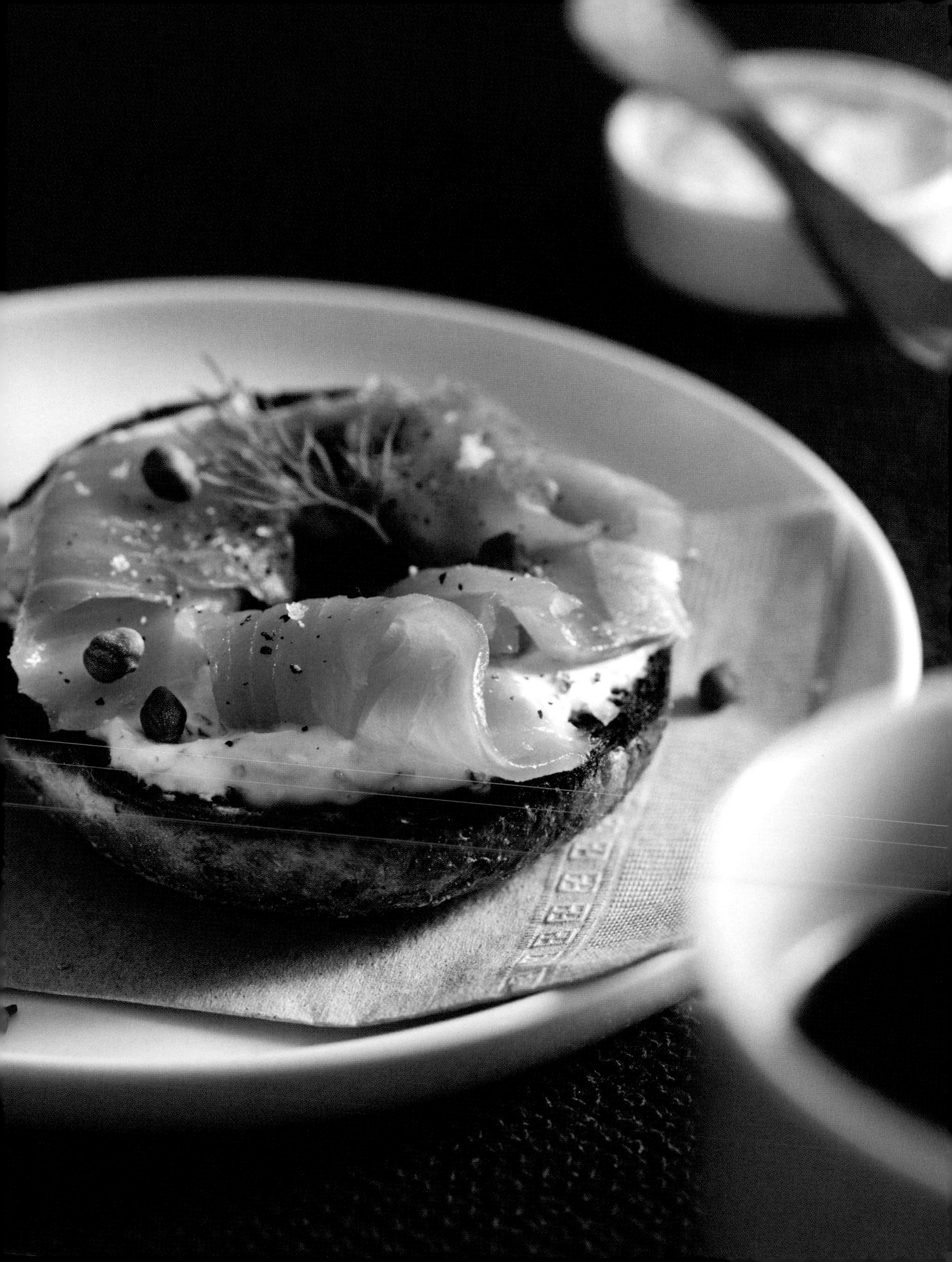

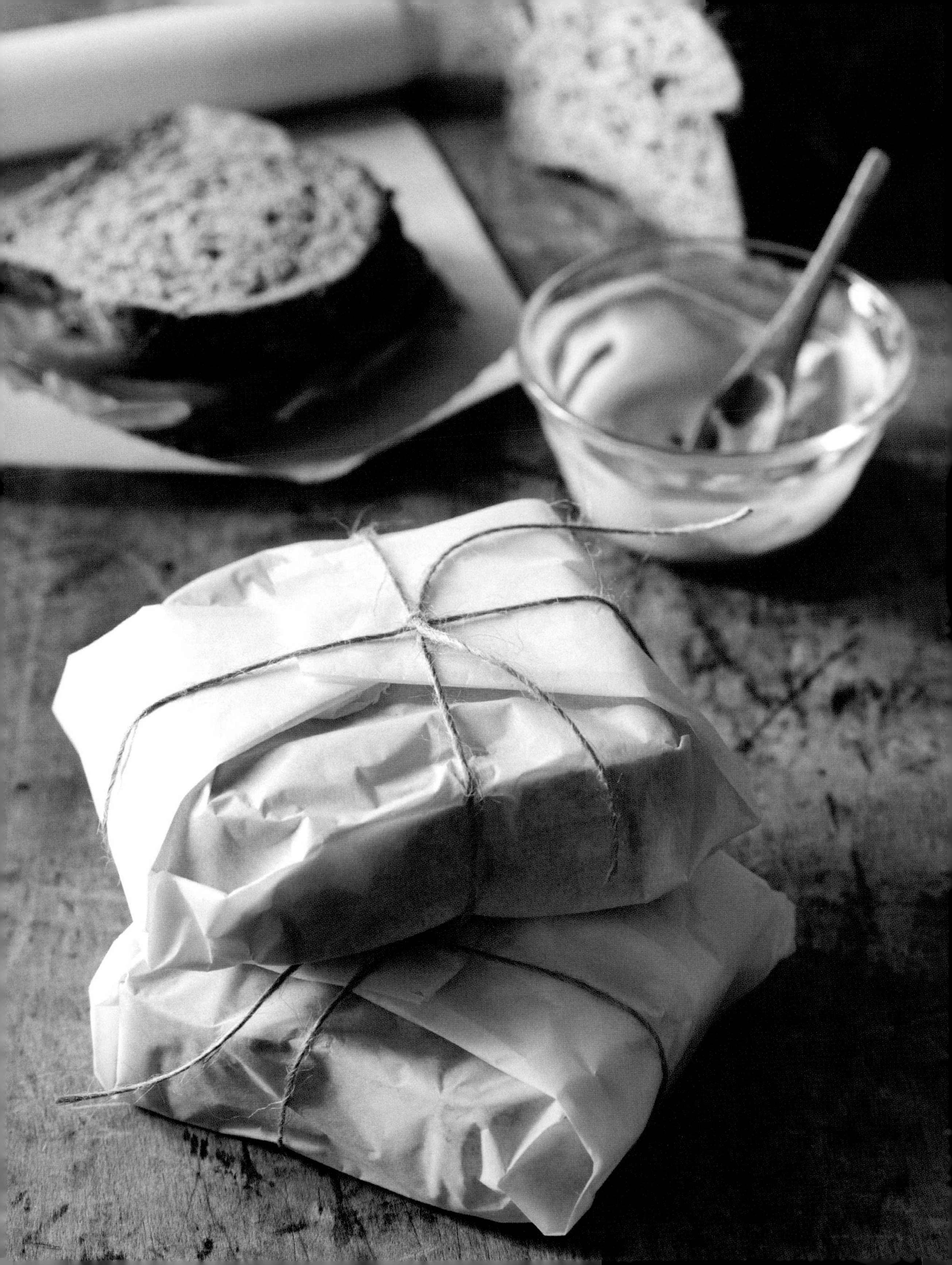

# SANDWICHES SOUPS AND SUBS

Not many men we know would be happy to live without sandwiches or subs. These are the ultimate convenience foods, and a great choice for a brown-bag lunch. They're easy, convenient and require little prep time. In the end they taste good and leave you satisfied. What man would pass up on this win-win opportunity? As for soup, a big bowl at the end of a hard-working day fills those empty places and warms you up at the same time. Can you say "feels like home"?

# BRING HOME THE BACON
## . . . LETTUCE AND TOMATO

The BLT is a mainstay of diners everywhere. Practically everyone loves them, and now you can enjoy a good BLT while Eating Clean. Enjoy!

**WHAT YOU'LL NEED »**

4 slices turkey bacon

1 tsp / 5 ml mustard powder

1 tsp / 5 ml curry powder

1 tsp / 5 ml red pepper flakes

2 slices sprouted-grain bread

1-2 leaves romaine lettuce, rinsed

3 slices grilled tomato

**HOW TO MAKE IT »**

1. Preheat oven to 375°F/ 190°C.
2. Prepare a baking sheet with parchment paper and place a cooling rack on top – this will catch all of the grease from the bacon, which can then be drained away. Conversely, you can use a broiling pan.
3. Mix mustard powder, curry powder and red pepper flakes. Sprinkle over top of the bacon, then flip and do the other side.
4. Place the bacon in the oven for 15 minutes, or until preferred crispiness is reached.
5. While bacon is cooking, toast the bread and grill the tomatoes. Heat a skillet with a little olive oil. Place sliced tomatoes in the hot skillet – you do not want to overcook them, just warm them.
6. Assemble your sandwich by placing lettuce and tomato onto a slice of toasted bread, then top with seasoned bacon and finally place the last slice of toasted bread.

### HOMEMADE DIJON MUSTARD

**WHAT YOU'LL NEED »**

3 Tbsp / 45 ml **yellow mustard seed**

2½ Tbsp / 37 ml **brown mustard seed**

⅓ cup / 90 ml **rice vinegar**

1 minced **shallot**

Pinch **allspice**

¾ tsp / 4 ml **sea salt**

½ tsp / 2½ ml freshly ground **black pepper**

**HOW TO MAKE IT »**

1. Combine all ingredients and refrigerate overnight.
2. Transfer to a blender and process until it has reached the desired texture and thickness.
3. Store for up to 2 weeks.

**NUTRITIONAL VALUE FOR ONE SANDWICH WITH 1 TBSP DIJON MUSTARD:**

Calories: 278 | Calories from Fat: 39 | Total Fat: 4.5 g | Saturated Fat: 0 g | Total Carbs: 35.5 g | Fiber: 8.5 g | Protein: 22 g | Sodium: 800 mg | Cholesterol: 60 mg

**Preparation time:** 5 minutes
**Cooking time:** 15 minutes
**Yield:** 1 sandwich

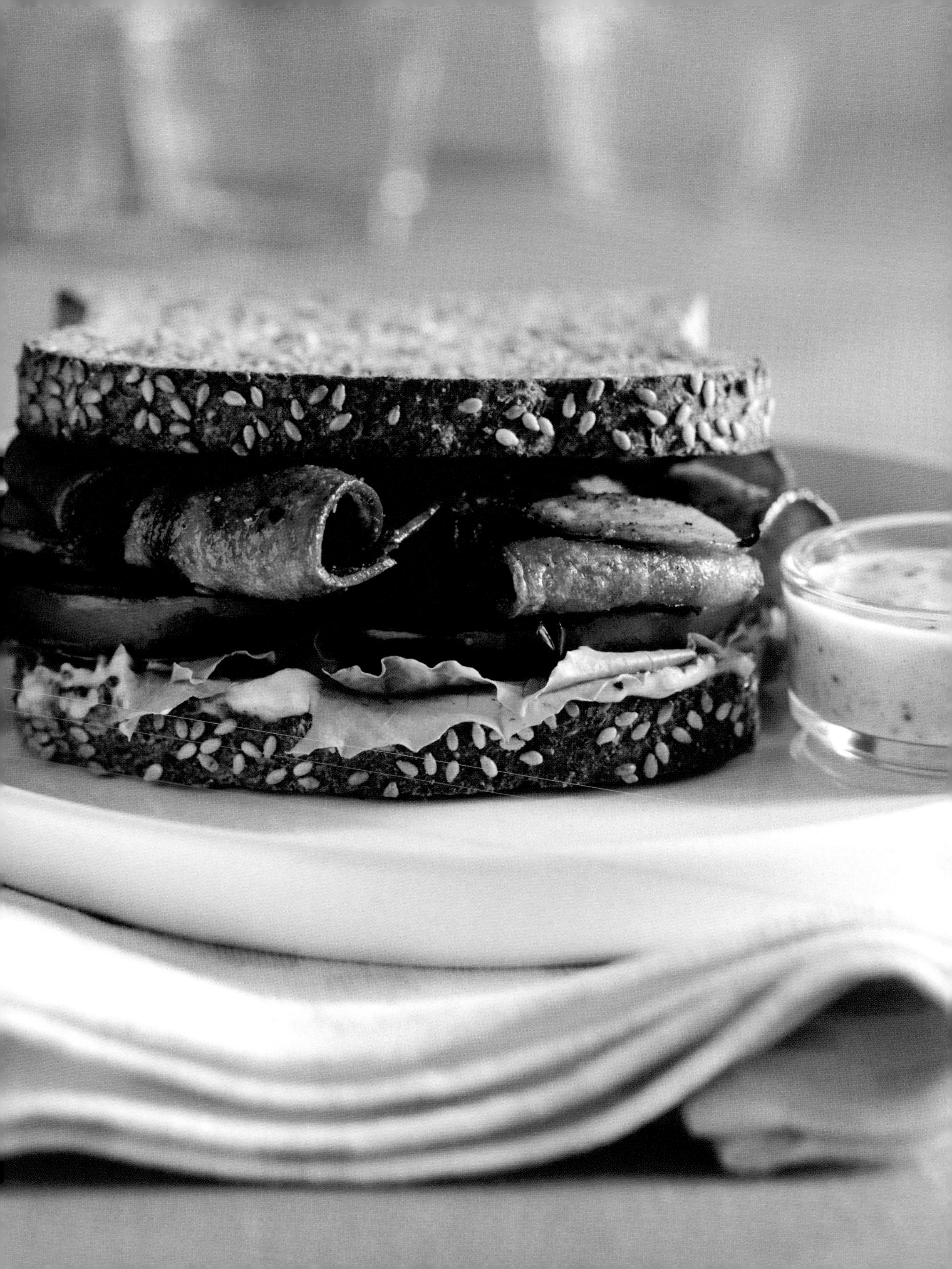

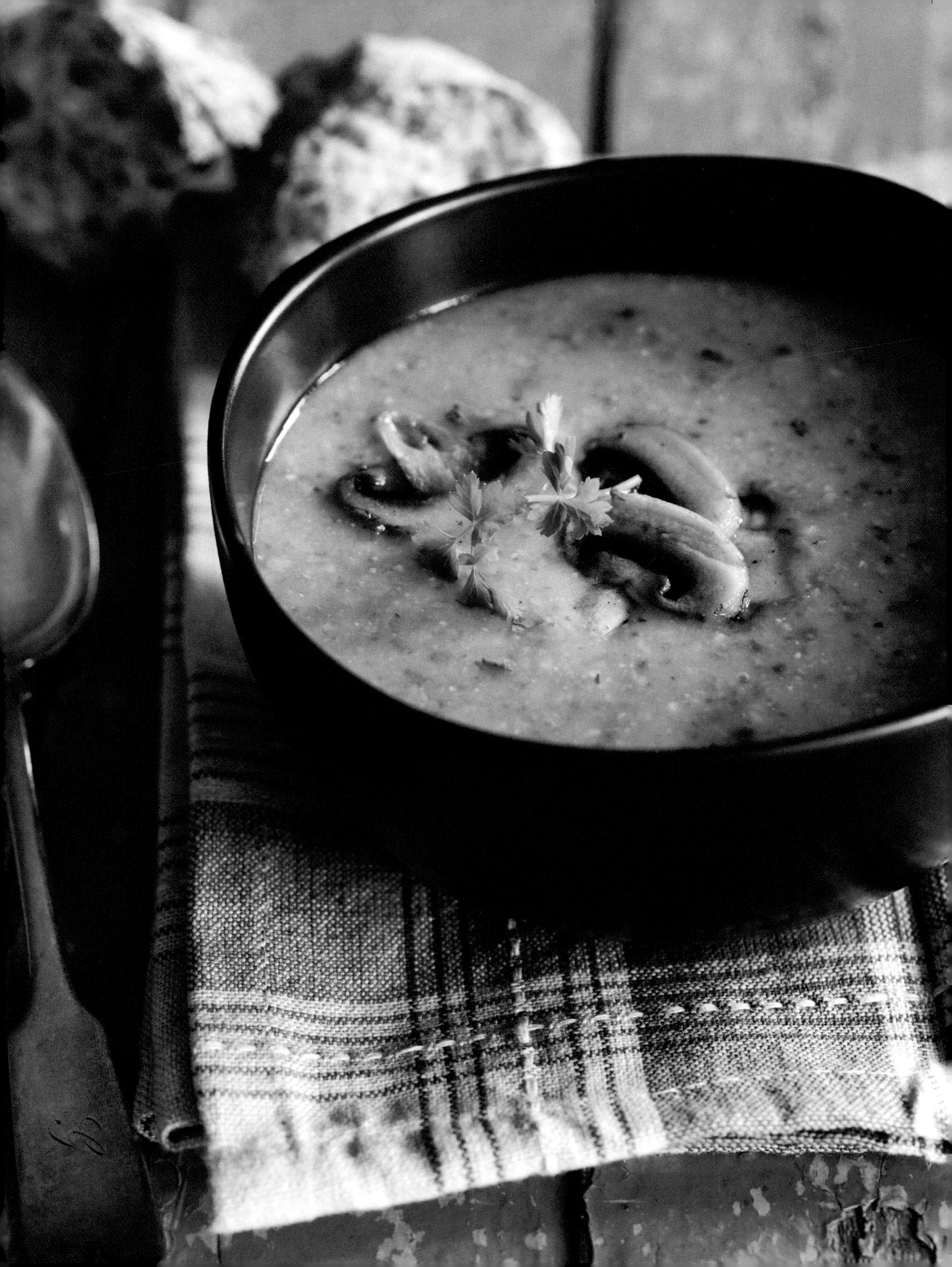

# GUYS DON'T TURN TO MUSH-ROOM SOUP

There are few foods as satisfying as a creamy-textured mushroom soup. The bachelor's ubiquitous food staple, it can be eaten on its own, or you can use it to liven up other foods as a sauce. Yum!

### WHAT YOU'LL NEED»

1 Tbsp / 15 ml best-quality olive oil
½ cup / 120 ml onion, chopped
3 strips cooked turkey bacon, chopped
½ cup / 120 ml spelt flour
6 cups / 1½ L chicken broth
1 small packet of low-sodium chicken bouillon
1 lb / 454 g mushrooms, thinly sliced
1¼ lb / 575 g all-purpose potatoes, peeled and chopped
1 Tbsp / 15 ml red wine vinegar
½ cup / 120 ml almond milk
1 Tbsp / 15 ml chopped fresh parsley

### HOW TO MAKE IT»

1. Splash olive oil into a large saucepan or Dutch oven and sauté onion and bacon over medium heat about 2 to 3 minutes, or until the onion is golden.
2. Add mushrooms and cook, stirring, for 8 minutes. Add the flour and cook for 1 minute, stirring all the while.
3. Stir broth and bouillon granules into the saucepan. Add potatoes and red wine vinegar. Simmer for 15 minutes or until the potatoes are tender.
4. Use a hand-held food processor to purée the soup mixture right in the pot. Stir in the almond milk.
5. Gently reheat.
6. Spoon into bowls and garnish with chopped parsley.

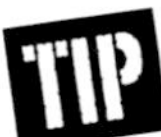


**In need of comfort food? Pour soup overtop two slices of toasted 100% rye bread or hearty whole-grain bread of your choice.**

**NUTRITIONAL VALUE FOR ONE CUP:**
Calories: 191 | Calories from Fat: 29 | Total Fat: 3 g | Saturated Fat: 0.5 g | Total Carbs: 32.5 g | Fiber: 4 g | Protein: 10 g | Sodium: 787 mg | Cholesterol: 2 mg

**Preparation time:** 15 minutes
**Cooking time:** 35 minutes
**Yield:** 6 cups

# WRAP YOU UP IN CURRIED CHICKEN LOVE

**WHAT YOU'LL NEED»**

3 Tbsp / 45 ml best-quality olive oil

4 boneless skinless chicken breasts (about 5 oz / 130 g each)

Sea salt, to taste

Freshly ground black pepper, to taste

½ cup / 120 ml yogurt cheese (see page 222)

1 tsp / 5 ml curry powder

Fresh lemon juice from ½ of a lemon

1 cup / 240 ml brown rice

¼ cup / 60 ml sundried tomatoes, chopped

Handful of fresh basil

4 x 7-inch / 18 cm Ezekiel or brown-rice wraps

**Preparation time:** 15 minutes
**Cooking time:** 45 minutes
**Yield:** 4 wraps

**NUTRITIONAL VALUE FOR ONE WRAP:**
Calories: 311 | Calories from Fat: 55 | Total Fat: 6 g | Saturated Fat: 0.6 g | Total Carbs: 34 g | Fiber: 5 g | Protein: 32.5 g | Sodium: 426 mg | Cholesterol: 61 mg

**HOW TO MAKE IT»**

1. Preheat the oven to 400°F / 205°C.
2. Heat the oil in a large ovenproof skillet over medium-high heat until it just begins smoking.
3. Sprinkle salt and pepper on both sides of the chicken breasts. Put the breasts in the skillet in a single layer, and brown for two minutes on each side. Put the skillet in the oven and roast until the chicken is just cooked through, about 15 minutes.
4. Remove from the oven and cool. Lower the oven to 375°F / 190°C. Place one cup rice and two cups water into a casserole dish. Splash some olive oil in to keep the rice from sticking to the sides. Place in oven. The rice will take about 40 to 45 minutes to cook.
5. Dice the chicken and put it into a large bowl. Add curry powder and lemon juice and mix well.
6. Spread the yogurt cheese on all four wraps. Spoon the curried chicken in the center of each wrap.
7. Divide the sundried tomatoes, rice and basil between the four wraps. Season with salt and pepper. To wrap, fold the two opposite edges into the center and roll.
8. Cut the wrap on the diagonal in the center, and hold it together with toothpicks.

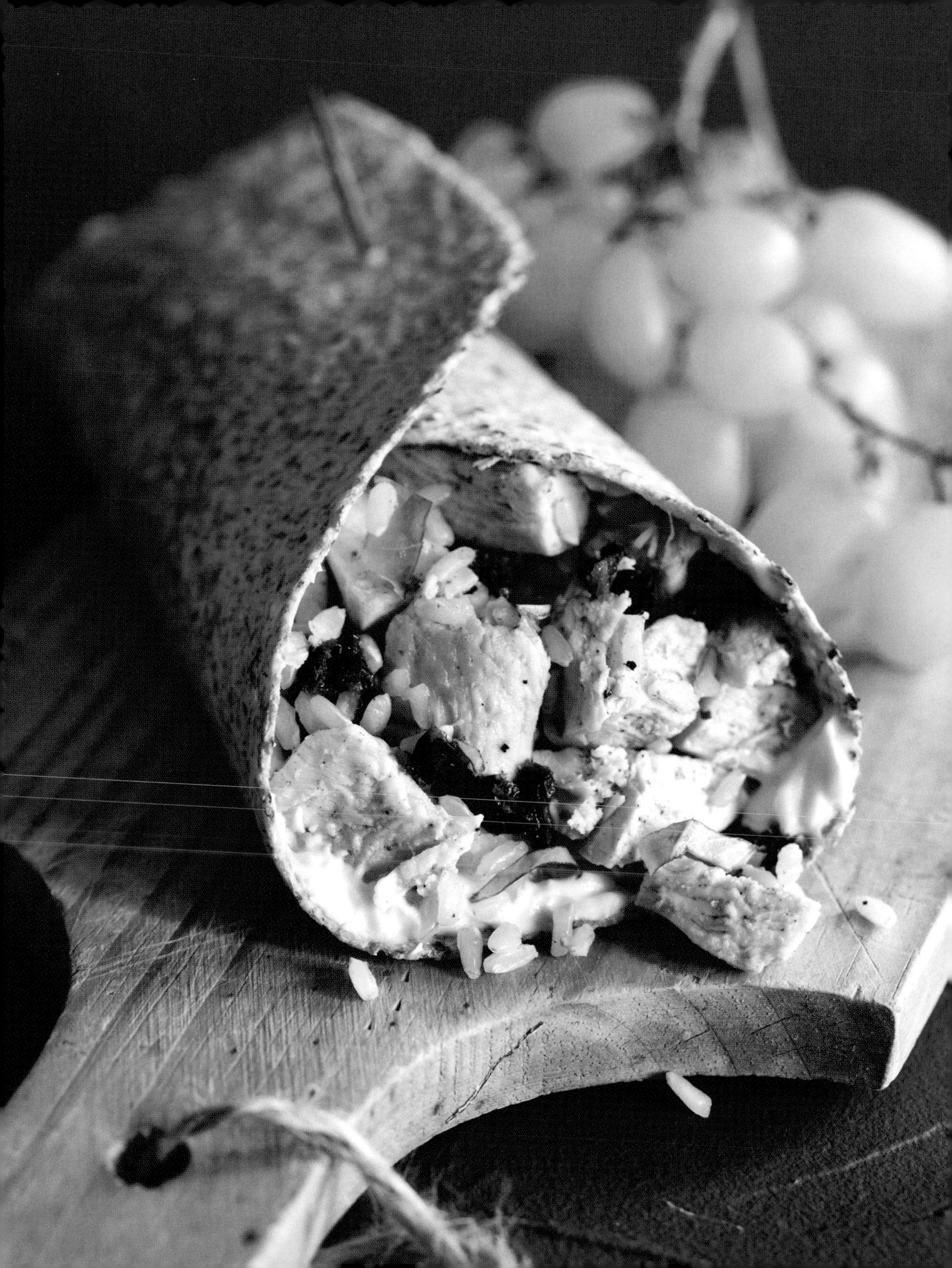

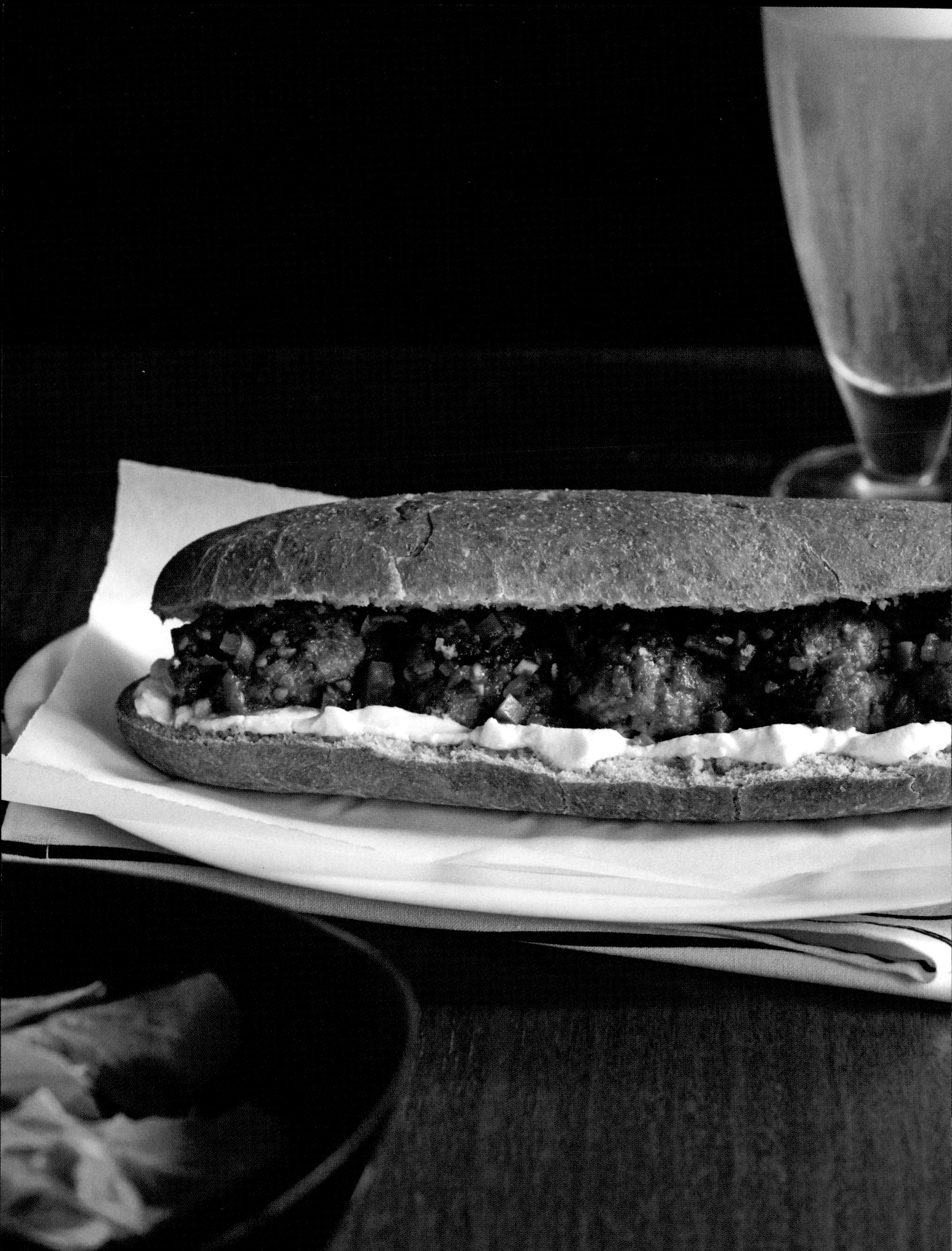

# THIRD-BASE TURKEY-BALL SUB

This sloppy sandwich is a favorite at sub shops everywhere, but most versions offer loads of saturated fat and little nutrition. Enjoy the pleasurable messiness, and make sure you have plenty of napkins on hand!

### WHAT YOU'LL NEED »

2 lb / 900 g lean ground turkey breast
½ cup / 120 ml ground almonds
1 large onion, chopped
1 garlic clove, minced and pressed
½ cup / 120 ml Tomato Hot and Spicy Sauce (recipe below)
4 sprouted-grain submarine-style buns
½ cup / 120 ml yogurt cheese (see page 222)

### HOW TO MAKE IT »

1. Preheat oven to 350°F / 177°C. Prepare a casserole dish with olive oil.
2. Mix together the turkey, ground almond, onion and garlic in a large bowl. Mix well.
3. Roll the mixture into golf-ball sized turkey-balls. Place the turkey-balls into the casserole dish and place in the oven for 25 minutes.
4. Remove the meat from the oven, drain excess juices and pour in tomato sauce. Place back into the oven at 150°F / 65°C to stay warm.
5. Slice the buns in half lengthwise. Scoop some of the bread out of one half to form a shallow trench.
6. Spread a thick layer of yogurt cheese on the other side of the bun, and sprinkle with sea salt and ground pepper.
7. Spoon the turkey-balls and sauce into the trench and top with the other half bun.

**Preparation time:** 10 minutes
**Cooking time:** 30 minutes
**Yield:** 4 sandwiches

## TOMATO HOT & SPICY SAUCE

### WHAT YOU'LL NEED »

1 **onion**, chopped
1 **bell pepper**, chopped
1 or 2 fresh **green chilies**, seeds removed and chopped
3 cups / 720 ml canned **tomatoes**, in juice
¼ cup / 60 ml best-quality **olive oil**
2 Tbsp / 30 ml chopped **fresh cilantro**
1 tsp / 5 ml **cumin seeds**
1 tsp / 5 ml **coriander seeds**
2 Tbsp / 30 ml **dried basil**
Freshly ground **black pepper** to taste

### HOW TO MAKE IT »

**1.** In a heavy pan, sauté the onions and garlic in the olive oil for about 10 minutes on medium heat, until translucent. Stir often to prevent sticking.
**2.** Drain the tomato juice into the sautéing onions. Add the chopped bell pepper and chilies.
**3.** Chop the tomatoes with a knife right in the can and add them to the onions, peppers and chilies.
**4.** Add the cilantro, cumin, coriander, basil and pepper. Simmer uncovered for about 15 minutes, until the sauce has thickened. Add sea salt and black pepper to taste.

**Preparation time:** 5 minutes
**Cooking time:** 30 minutes
**Yield:** 3 cups

**NUTRITIONAL VALUE FOR ONE SANDWICH:**
Calories: 654 | Calories from Fat: 257 | Total Fat: 29 g | Saturated Fat: 6 g | Total Carbs: 45 g | Fiber: 8.5 g | Protein: 55 g | Sodium: 444 mg | Cholesterol: 179 mg

# MEGA-MUSCLES MINESTRONE SOUP

Soup makes a great meal, combining all the nutrients in one dish. Minestrone is usually a nutritious choice, and the addition of bison sausages makes this one even better by giving you protein along with your veggies and pasta carbs. Eat this after your workout to refuel your muscles!

### WHAT YOU'LL NEED»

1 Tbsp / 15 ml best-quality olive oil
1 cup / 240 ml leeks, rinsed and chopped
4 bison sausages, cut into ¼-inch rounds
2 garlic cloves, minced or pressed
2 cups / 480 ml cabbage, rinsed and shredded
1½ cups / 360 ml zucchini, rinsed and quartered
1 large carrot, peeled and sliced
6 cups / 1½ L chicken broth
1 x 14 oz / 398 ml can Italian-style stewed tomatoes, undrained, coarsely chopped,
2 chicken breasts, cooked and cubed
⅓ cup / 80 ml rice vinegar
2 cups / 480 ml fresh tomatoes, chopped
1 Tbsp / 15 ml oregano
1 sprig of fresh thyme
3 bay leaves
⅛ tsp / ½ ml freshly ground black pepper
½ cup / 120 ml whole-wheat macaroni pasta

### HOW TO MAKE IT»

1. Heat olive oil over medium-high heat in a saucepan. Add the leeks, bison sausage, garlic and cabbage, and sauté for 10 minutes.
2. Add the remaining ingredients, except the pasta. Bring to a boil, cover, reduce heat and simmer for 5 to 10 minutes
3. Add pasta to soup and cook for an additional 10 minutes or until pasta is done, stirring occasionally. Serve hot.

**NUTRITIONAL VALUE FOR ONE CUP:**
Calories: 224 | Calories from Fat: 76 | Total Fat: 9 g | Saturated Fat: 3 g | Total Carbs: 18 g | Fiber: 2.5 g | Protein: 20 g | Sodium: 1000 mg | Cholesterol: 1 mg

**Preparation time:** 15 minutes
**Cooking time:** 30 minutes
**Yield:** 8 cups

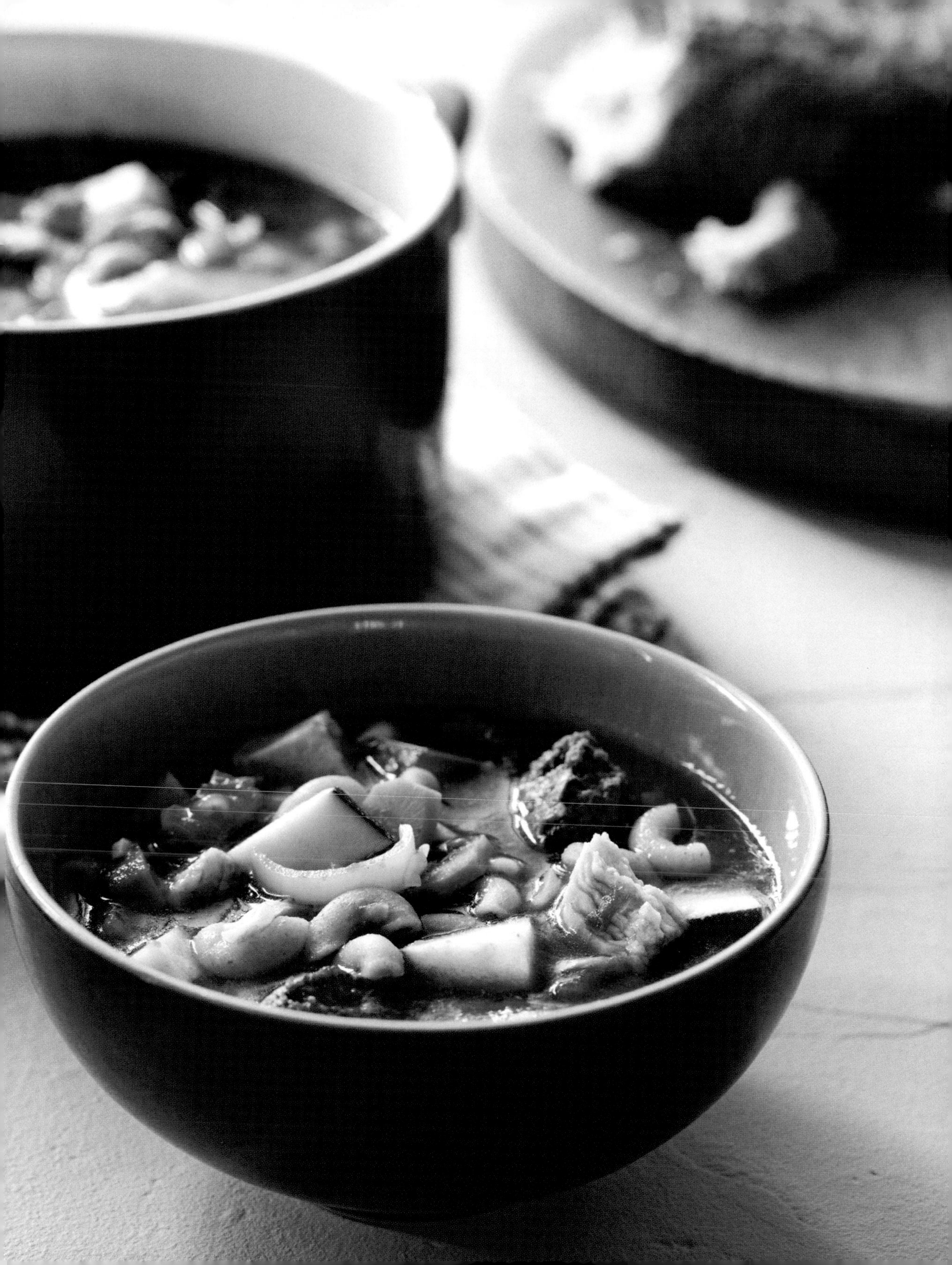

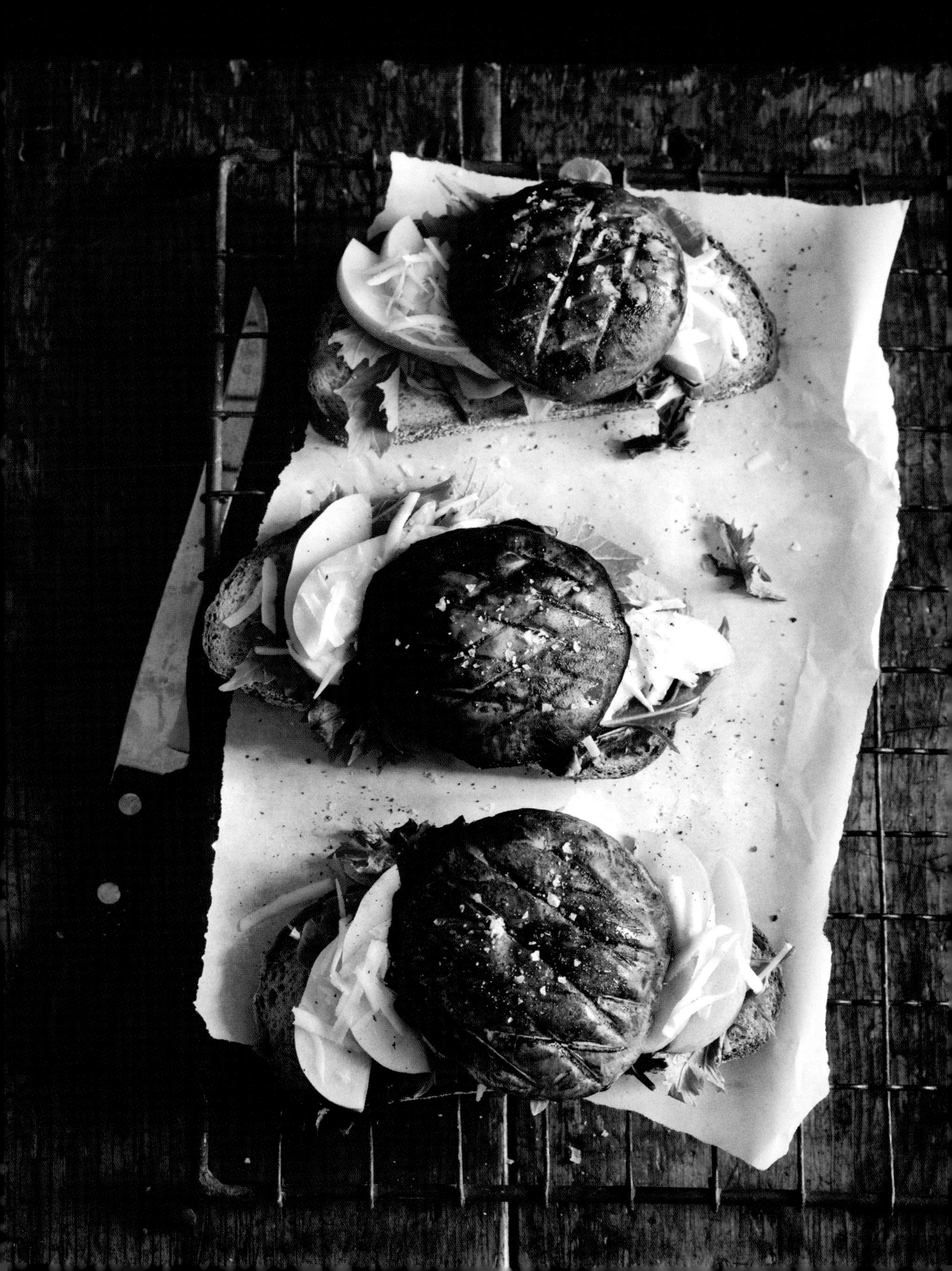

# BIG FELLO PORTOBELLO
## OPEN-FACED SANDWICH

Portobellos are the manliest of mushrooms – big, meaty and flavorful, they are a wonderful replacement if you're trying to cut down on your meat consumption. Try this sandwich for a healthy burger alternative.

### WHAT YOU'LL NEED»

2 Tbsp / 30 ml balsamic vinegar
¼ cup / 60 ml best-quality olive oil
½ tsp / 2½ ml freshly ground black pepper
4 large Portobello mushroom caps
4 thick slices of sprouted-grain rye bread, toasted
2 cups / 480 ml grated almond cheese (available in natural-food stores)
1 or 2 pears, sliced into 12 thin slices
2 cups / 480 ml of mixed spring greens

**TIP Are you a meat lover? Try this open-faced sandwich with a lean-ground turkey burger patty or a grilled bison steak.**

**Marinade time:** 30 minutes
**Preparation time:** 10 minutes
**Cooking time:** 10 minutes
**Yield:** 4 sandwiches

**NUTRITIONAL VALUE FOR ONE SANDWICH:**
Calories: 305 | Calories from Fat: 67 | Total Fat: 7.5 g | Saturated Fat: 1 g | Total Carbs: 36 g | Fiber: 9 g | Protein: 25 g | Sodium: 518 mg | Cholesterol: 10 mg

### HOW TO MAKE IT»

*Remember this is an open-faced sandwich, only one slice of bread per serving!*

1. Put the balsamic vinegar, olive oil, salt, pepper and Portobello mushroom caps in a large sealed bag. Make sure the caps are completely coated in the marinade. Seal the bag and place in the refrigerator for at least 30 minutes but preferably several hours or overnight.
2. Heat the grill or broiler to medium-high. Once the grill is heated, drain the marinade from the mushrooms and place mushroom caps on the grill. Cook for approximately five minutes on each side, but make sure they don't get overdone. Remove caps from the grill.
3. Set toasted bread slices on a baking sheet. Place ½ cup / 120 ml of mixed greens on each piece of toasted rye bread, then three pear slices on each sandwich. Top with ½ cup / 120 ml of grated almond cheese, and finally place the grilled mushroom cap over the cheese. Sprinkle with sea salt and freshly ground black pepper.
4. Return to grill or broiler until cheese melts.

SHE GRILLED ME
# SALMON SANDWICH

If you think a salmon sandwich means salmon from a can mixed with some mayo, think again! Here's a salmon sandwich that will become your new standard.

### WHAT YOU'LL NEED»

1 lb / 454 g salmon fillet, cut into four portions
8 tsp / 40 ml black peppercorns, divided
1 avocado, peeled and pitted
4 large pieces of romaine lettuce, rinsed
2 plum tomatoes, washed and thinly sliced
½ cup / 120 ml thinly sliced red onion
Fresh lemon juice from ½ of a lemon
2 Tbsp / 30 ml best-quality olive oil
4 sprouted-grain kamut bagels, cut in half and toasted

### HOW TO MAKE IT»

1. Oil the grill rack and preheat grill to high.
2. Rub the salmon in the peppercorns – 2 tsp / 10 ml on each fillet. Grill until cooked through, about 3 to 4 minutes per side.
3. Mash together the avocado, oil and lemon juice.

To assemble the sandwich, spread the avocado mixture on the bottom half of the bagel. Top with the salmon, tomato, onion and lettuce. Sprinkle some sea salt and fresh ground black pepper for flavor.

**NUTRITIONAL VALUE FOR ONE SANDWICH:**
Calories: 522 | Calories from Fat: 241 | Total Fat: 27 g | Saturated Fat: 4.5 g | Total Carbs: 37 g | Fiber: 10 g | Protein: 32 g | Sodium: 732 mg | Cholesterol: 67 mg

**Preparation time:** 15 minutes
**Cooking time:** 6 – 8 minutes
**Yield:** 4 sandwiches

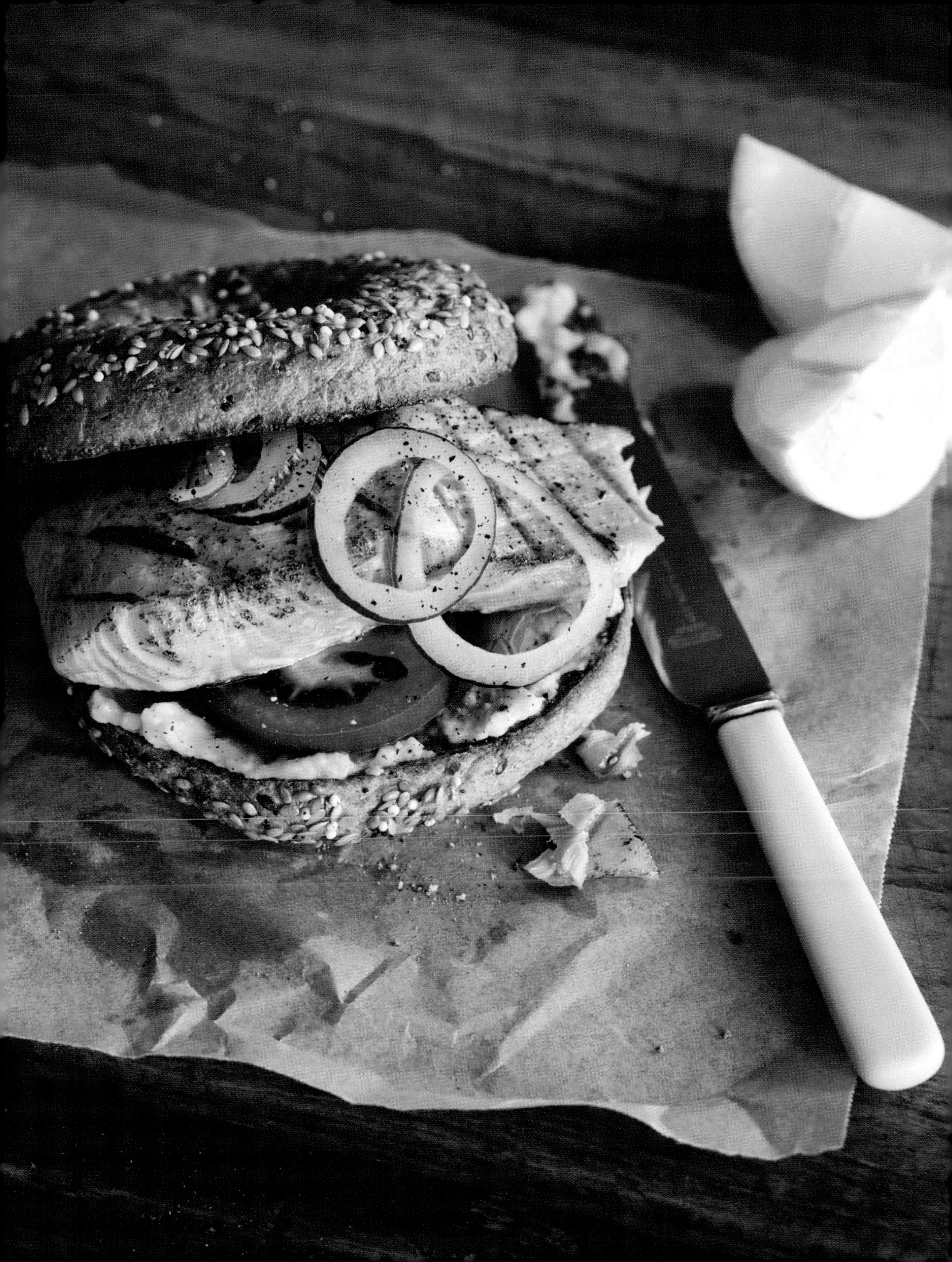

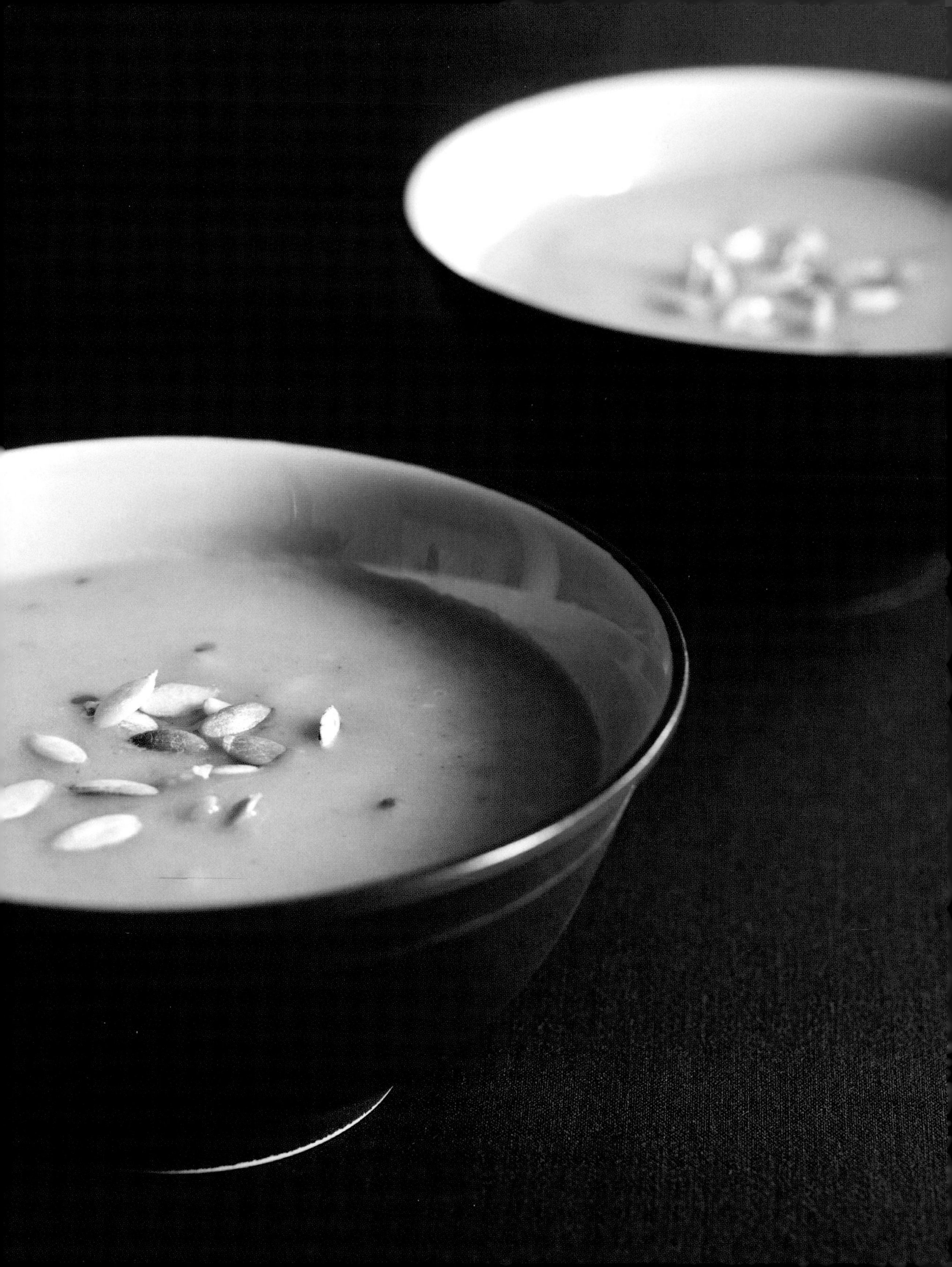

# PUMPKIN SOUP

And you thought pumpkin was good for only pies or jack-o-lanterns! Try pumpkin in this soup to get tons of fall flavor along with the nutrients this superfood offers.

### WHAT YOU'LL NEED»

2 Tbsp / 30 ml best-quality olive oil
1 cup / 240 ml leeks, whites only, well-washed and thinly sliced
6 cups / 960 ml low-sodium chicken broth
1½ cups / 360 ml fresh pumpkin, peeled and seeded, cut into 1-inch / 2½-cm cubes
2 large Yukon gold potatoes, peeled and quartered
2 garlic cloves, pressed or minced
1 tsp / 5 ml ginger, freshly grated
1 tsp / 5 ml fresh thyme, crumbled
1 Tbsp / 15 ml curry powder
1 Tbsp / 15 ml red pepper flakes
½ tsp / 2½ ml ground coriander
Sea salt

### HOW TO MAKE IT»

1. Add olive oil to a small frying pan and sauté leeks until softened. In a large saucepan add the broth, sautéed leeks, potato and pumpkin. Bring to a boil, then reduce heat and cook for 30 minutes and until the potatoes are soft.
2. Add garlic, ginger, thyme, curry powder, red pepper flakes and coriander. Simmer for another 15 minutes. Using a hand blender, purée soup mixture until uniformly smooth. Add sea salt as desired. Serve hot! Garnish with pumpkin seeds.

**NUTRITIONAL VALUE FOR ONE CUP:**
Calories: 239 | Calories from Fat: 32 | Total Fat: 6 g | Saturated Fat: 1 g | Total Carbs: 32 g | Fiber: 4 g | Protein: 6 g | Sodium: 96 mg | Cholesterol: 0 mg

**Preparation time:** 15 minutes
**Cooking time:** 50 minutes
**Yield:** 6 cups

# MR. BIG'S FRESH FIG AND PORK LOIN SANDWICH

**WHAT YOU'LL NEED»**

1 x 100% rye submarine bun, cut lengthwise in half

½ cup / 120 ml basil pesto

½ cup / 120 ml raw spinach

4 thin slices cooked pork loin

3 fresh, ripe, purple or green figs, cut into slices

2 Tbsp / 30 ml lemon juice

Freshly ground black pepper to taste

**HOW TO MAKE IT»**

1. Place your bun in the oven on a very low heat – 150°F / 65°C – to toast.
2. Prepare basil pesto, cut figs and slice the pork loin.
3. In a small bowl mix the lemon juice and black pepper.
4. Remove your bun from the oven and spread the basil pesto, thickly covering both sides. Arrange the spinach and figs on one half of the bun. Place your sliced loin on top and drizzle the lemon juice / black pepper mixture over top. Close the sandwich and cut on the diagonal.

**NUTRITIONAL VALUE FOR ONE SANDWICH:**

Calories: 438 | Calories from Fat: 112 | Total Fat: 12.5 g | Saturated Fat: 4 g | Total Carbs: 53 g | Fiber: 7 g | Protein: 31 g | Sodium: 685 mg | Cholesterol: 67 mg

**Preparation time:** 15 minutes
**Cooking time:** 0 minutes
**Yield:** 1 sandwich

## BASIL PESTO

**WHAT YOU'LL NEED»**

1 cup / 240 ml **basil leaves**

1 **sweet red pepper**, chopped

1 **garlic clove**, pressed or minced

1 Tbsp / 15 ml **pumpkin seeds**, toasted

1 tsp / 5 ml **sea salt**

**HOW TO MAKE IT»**

**1.** Rinse and drain the basil leaves

**2.** In a blender purée the basil, red pepper, garlic, pumpkin seeds and salt until smooth. Scrape the side every so often with a rubber spatula.

**3.** Transfer to re-sealable container.

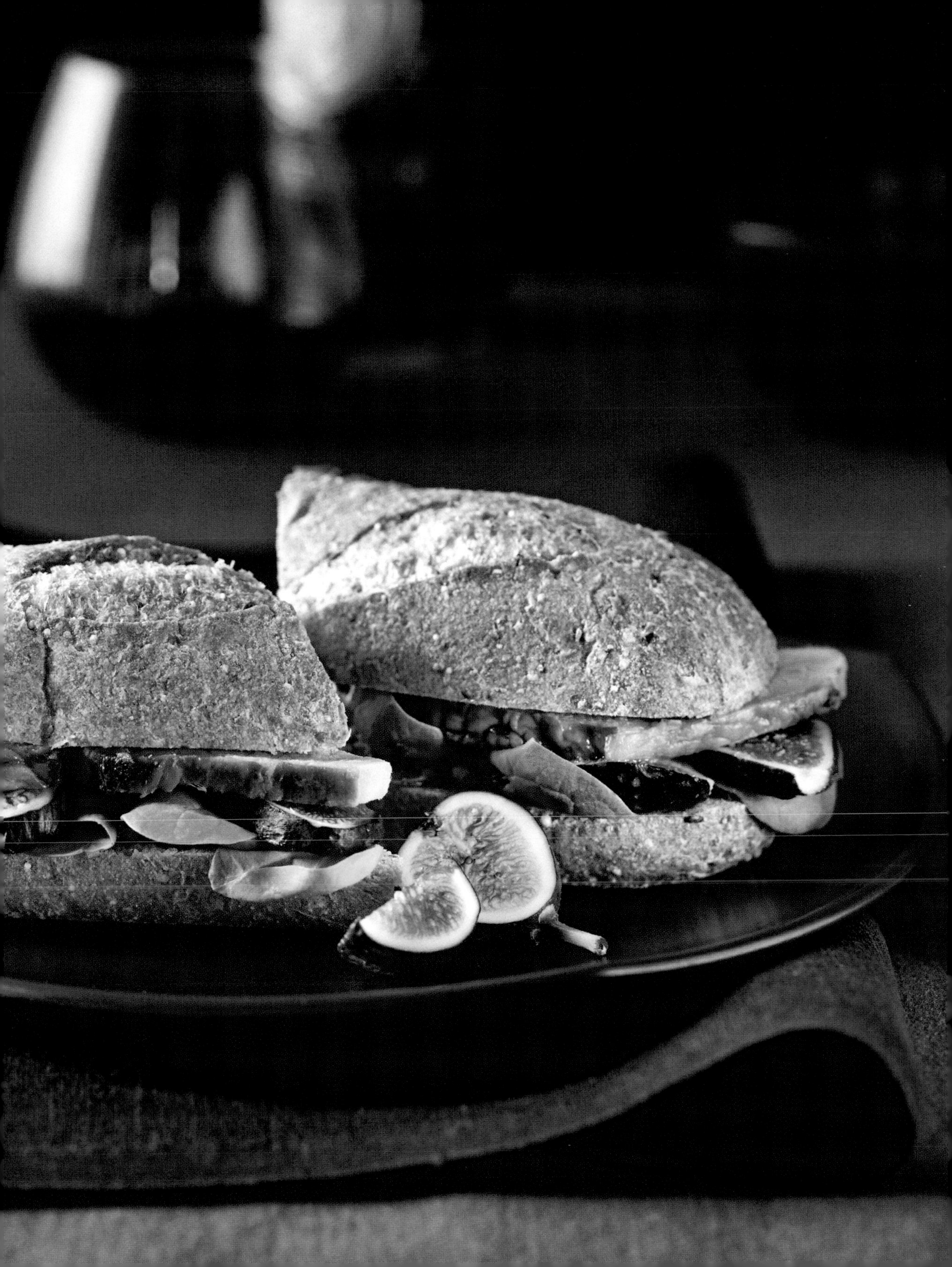

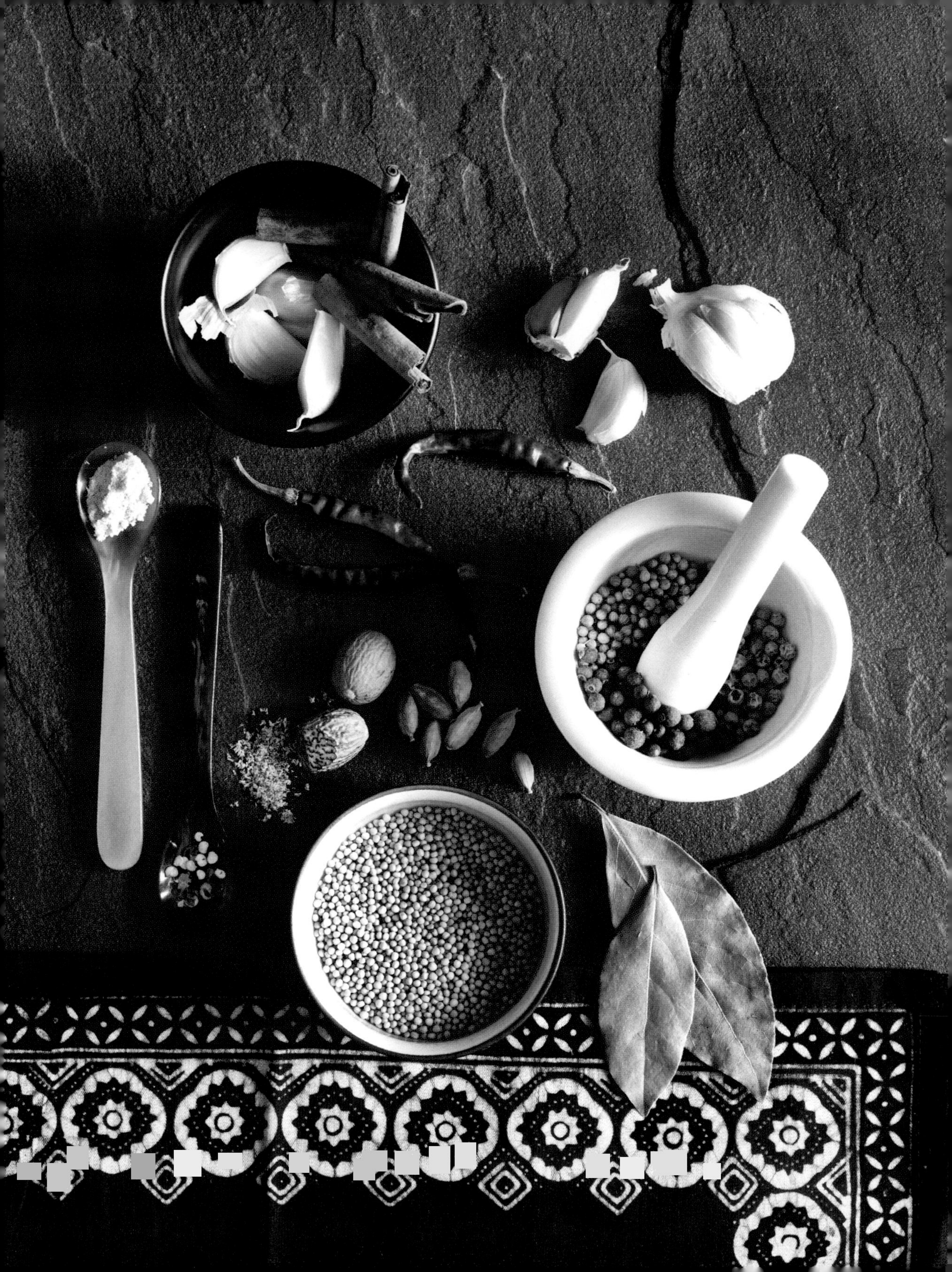

# AROUND THE WORLD

After sampling a few recipes from this section you will never again say eating well is boring. And if you create one or two of these dishes to share with others, they will never guess you're being health conscious ... they will think you've been secretly taking courses on international cooking. Treat your guests to flavors that hail from East Asia to India to Africa to the Caribbean and Mexico.

# BHOONA

For those who like foods spicy and sweet, this bhoona is a great choice. Cooking the spices in the oil both enhances and mellows their flavor, and the purée that includes pineapples and coconut milk – heavenly. Serve over brown rice for a satisfying feast.

**WHAT YOU'LL NEED»**

2 lbs / 900 g chicken, lamb or beef, cut into 2-inch / 5-cm cubes
2 tomatoes
2 onions
½ fresh pineapple, peeled and cubed
4 garlic cloves
¼ cup / 60 ml rice vinegar
4 Tbsp / 60 ml best-quality olive oil, divided
1 cup / 240 ml unsweetened coconut milk
1 tsp / 5 ml garam masala
1 tsp / 5 ml coriander powder
½ tsp / 2½ ml chili pepper
½ tsp / 2½ ml turmeric

**TIP** 1. Serve with brown rice.
2. For a hungry-man-sized meal, grab a large brown-rice wrap, place two scoops of brown rice down the center and pour the Bhoona over top. Roll up the wrap and dip into hot sauce, apple butter or yogurt.

**NUTRITIONAL VALUE FOR ONE-CUP SERVING:**
Calories: 410 | Calories from Fat: 197 | Total Fat: 22 g | Saturated Fat: 9 g | Total Carbs: 19 g | Fiber: 2 g | Protein: 39 g | Sodium: 800 mg | Cholesterol: 97 mg

**HOW TO MAKE IT»**

**1.** Purée the tomato, onion, pineapple and garlic with the vinegar.
**2.** Heat 2 Tbsp / 30 ml olive oil in a large deep saucepan over medium flame, until it bubbles and just starts to turn light brown. Quickly add the spices and some salt to taste. Stir to blend.
**3.** Add the vegetables and pineapple mixture to the pan, increase heat to medium high and boil for several minutes. Reduce heat to simmer.
**4.** Heat the remaining oil in another frying pan. Add the cubed meat once the oil is hot. Cook until the outside is seared, but do not cook through.
**5.** Add the seared meat to the vegetable and pineapple mixture. Keep it simmering. Stir occasionally. Cook until the same sauce begins to "stick" at the bottom of the pot, or for about an hour. Keep the lid set slightly to the side so moisture can escape.
**6.** Add the coconut milk and continue to cook at a simmer, again until the sauce starts to stick slightly to the bottom after stirring.

**Preparation time:** 35 minutes
**Cooking time:** 70 minutes
**Yield:** 5 cups

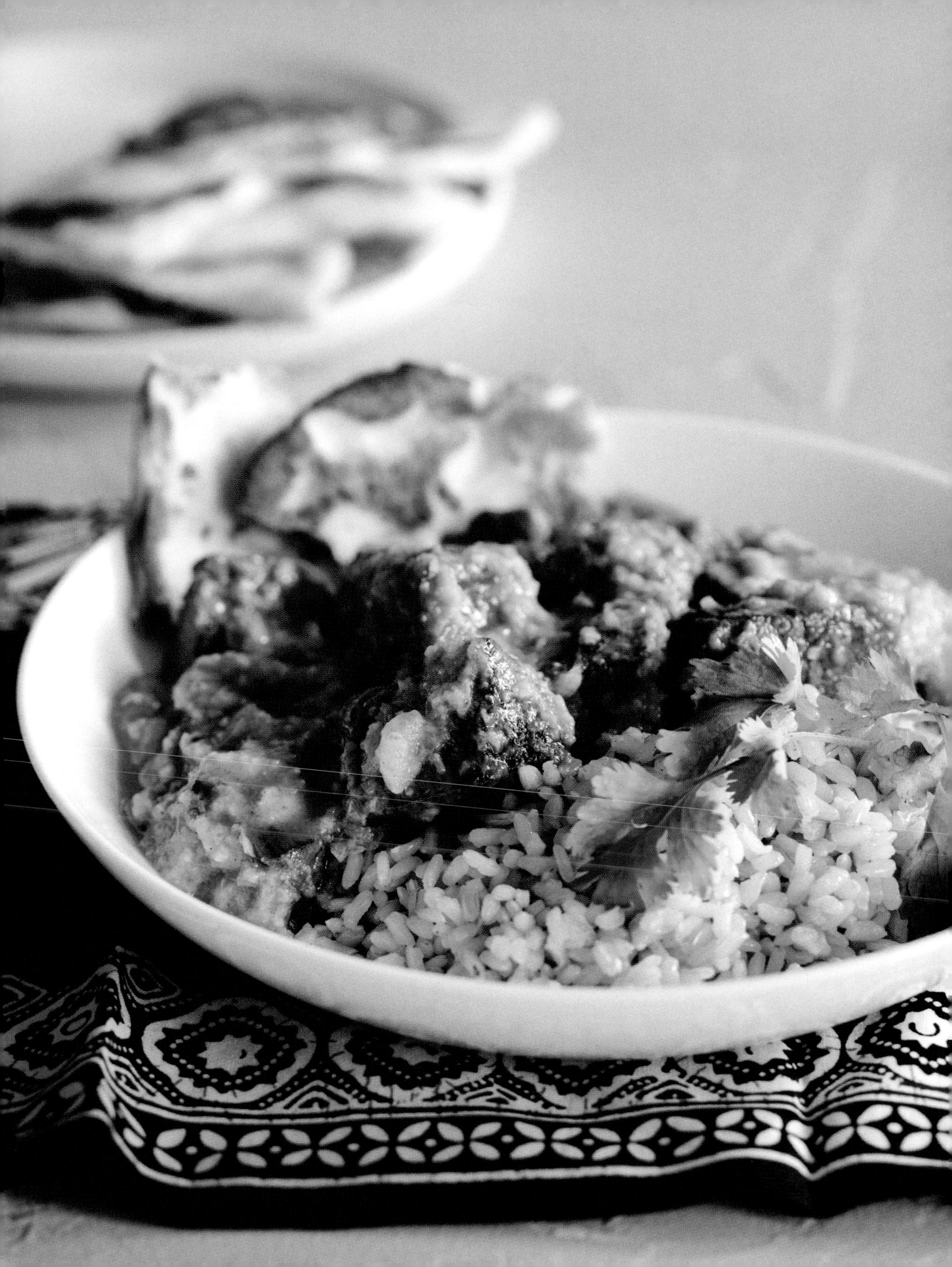

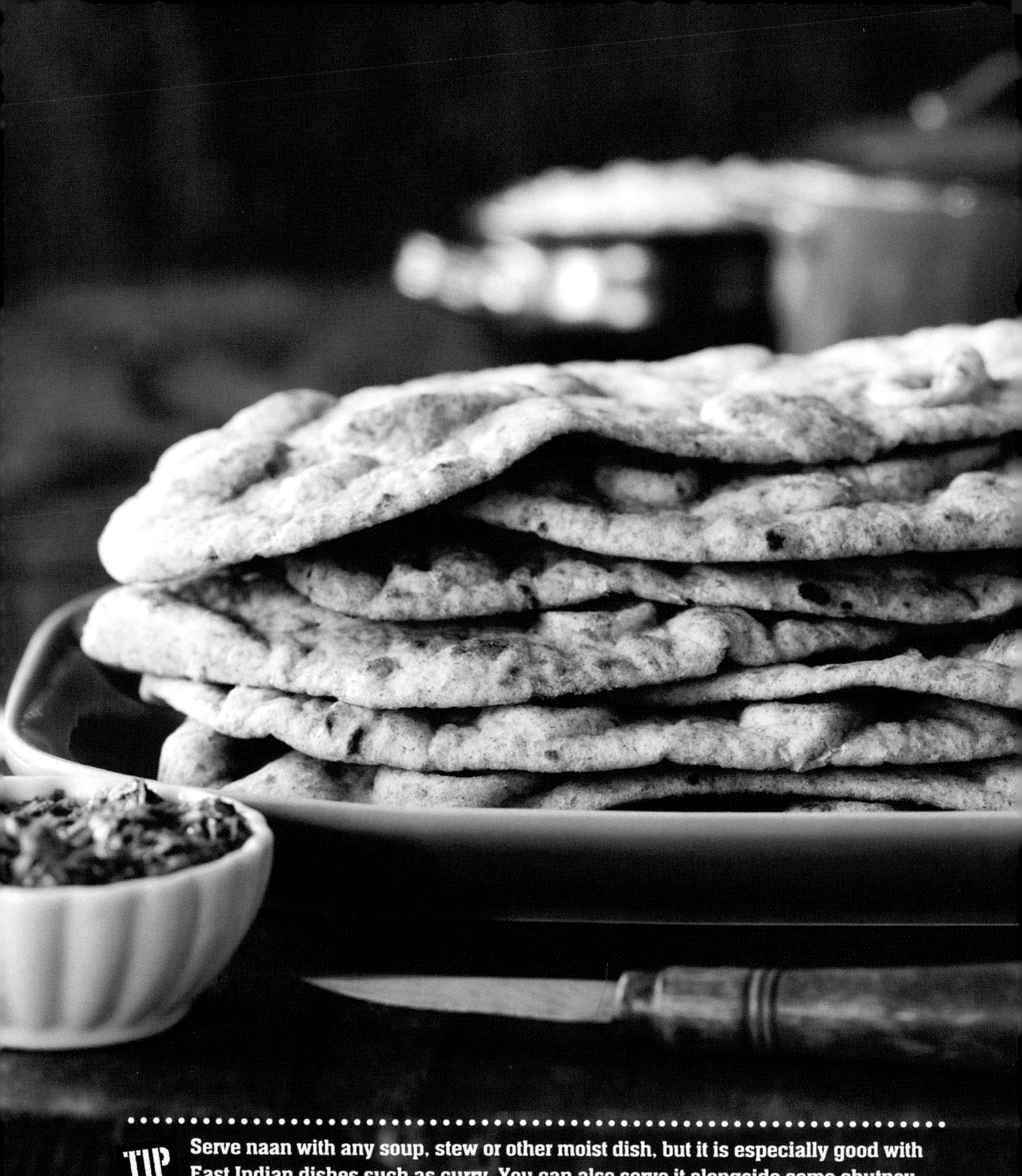

**TIP** Serve naan with any soup, stew or other moist dish, but it is especially good with East Indian dishes such as curry. You can also serve it alongside some chutney, such as the coriander chutney on page 221.

# CLEAN-EATING NAAN BREAD

The flavor of naan is wonderful. This light, fluffy bread can be purchased virtually everywhere, but baking a batch of fresh naan is a delightful activity that unleashes the unmistakable aroma of home. Adding garlic to this multi-tasking bread not only adds flavor but also essential nutrients that help fight disease.

### WHAT YOU'LL NEED»

2 cups / 480 ml spelt flour (Any whole-grain flour is fine to use. Choose whichever you prefer, but reach for unrefined flour at all times)
Pinch baking powder
1 Tbsp / 15 ml dry yeast
2 Tbsp / 30 ml plain yogurt
2 Tbsp / 30 ml Sucanat or agave nectar, divided
½ cup / 120 ml warm water
1 Tbsp / 15 ml best-quality olive oil
Sea salt
3 garlic cloves, minced

### HOW TO MAKE IT»

**1.** In a medium-sized mixing bowl place flour, baking powder, and sea salt. Mix thoroughly.

**2.** In a smaller bowl combine yeast and warm water. Set in a warm place and wait for the surface to appear slightly foamy. This will take about 5 minutes.

**3.** In a separate bowl, mix oil, sugar and yogurt. Add the yeast and yogurt mixture to the flour. Press your knuckles into the dough until it resembles a uniform dough. If the dough is too sticky, add a tablespoon or two of flour and knead well. If your dough is too dry, add a small amount of water to improve it.

**4.** Dampen a clean kitchen towel and place it over the bowl. Place the bowl in a warm place, like near a sunny window, and allow the yeast to do its work. Rising takes about 4 hours.

**5.** Preheat oven to 450°F / 232°C, and prepare a baking sheet with parchment paper. If you have a pizza stone, use this instead.

**6.** Remove the towel from the bowl and knead the dough for about 3 minutes. Sprinkle a few tablespoons of flour on a clean, dry countertop.

**7.** Break the dough into five evenly sized balls. Work some garlic and sea salt into each ball. Using a lightly floured rolling pin, roll each ball into a long oval shape. Don't roll your dough too thinly or the naan will turn out more like a cracker than bread.

**8.** Place each rolled-out naan onto the baking sheet and bake for 3 to 5 minutes. Remove from the oven when you see that the bread is puffy and lightly golden. You can keep the naan warm by wrapping it in a large sheet of foil until you are ready to serve it.

**NUTRITIONAL VALUE FOR ONE PIECE OF NAAN:**
Calories: 205 | Calories from Fat: 33 | Total Fat: 3.7 g | Saturated Fat: 0.5 g | Total Carbs: 38.5 | Fiber: 6 g | Protein: 8 g | Sodium: 151 mg | Cholesterol: 0 mg

**Rising time:** 3 – 4 hours
**Preparation time:** 40 minutes
**Cooking time:** 3 – 5 minutes
**Yield:** 5 servings

# SENEGALESE MAFÉ

**WHAT YOU'LL NEED»**

**Senegalese spice mix:**

1 Tbsp / 15 ml thyme

1 tsp / 5 ml sea salt

1 tsp / 5 ml red and black pepper

1½ lb / 675 g beef tenderloin, cut into cubes

4 Tbsp / 60 ml peanut oil

1 medium green pepper, coarsely chopped

1 medium onion, coarsely chopped

4 garlic cloves, minced or pressed

1 x 16 oz / 500 ml can of low-sodium beef broth

1 x 8 oz / 240 ml can of tomato sauce

1 squash, peeled and cubed

4 carrots, peeled and cut into chunks

1 sweet potato, peeled and cubed

½ cup / 120 ml natural peanut butter

**Marination time:** 30 minutes
**Preparation time:** 30 minutes
**Cooking time:** 50 minutes
**Yield:** 8 cups

**NUTRITIONAL VALUE FOR ONE-CUP SERVING WITHOUT RICE:**

Calories: 383 | Calories from Fat: 185 | Total Fat: 20 g | Saturated Fat: 4 g | Total Carbs: 19 g | Fiber: 4 g | Protein: 30 g | Sodium: 485 mg | Cholesterol: 56 mg

**HOW TO MAKE IT»**

**1.** About 30 minutes before cooking, prepare the spice mix. Combine red and black pepper, thyme and salt. Mix well. Rub this spice mixture into the meat and let sit for 30 minutes before cooking.

**2.** Place the chopped onions, garlic and green pepper into a food processor and grind coarsely.

**3.** Pour oil into a saucepan over medium-high flame. Let the oil coat the entire pan. Turn down the heat a little and pour the meat and spices into the oil, stirring so pieces do not burn and the meat is browned evenly.

**4.** Add the broth, stir in the ground veggies, tomato sauce, and chili pepper. Add water so the liquid just covers the tenderloin.

**5.** Simmer stew until the tenderloin is cooked the entire way through.

**6.** In a small bowl, combine the peanut butter with about ½ cup / 120 ml of hot broth from the stew. Using a whisk, stir the peanut butter / broth mixture until it's smooth and liquid. Pour the mixture back into the pot with the rest of the stew.

**7.** Add the sweet potato chunks, carrot and squash. Simmer on low heat until the oil from the peanut butter rises to the top of the stew – 30 minutes.

**8.** Serve over brown rice.

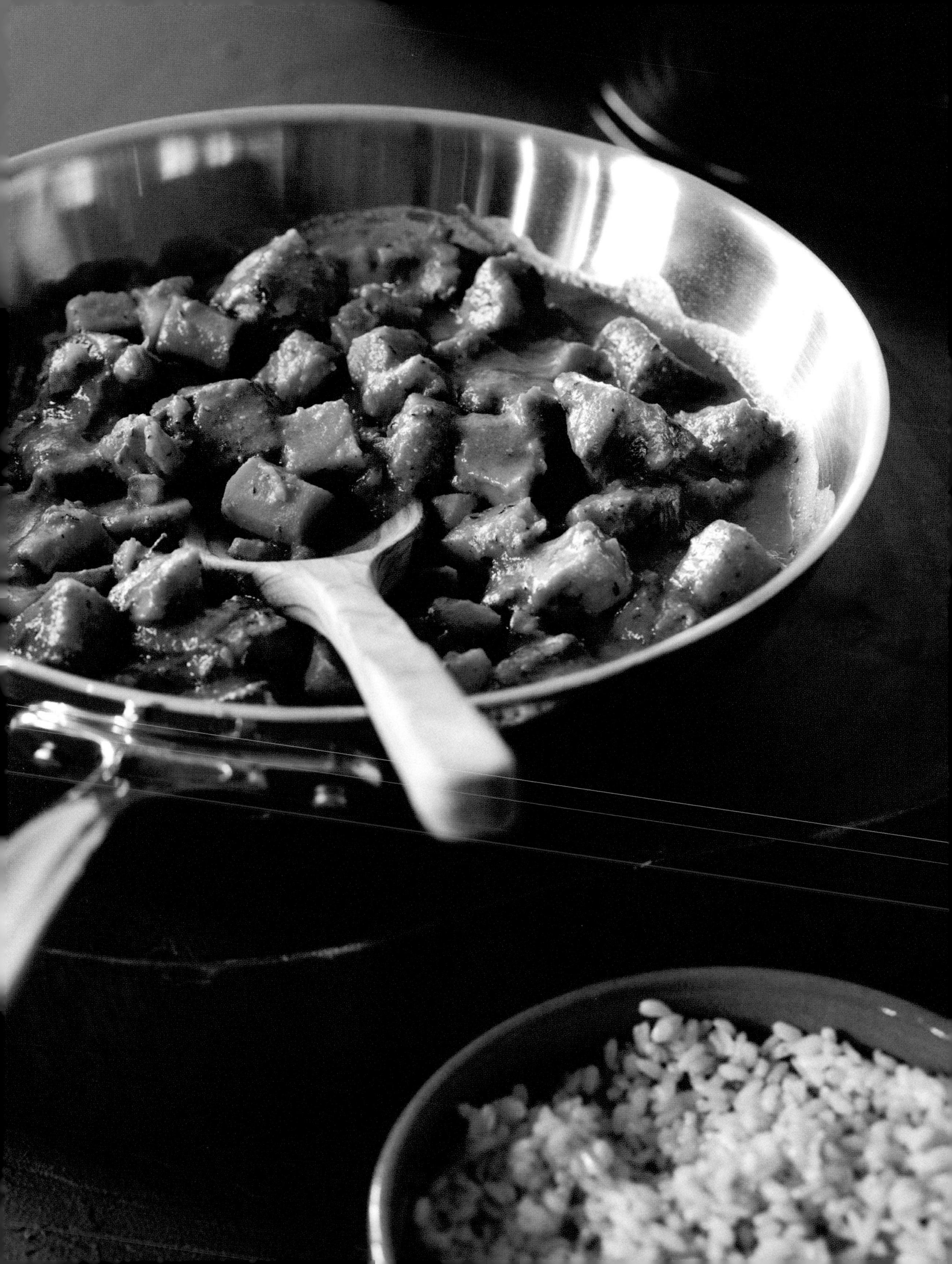

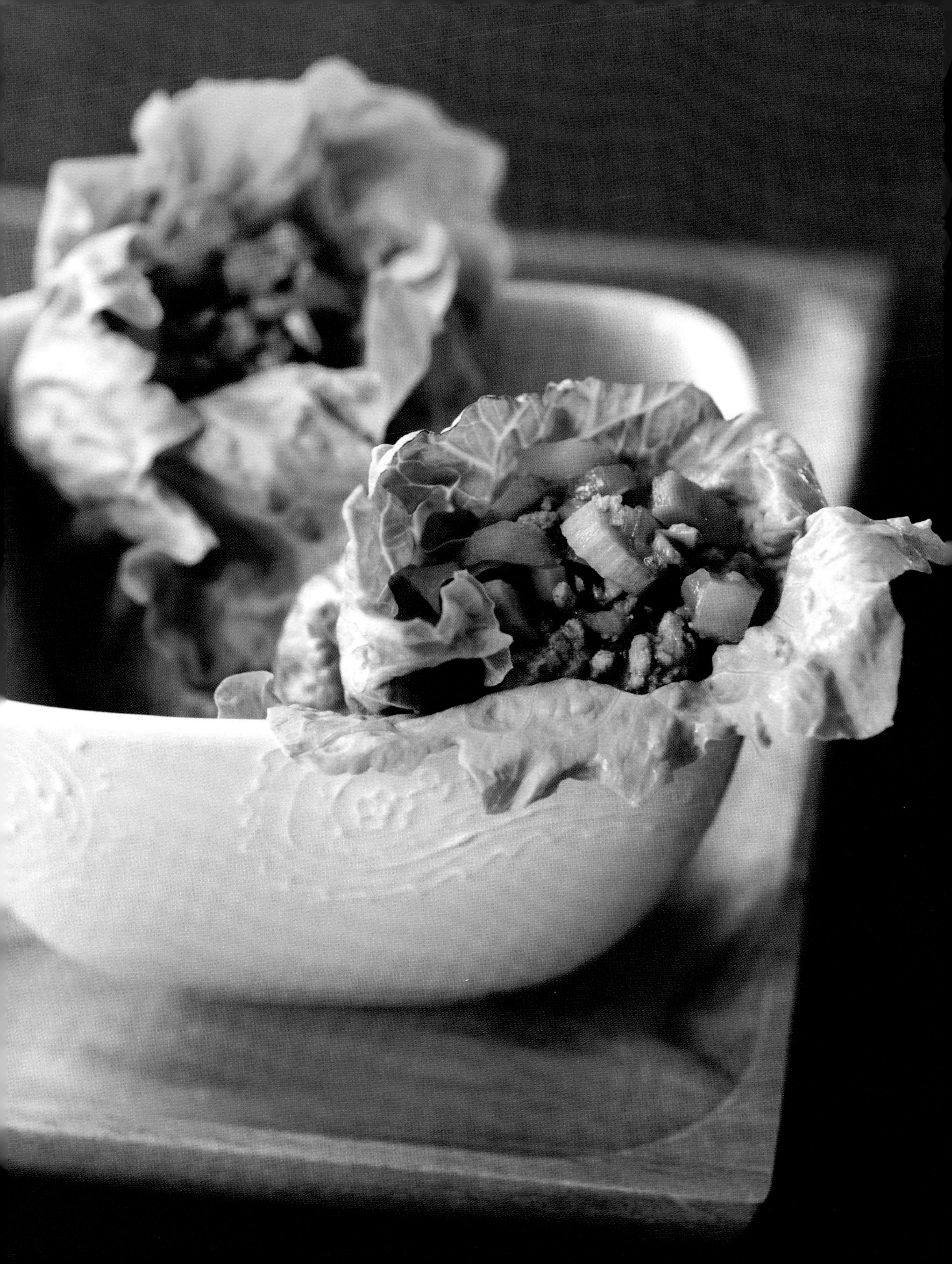

# RAINBOW CRYSTAL WRAP

Rainbow crystal is the poetic term used for simple lettuce in China. Using lettuce as a wrap instead of bread is a novel idea, and the texture provides an interesting balance for the food wrapped inside.

### WHAT YOU'LL NEED»

1 Tbsp / 15 ml sesame oil

1½ cups / 360 ml chopped Vidalia or other sweet onion

1 garlic clove, pressed or minced

1½ cups / 360 ml chopped celery

¾ cup / 180 ml carrots, peeled and diced

1 x 10-oz / 285 g can water chestnuts, peeled and coarsely chopped

1 cup / 240 ml coarsely chopped mushrooms, shiitake, oyster or enoki

1½ cups / 360 ml lean ground turkey breast, cooked

⅓ cup / 80 ml hoisin sauce

Sea salt, to taste

Freshly ground black pepper, to taste

12 large leaves iceberg lettuce, rinsed

### HOW TO MAKE IT»

**1.** In a large skillet, heat oil on medium-high. Add onions. Cook, stirring, for 3 minutes. Stir in garlic and cook for 30 seconds. Add celery, carrots, water chestnuts and mushrooms. Cook, stirring, till tender but still crisp.

**2.** Add ground turkey, Cook, stirring, for 3 minutes. Stir in the hoisin sauce. Season with salt and pepper.

**3.** Lay lettuce leaves on plate.

**4.** Place ¼ to ½ cup of mixture in the middle of each lettuce leaf, and fold lettuce around the mixture like a burrito.

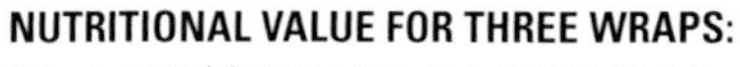

**NUTRITIONAL VALUE FOR THREE WRAPS:**

Calories: 287 | Calories from Fat: 45 | Total Fat: 5 g | Saturated Fat: 1 g | Total Carbs: 37 g | Fiber: 5.5 g | Protein: 25 g | Sodium: 400 mg | Cholesterol: 53 mg

**Preparation time:** 10 minutes
**Cooking time:** 5 minutes
**Yield:** 12 wraps

# BISON AND BROCCOLI

East meets West in this dish that combines the healthy high-protein goodness of this big North American beast with the distinctive flavors of China.

### WHAT YOU'LL NEED»

2 tsp / 10 ml of peanut oil
1-inch / 10 ml fresh ginger, peeled and diced
2 scallions, sliced thinly
2 garlic cloves, pressed or minced
½ tsp / 2½ ml red pepper flakes, crushed
Zest of one orange
½ lb / 227 g bison steaks, sliced thinly with no visible fat
2 cups / 480 ml fresh broccoli
1 red bell pepper, chopped
2 Tbsp / 30 ml low-sodium soy sauce
2 Tbsp / 30 ml rice wine vinegar
½ cup / 120 ml Tsingtao beer
1 Tbsp / 15 ml spelt flour
1 Tbsp / 15 ml water

**NUTRITIONAL VALUE FOR ONE SERVING:**
Calories: 372 | Calories from Fat: 97 | Total Fat: 11 g | Saturated Fat: 3 g | Total Carbs: 25 g | Fiber: 5 g | Protein: 40 g | Sodium: 1000 mg | Cholesterol: 97 mg

### HOW TO MAKE IT»

**1.** Heat oil in a large saucepan on medium high. Add the ginger, scallions and garlic. Stir until fragrant; about 30 seconds. Add red pepper flakes and orange zest. Cook 20 seconds longer.
**2.** Place bison strips in the pan and cook until lightly browned, about 2 minutes.
**3.** Add the broccoli and bell pepper. Heat, stirring, until soft but still crunchy (about 1 minute).
**4.** Pour in soy sauce, vinegar and beer. Bring to a boil, stirring constantly. Mix together the spelt flour and water and add to the mixture in the pan. Stir and cook until thick, about 15 minutes. Remove from heat and let stand for about 1 minute before serving.
**5.** Serve over rice or udon noodles.

**Preparation time:** 20 minutes
**Cooking time:** 20 minutes
**Yield:** 2 servings

### COOKING WITH BEER

TIP

➤ Beer has a lot in common with the foods we eat. It contains barley, herbs, water and yeast. It enhances the flavor of other ingredients, creates a delicious broth, and lends an earthy richness to whatever you are whipping up.

➤ Try adding beer to any broth, soup, gravy or marinade. Look for organic beers and those from local breweries for added interest.

➤ Splash it on soup, on grilled meats or in sautées.

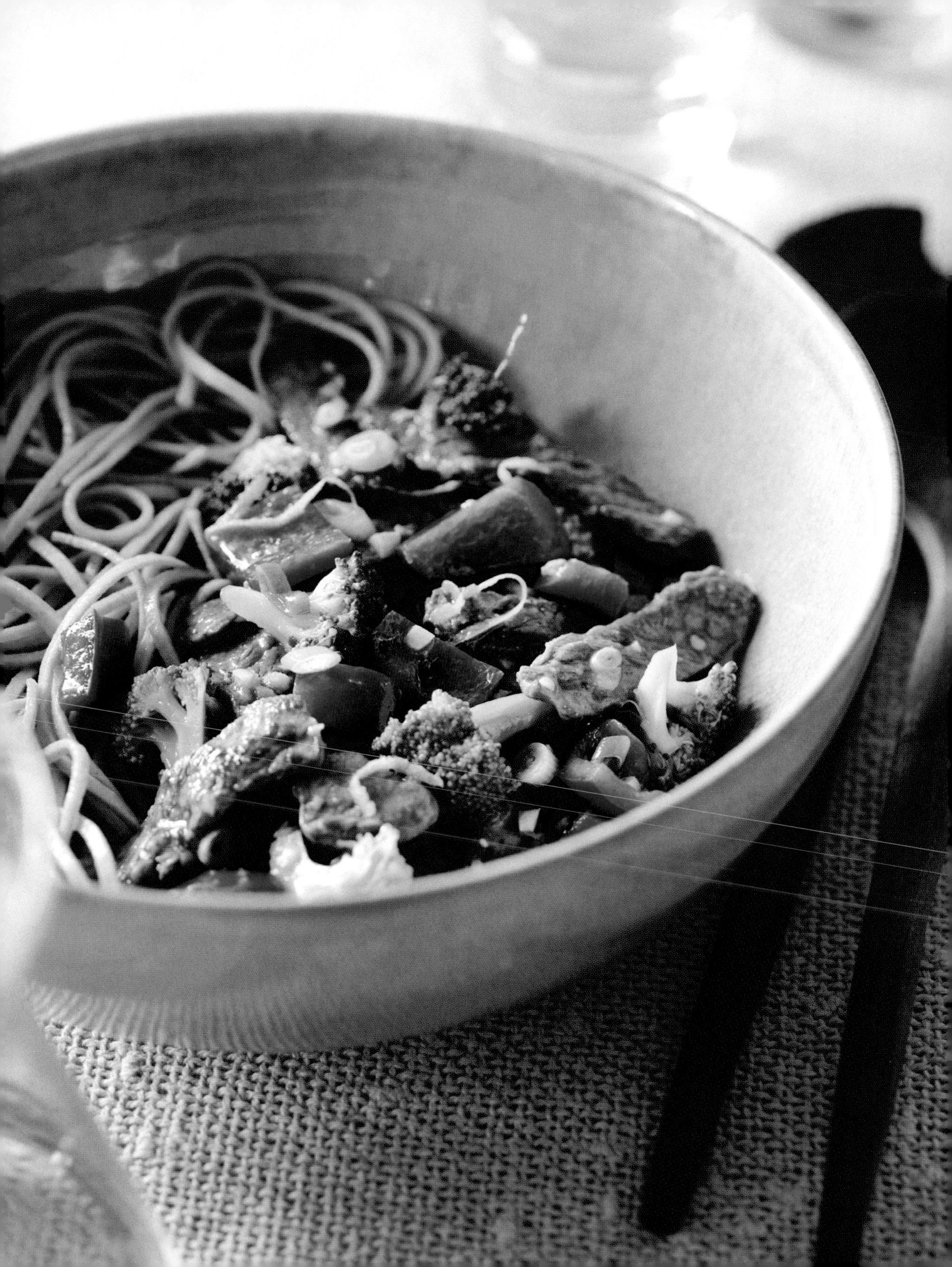

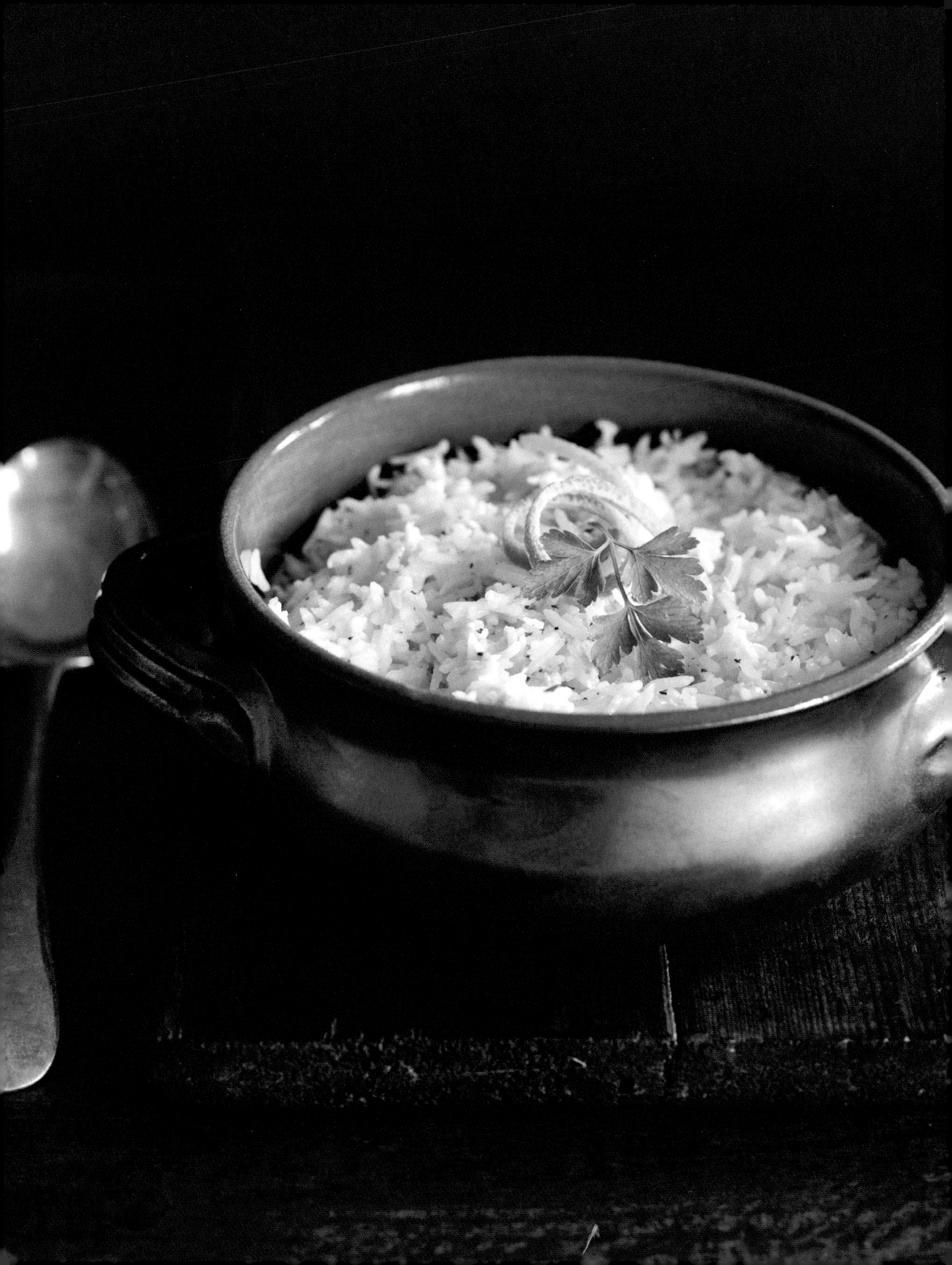

# COCONUT RICE

Ideal with Thai food, this creamy dish makes the perfect accompaniment for most spicy fare.

**WHAT YOU'LL NEED»**

1½ cups / 360 ml water

1 cup / 240 ml unsweetened coconut milk

1 cup / 240 ml shredded coconut

Zest of one orange

2 tsp / 10 ml cinnamon

1¼ cups / 300 ml jasmine or long-grain rice

**HOW TO MAKE IT»**

**1.** Place water and coconut milk in a saucepan and bring to a boil.

**2.** Add the rice, return to a boil, then reduce to medium-low heat and stir well.

**3.** Cover and cook for about 10 minutes.

**4.** Add the shredded coconut, orange zest and cinnamon, and cook for 5 more minutes.

**5.** Remove from heat and set aside, covered, for 5 minutes. Drain and fluff with fork.

**NUTRITIONAL VALUE FOR HALF-CUP SERVING:**
Calories: 277 | Calories from Fat: 141 | Total Fat: 15 g | Saturated Fat: 12 g | Total Carbs: 34 g | Fiber: 4 g | Protein: 5 g | Sodium: 0 mg | Cholesterol: 0 mg

**Preparation time:** 2 minutes
**Cooking time:** 15 minutes
**Yield:** 3 cups

# ORANGE-MANGO CASHEW CHICKEN

We love the combination of flavors and textures in this dish – the crunchy cashews with the slippery noodles, the sweet mango with the zesty ginger. Remember to make enough for lunch tomorrow!

**WHAT YOU'LL NEED»**

1 cup / 240 ml frozen shelled edamame
1 cup / 240 ml water
2 cups / 480 ml rice noodles
2 tsp / 10 ml dark sesame oil
1 medium onion, chopped
1 lb / 454 g boneless skinless chicken breast, cut into strips
½ cup / 120 ml raw cashews
2 garlic cloves, pressed or minced
1 Tbsp / 15 ml fresh ginger, peeled and minced
Zest of one orange
1 mango, peeled and cubed
½ cup / 120 ml low-sodium chicken stock
2 Tbsp / 30 ml low-sodium soy sauce
1 Tbsp / 15 ml unpasteurized honey

**HOW TO MAKE IT»**

**1.** Place edamame in a colander and rinse with cool water. Set aside.

**2.** Soak rice noodles in cold water till ready to use. Have pot of boiling water on hand to cook noodles for one minute only when ready to serve. Remove from water quickly when done.

**3.** Heat sesame oil in a large nonstick skillet. Add the chopped onion. Cook gently, stirring occasionally, for about 5 minutes. Add the garlic and cook for 2 to 3 minutes more, until the onion is translucent.

**4.** Add the chicken breast, cashews, orange zest, mango and ginger to the pan. Cook, stirring frequently, until chicken is cooked through.

**5.** Stir in chicken broth, soy sauce and honey. Add the thawed edamame and cook for another few minutes, until the edamame is tender. Serve over hot rice noodles.

**NUTRITIONAL VALUE FOR ONE CUP WITHOUT NOODLES:**

Calories: 432 | Calories from Fat: 150 | Total Fat: 17 g | Saturated Fat: 3 g | Total Carbs: 44 g | Fiber: 5 g | Protein: 31 g | Sodium: 338 mg | Cholesterol: 49 mg

**Preparation time:** 10 minutes
**Cooking time:** 20 minutes
**Yield:** 5 cups

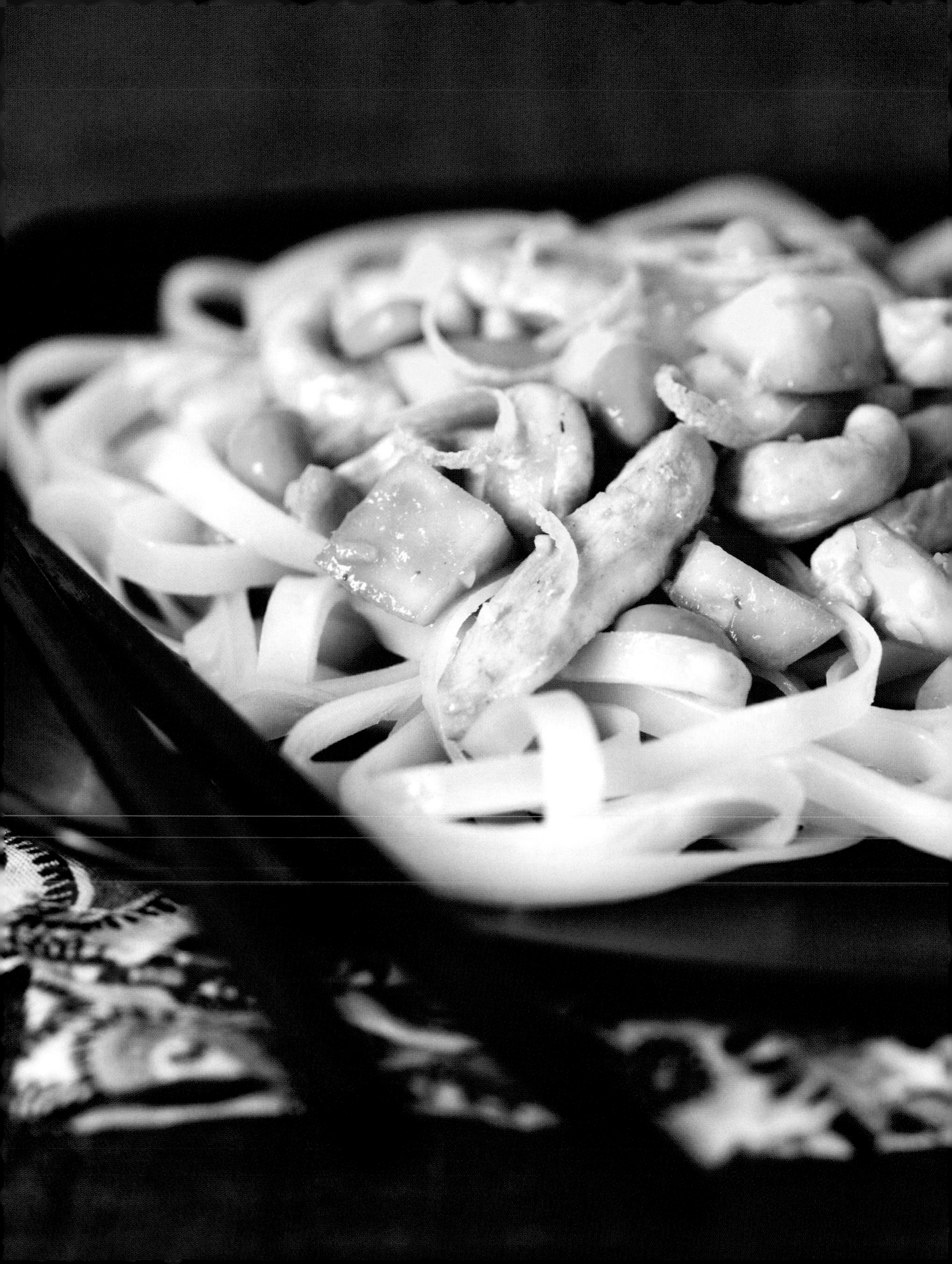

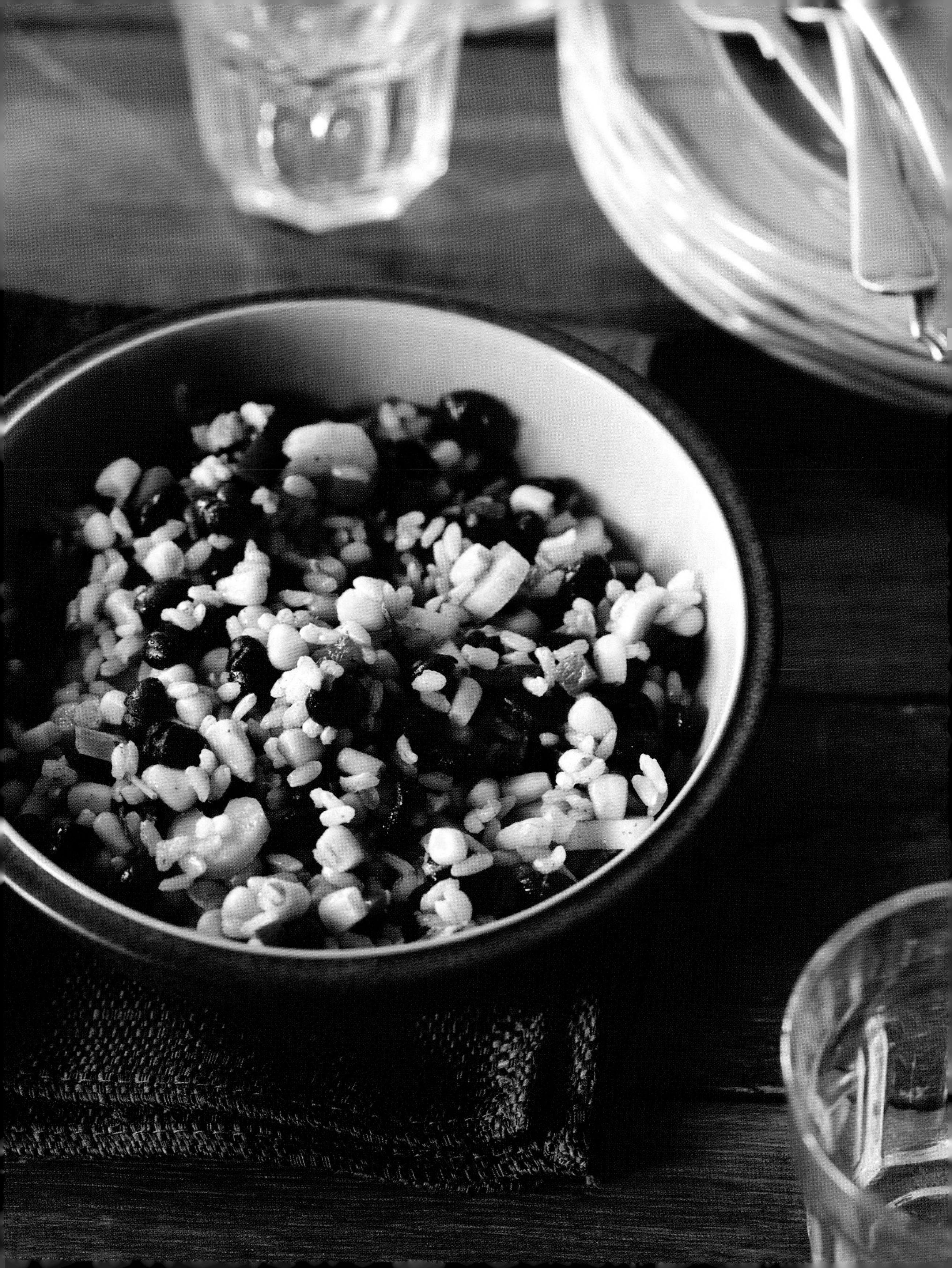

# BLACK BEANS AND RICE

Beans and rice is a common dish throughout the world, and with good reason! This combination of food provides complete protein and lots of inexpensive nutrition. This can be a meal in itself, or you can eat alongside your favorite protein. Enjoy!

**WHAT YOU'LL NEED»**

2 cups / 480 ml brown rice, cooked
1 x 19 oz / 540 ml can black beans
½ cup / 120 ml chopped red bell pepper
½ cup / 120 ml chopped celery
1 cup / 240 ml fresh or canned corn kernels
½ cup / 120 ml fresh parsley, chopped
2 Tbsp / 30 ml chives, chopped
2 Tbsp / 30 ml best-quality olive oil
2 tsp / 10 ml fresh thyme, minced
½ tsp / 2½ ml turmeric
½ tsp / 2½ ml paprika
½ tsp / 2½ ml sea salt
⅔ cup / 160 ml fresh lime juice
1 tsp / 5 ml hot sauce

**HOW TO MAKE IT»**

**1.** Combine all ingredients in a large bowl.
**2.** Mix well and adjust salt, lime juice and hot sauce to taste.
**3.** Serve!

**NUTRITIONAL VALUE FOR HALF-CUP SERVING:**
Calories: 110 | Calories from Fat: 26 | Total Fat: 3 g | Saturated Fat: 0.5 g | Total Carbs: 18 g | Fiber: 3 g | Protein: 3.6 g | Sodium: 254 mg | Cholesterol: 0 mg

**Preparation time:** 15 minutes
**Cooking time:** 0 minutes
**Yield:** 6 cups

# SHARK 'N BAKE

In Trinidad and Tobago, locals flock to roadside stands for this favorite. Made with shark meat, this meal is a great fish and chips alternative. If you can't find shark, try catfish or another firm-fleshed fish.

### WHAT YOU'LL NEED»

Juice from 2 fresh limes – set the unpeeled limes in a cup of hot water to release the juices more readily
1 lb / 454 g shark meat, cut into strips about 1 x 4 inches, or 2½ x 10 cm
1 clove garlic, minced
2 Tbsp / 30 ml chopped green onions
1 tsp / 5 ml finely chopped fresh thyme
1 tsp / 5 ml sea salt
2 cups / 480 ml spelt flour seasoned with 1 tsp / 5ml sea salt, 1 Tbsp / 15 ml black pepper and a pinch of red pepper flakes
Eat-Clean Cooking Spray (see below)

### EAT-CLEAN COOKING SPRAY

Cooking sprays such as Pam and others are very handy, but we have become concerned about the presence of isobutane as an ingredient. Our solution is to put healthy oils such as extra-virgin olive oil inside a spritz bottle, and simply spritz our pans and baking sheets when ready to use. Voilà! Healthy Eat-Clean cooking spray with no questionable ingredients.

### HOW TO MAKE IT»

**1.** Preheat oven to 350°F / 177°C.

**2.** Prepare baking sheet with a layer of parchment paper.

**3.** Place shark meat in a medium-sized glass bowl and cover with lime juice squeezed from fresh limes. Let sit for several minutes.

**4.** In a small bowl combine garlic, chives, thyme and sea salt and mix. Set aside.

**5.** In another medium bowl place flour and seasonings. Mix well and set aside.

**6.** Using paper towel, pat the shark meat dry. Dip each piece in the spice mixture first, then the flour mixture. Place on baking sheet.

**7.** Coat the seasoned shark pieces lightly with a mist of Eat-Clean Cooking Spray and bake in the oven for 15 minutes. Shark pieces should be golden brown and fairly firm to touch.

**8.** Serve in a warmed wrap or corn tortilla along with chopped fresh veggies and herbed yogurt cheese if desired.

**NUTRITIONAL VALUE FOR ONE SERVING WITHOUT WRAP, VEGGIES OR YOGURT CHEESE:**
Calories: 203 | Calories from Fat: 48 | Total Fat: 5.4 g | Saturated Fat: 1.1 g | Total Carbs: 12.5 g | Fiber: 2 g | Protein: 26 g | Sodium: 484 mg | Cholesterol: 58 mg

**Preparation time:** 10 minutes
**Cooking time:** 15 minutes
**Yield:** 4 servings

**TIP** Shark and Bake is usually served with a "bake," which is a thin, fried bread – not exactly Clean! But you can serve the shark in small, warmed wraps or corn tortillas for a healthy alternative.

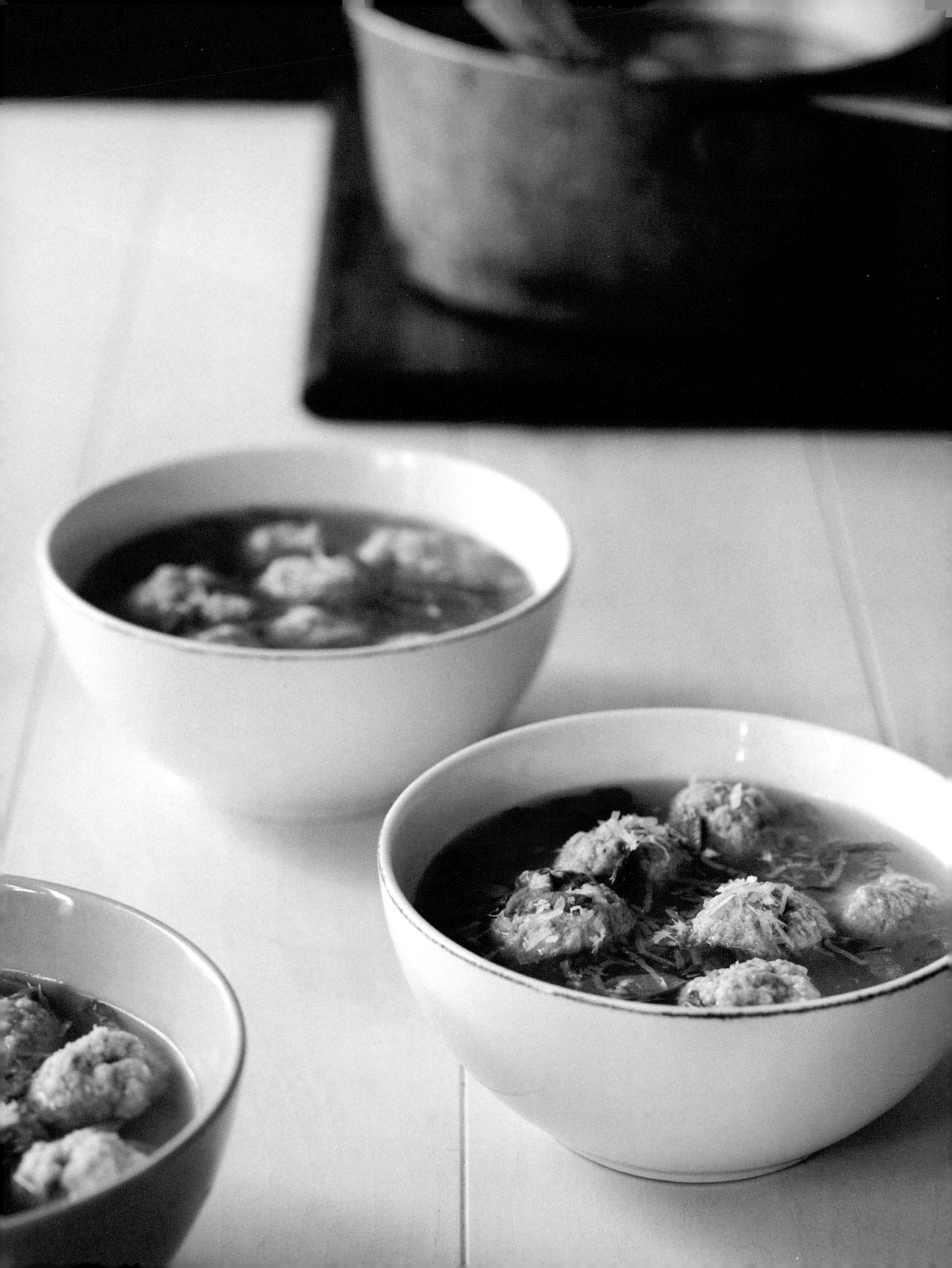

# ITALIAN WEDDING SOUP

You don't have to be either Italian or getting married to enjoy this delicious soup. Its ancestry is from southern Italy, though the soup itself actually hails from the Italian districts of Northeastern US.

**WHAT YOU'LL NEED»**

1 lb / 454 g extra-lean ground turkey breast
2 eggs, beaten
¾ cup / 180 ml oat bran
3 Tbsp / 45 ml freshly grated parmesan cheese, divided
2 Tbsp / 30 ml minced fresh basil
3 Tbsp / 45 ml minced onion
8 cups / 2 L low-sodium chicken stock
2 cups / 480 ml spinach, rinsed, packed and thinly chopped
¾ cup / 180 ml diced carrots

**HOW TO MAKE IT»**

**1.** In a medium bowl, combine the turkey, eggs, oat bran, 2 tablespoons of parmesan cheese, basil and onion. Shape mixture into ¾-inch / 2-cm balls and set aside.

**2.** In a large stockpot, heat chicken broth to boiling. Stir in spinach, carrots and meatballs. Return to boil; reduce heat to medium. Cook, stirring frequently, at a slow boil for 10 minutes – until the meatballs are no longer pink.

**3.** Serve hot with the rest of the parmesan cheese sprinkled on top.

**NUTRITIONAL VALUE FOR ONE CUP OF SOUP:**
Calories: 153 | Calories from Fat: 61 | Total Fat: 7 g | Saturated Fat: 2 g | Total Carbs: 9 g | Fiber: 2 g | Protein: 17 g | Sodium: 609 mg | Cholesterol: 85 mg

**Preparation time:** 40 minutes
**Cooking time:** 30 – 40 minutes
**Yield:** 8 cups

# ROPA VIEJA

The name of this Cuban dish translates into "old clothes." The story goes that a man was so poor he could not feed his family. He went to his closet, shredded his clothes and cooked them, and his love for his family transformed the clothes into this tasty, meaty dish. We've made it a little more nutritious by adding some peppers and carrots. Enjoy our Clean version of this traditional Cuban dish with brown rice, or for some real Caribbean flavor, try it with Black Beans and Rice (page 261).

### WHAT YOU'LL NEED»

3 lbs / 1,350 g flank steak, trimmed
8 cups / 2 L beef broth
2 cups / 480 ml coarsely chopped carrots
1 bay leaf
6 garlic cloves, pressed or minced
1 tsp / 5 ml dried oregano
1 tsp / 5 ml sea salt
¼ tsp / 1¼ ml whole black peppercorns
2 green bell peppers, cut into strips
2 red bell peppers, cut into strips
2 yellow bell peppers, cut into strips
2 large carrots, sliced
1 red onion, sliced
2 chilies, minced
4 Tbsp / 60 ml best-quality olive oil, separated
1 x 14 oz / 398 ml can diced tomatoes
3 Tbsp / 45 ml tomato paste
1 tsp / 5 ml ground cumin
½ cup / 120 ml chopped fresh parsley

**Preparation time:** 30 minutes
**Cooling time:** 30 minutes
**Cooking time:** 2 hours
**Yield:** 10 cups

**NUTRITIONAL VALUE FOR ONE-CUP SERVING WITHOUT RICE:**

Calories: 291 | Calories from Fat: 102 | Total Fat: 11 g | Saturated Fat: 4 g | Total Carbs: 8 g | Fiber: 2 g | Protein: 38 g | Sodium: 179 mg | Cholesterol: 86 mg

### HOW TO MAKE IT»

**1.** Combine meat, broth, carrots, bay leaf, oregano, salt, pepper and half of the garlic in a large saucepan. Simmer, uncovered, for 1½ hours or until beef is tender. Remove from heat and let cool for 30 minutes.

**2.** Remove meat from the liquid and set aside. Strain solids from liquid through a strainer. Return liquid to pot and simmer until reduced to 3 cups – about 30 minutes. Discard solids and chill liquid in the refrigerator.

**3.** In a large saucepan heat 2 Tbsp / 30 ml olive oil over moderate heat and cook green bell peppers, chilies and onion, stirring, until softened.

**4.** Meanwhile, pull the meat into shreds. Add the shredded meat to the onion mixture along with 2 cups / 480 ml of the simmered liquid, tomatoes with juice, tomato paste, cumin, parsley, salt, pepper and the rest of the garlic. Simmer, uncovered, for 20 minutes.

**5.** While meat is simmering, in a skillet sauté red and yellow bell peppers and carrots in 2 Tbsp / 30 ml olive oil over moderate heat, stirring occasionally, until softened. Stir peppers into stew with enough additional liquid to thin to desired consistency, and simmer uncovered for 5 minutes.

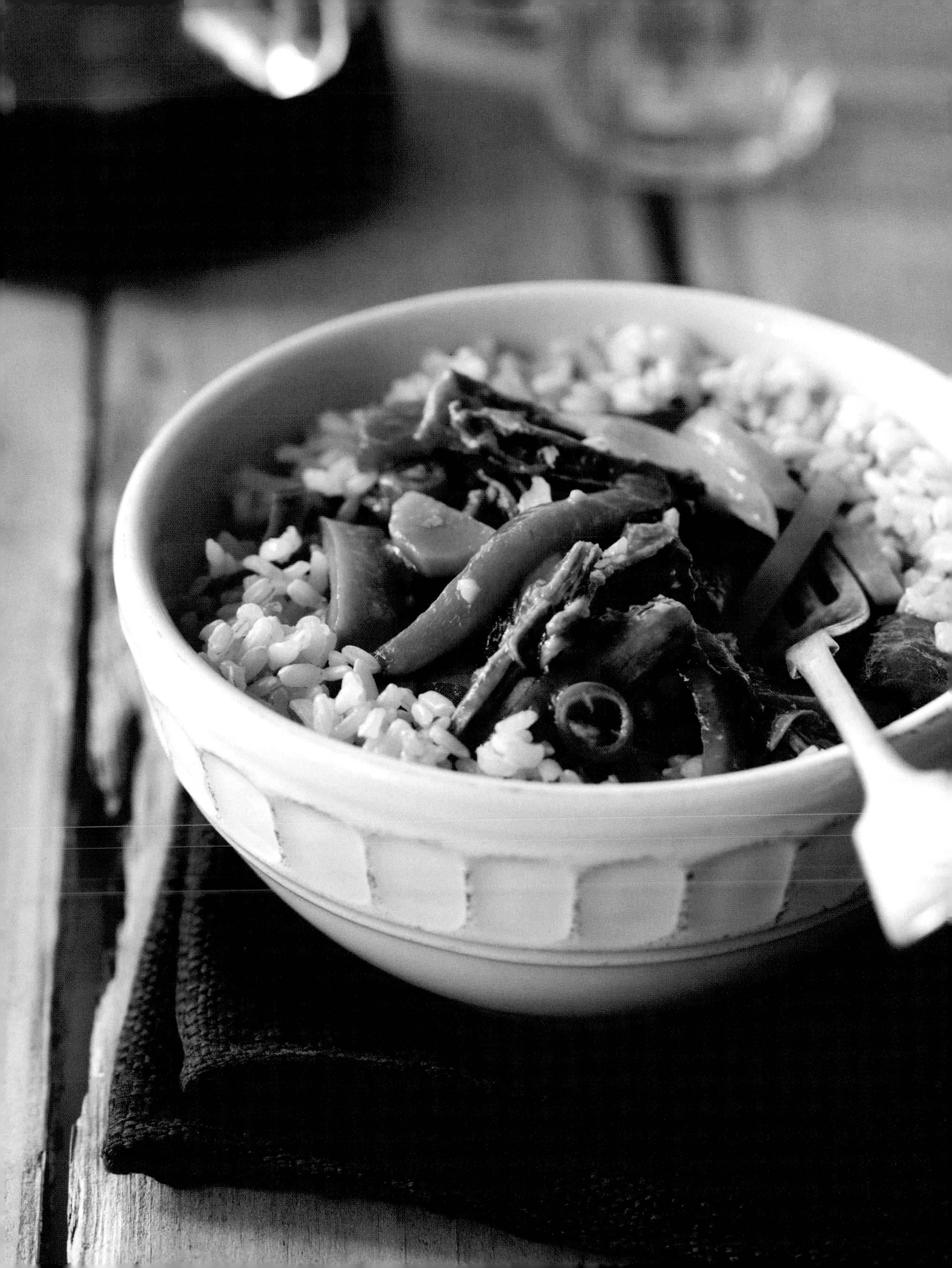

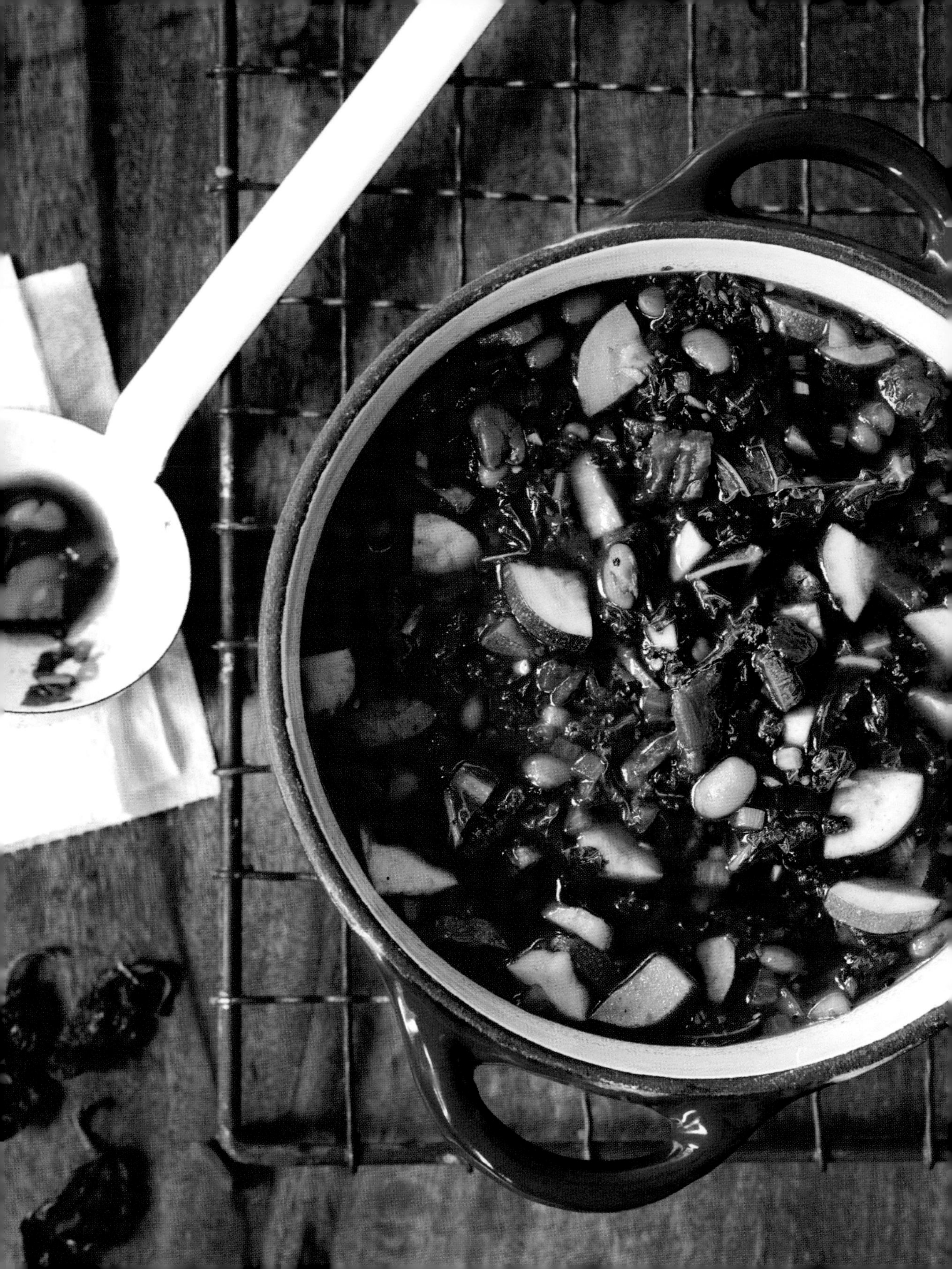

# MOLE MOLE SOUP

Most of us know mole as a Mexican sauce made with chilies, spices and chocolate. Here's a new idea – take the same sauce and turn it into a rich, spicy soup. Olé!

### WHAT YOU'LL NEED»

2 medium ancho chilies, wiped clean
1 dried chipotle chili, wiped clean
1 tsp / 5 ml cumin seeds, toasted and cooled
1 tsp / 5 ml dried oregano, crumbled
1 tsp / 5 ml cinnamon
1½ tsp / 7½ ml sea salt
2 medium onions, chopped
3 Tbsp / 45 ml best-quality olive oil
4 garlic cloves, pressed or minced
3 medium zucchini, quartered lengthwise and cut into ½-inch / 1-cm pieces
¾ lb / 340 g kale leaves, coarsely chopped
Zest of one orange
1 tsp / 5 ml agave nectar
1 oz / 30 ml unsweetened chocolate, finely chopped
1 x 14 oz / 398 ml can whole tomatoes, chopped – save juice
1¼ cups / 300 ml water
3 x 14 oz / 398 ml cans pinto beans

**NUTRITIONAL VALUE FOR ONE CUP:**
Calories: 268 | Calories from Fat: 73 | Total Fat: 8 g | Saturated Fat: 2 g | Total Carbs: 41 g | Fiber: 10 g | Protein: 11 g | Sodium: 766 mg | Cholesterol: 0 mg

### HOW TO MAKE IT»

**1.** Slit chilies lengthwise, then stem and seed. Heat a dry, heavy, medium-sized skillet over medium until hot. Open the chilies until they are flat, then toast, turning and pressing with tongs, until pliable and slightly changed in color, about 30 seconds. Chop into small pieces. Don't touch your eyes!

**2.** Pulse cumin seeds and chilies in a grinder until finely ground. Transfer to a small bowl and stir in the oregano, cinnamon and sea salt.

**3.** Heat oil in a large pot over medium-high heat. Add onions and cook, stirring occasionally, until translucent. Add garlic and cook, stirring, for 1 minute. Add chili mixture and cook, stirring, for 30 seconds. Stir in zucchini and kale and cook, covered, for 5 minutes. Add orange zest, agave nectar, tomatoes with their juice, and water. Simmer, covered, stirring occasionally, until vegetables are tender – about 15 to 20 minutes.

**4.** Stir in beans and simmer for 5 minutes. Season with salt.

**Preparation time:** 25 minutes
**Cooking time:** 50 minutes
**Yield:** 8 cups

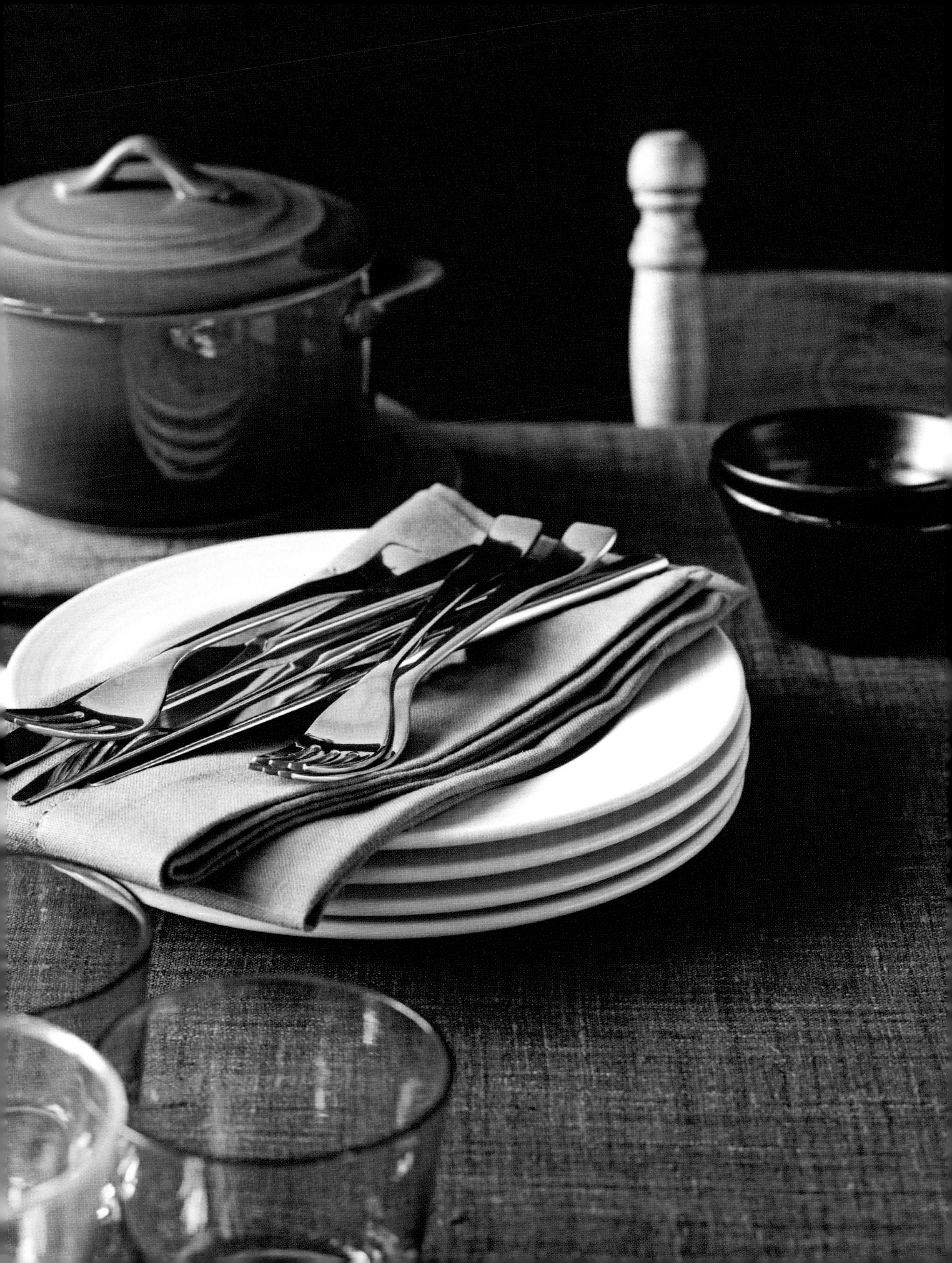

# DINNER

Real estate success is said to be determined by these three words: "Location, location, location!" In our opinion weight-loss success is determined by these three words: "Selection, selection, selection!" And to that end, we offer you dishes for every occasion, whether that means making a big pot of chili for you and the guys, a barbecued turkey (yes!) for the family or a lovely light pasta for a special evening.

# RISKY BUSINESS BBQ RIBS

There's nothing like digging into a rack of tender, juicy ribs, and doing them on the barbecue is best. You'll be licking your fingers after eating a helping of these!

### WHAT YOU'LL NEED»

2 lb / 908 g beef ribs

¼ cup / 60 ml agave nectar

2 Tbsp / 30 ml maple syrup

2 Tbsp / 30 ml unsulfured blackstrap molasses

1 tsp / 5 ml paprika

1 tsp / 5 ml coriander seed

1 tsp / 5 ml chili powder (not chili pepper!)

1 tsp / 5 ml oregano

½ tsp / 2½ ml sea salt

½ tsp / 2½ ml freshly ground black pepper

4 garlic cloves, pressed or minced

1½ cups / 360 ml low-sodium beef broth, divided

**Preparation time:** 10 minutes
**Cooking time:** 1¾ hours
**Yield:** 8 servings

**NUTRITIONAL VALUE FOR ONE SERVING:**
Calories: 290 | Calories from Fat: 127 | Total Fat: 5.6 g | Saturated Fat: 11.6 g | Total Carbs: 0.5 g | Fiber: 3 g | Protein: 28 g | Sodium: 162 mg | Cholesterol: 80 mg

### HOW TO MAKE IT»

1. Pre-heat barbecue to medium high.
2. Combine maple syrup, molasses, paprika, coriander, chili powder, oregano, salt, pepper and garlic in a large bowl. Stir in half of the broth.
3. Tear a piece of tinfoil that is long and wide enough to completely cover the meat if wrapped around. Lay ribs on top. Fold the foil up enough to make a tray or bowl around the meat, and pour maple syrup mixture over top of the ribs. Fold the foil up completely, securing the ends and top tight so no liquid can escape.
4. Reduce heat to medium low and place pouch on the grill. Close the lid and slowly braise for 1½ hours or to your liking – until ribs are tender.
5. Remove package from grill and open carefully to let steam escape. Remove ribs and place on a platter or baking sheet. Pour ½ cup / 120 ml of the cooking juices into a saucepan and bring to a boil. Remove from heat and stir in unused grilling sauce.
6. Place ribs right on the grill on medium-high heat until ribs are glazed about 10 minutes – turning and glazing with grilling sauce mixture until the sauce is gone.
7. Cut the ribs into eight pieces.

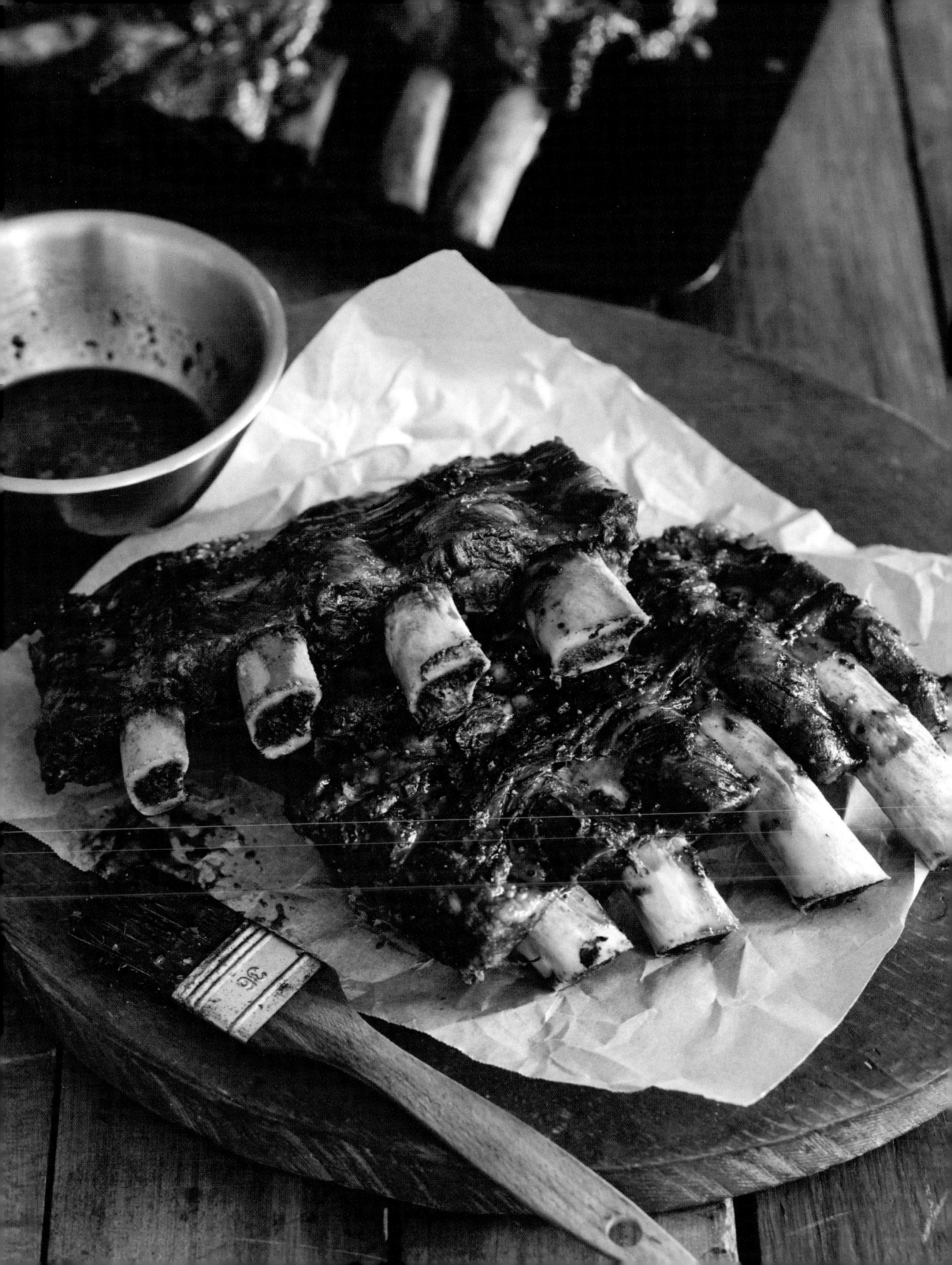

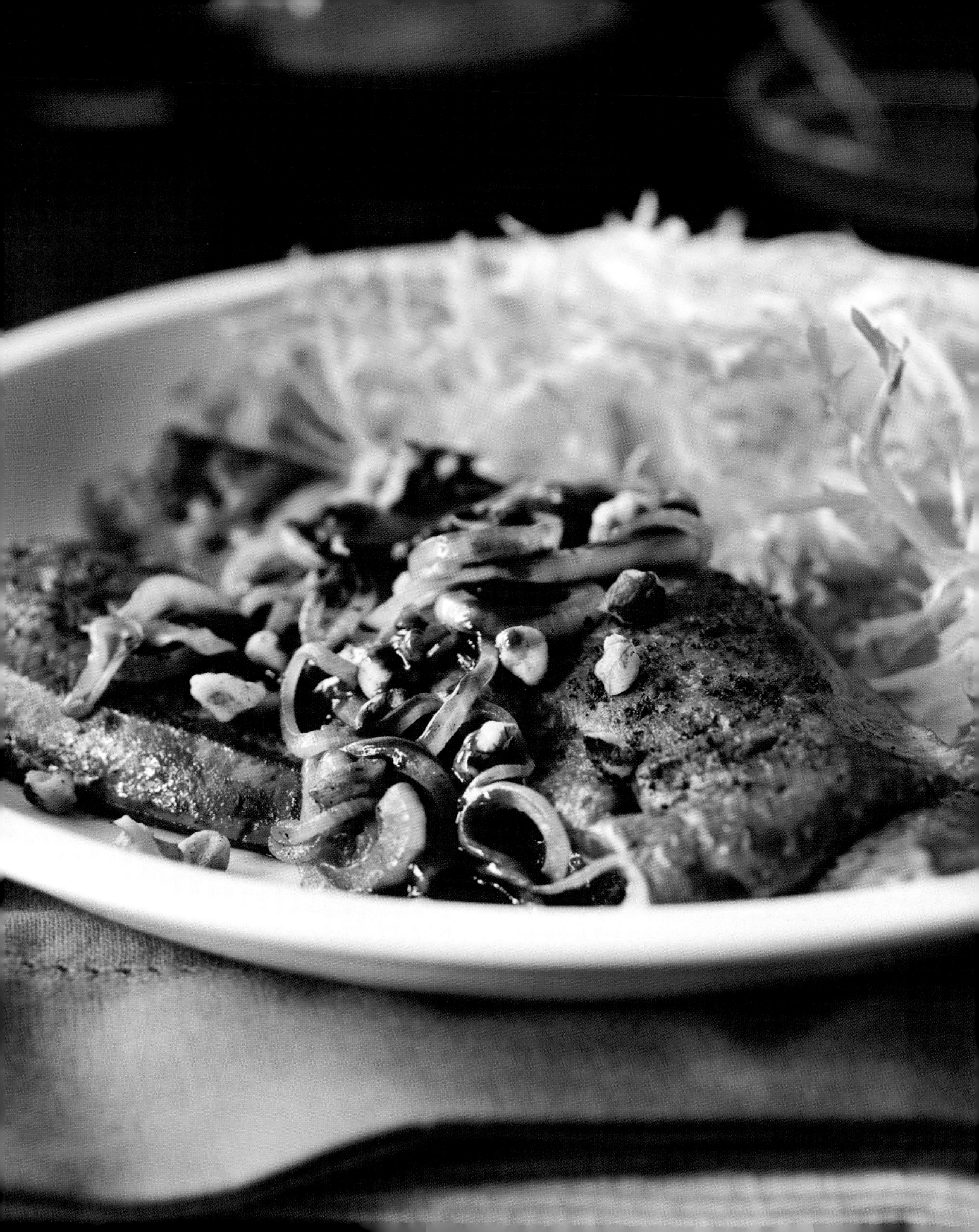

# LIVER AND CARAMELIZED ONIONS

Lots of men love a hefty plate of liver and onions. It is such a favorite it appears on practically every diner (that's diner, not dinner) menu. Here is a Clean recipe for your very own kitchen – with healthy fats from walnuts and olive oil instead of the thick blobs of trans fats normally used in diners!

### WHAT YOU'LL NEED »

¼ cup / 60 ml chopped walnuts
2 Tbsp / 30 ml best-quality olive oil, divided
1 large onion, thinly sliced
¼ tsp / 1½ ml ground cloves, divided
½ lb / 225 g beef calf liver
¼ cup / 60 ml balsamic vinegar
1 Tbsp / 15 ml butter
Sea salt
Freshly ground black pepper

**Preparation time:** 15 minutes
**Cooking time:** 20 minutes
**Yield:** 2 servings

**NUTRITIONAL VALUE FOR ONE SERVING:**
Calories: 494 | Calories from Fat: 271 | Total Fat: 30 g | Saturated Fat:7 g | Total Carbs: 16 g | Fiber: 2 g | Protein: 28 g | Sodium: 273 mg | Cholesterol: 644 mg

### HOW TO MAKE IT »

1. Stir walnuts in a large skillet over medium heat until slightly darker in color – about 2 minutes. Transfer nuts to a small bowl and set aside.
2. Melt 1 tablespoon of olive oil in same skillet over medium heat. Add onion and sauté until golden brown – about 10 minutes. If you love onions don't hold back – we say one, but cut up as many as you like. They taste incredible caramelized this way.
3. Add half the ground cloves and sauté for a minute longer. Season with sea salt and fresh black pepper to taste. Transfer onions to a plate using a slotted spoon. This allows the oil to drip out.
4. Melt remaining tablespoon of olive oil along with the butter in the same skillet over medium-high heat
5. Sprinkle liver with remaining cloves, salt and pepper. Add liver to the skillet and cook until brown on outside but still pink in the center, about 2 minutes per side. Transfer liver to two plates. Add balsamic vinegar, walnuts and onion to same skillet and cook, stirring, for 1 minute. Spoon onion mixture on top of liver. Serve and enjoy!

# LAZY SUNDAY VENISON STEW

This tasty and low-fat dish is perfect for a lazy Sunday. Prep all the ingredients early in the day and let it cook while you relax. Double the recipe and store extra in smaller containers in the freezer and you have an instant dinner ready for another lazy day.

### WHAT YOU'LL NEED »

4 large venison steaks
2 Tbsp / 30 ml best-quality olive oil
1 yellow onion, peeled and cubed
1 leek, chopped, tough dark ends removed
2 celery stalks, chopped
4 garlic cloves, pressed or minced
2 Tbsp / 30 ml dried thyme
1 Tbsp / 15 ml sea salt
2 Tbsp / 30 ml freshly ground black pepper
4 sweet potatoes, peeled and cubed
1 large handful of white button mushrooms
2 jalapeno peppers, seeded and chopped finely
5 carrots, chopped into chunks
Enough low-sodium beef broth to cover the vegetables

### HOW TO MAKE IT »

1. Cut the venison into bite-sized pieces. Heat oil in a large stockpot on medium heat. Brown venison pieces lightly.
2. Add onion, leek, celery and garlic, drizzling in a little more oil if needed. Stir well. When onions turn translucent, add the thyme, sea salt and black pepper.
3. Add the sweet potatoes, mushrooms, jalapeno peppers and carrots to the stockpot. Add the broth. Bring to a boil and let simmer for two hours while you watch the game.
4. Serve over brown rice, or warm some crusty whole-grain bread in the oven and serve alongside.

**NUTRITIONAL VALUE FOR TWO-CUP SERVING:**
Calories: 250 | Calories from Fat: 85 | Total Fat: 9.5 g | Saturated Fat: 3 g | Total Carbs: 25 g | Fiber: 5 g | Protein: 17.5 g | Sodium: 907 mg | Cholesterol: 54 mg

**Preparation time:** 40 minutes
**Cooking time:** 2 hours
**Yield:** 7 servings

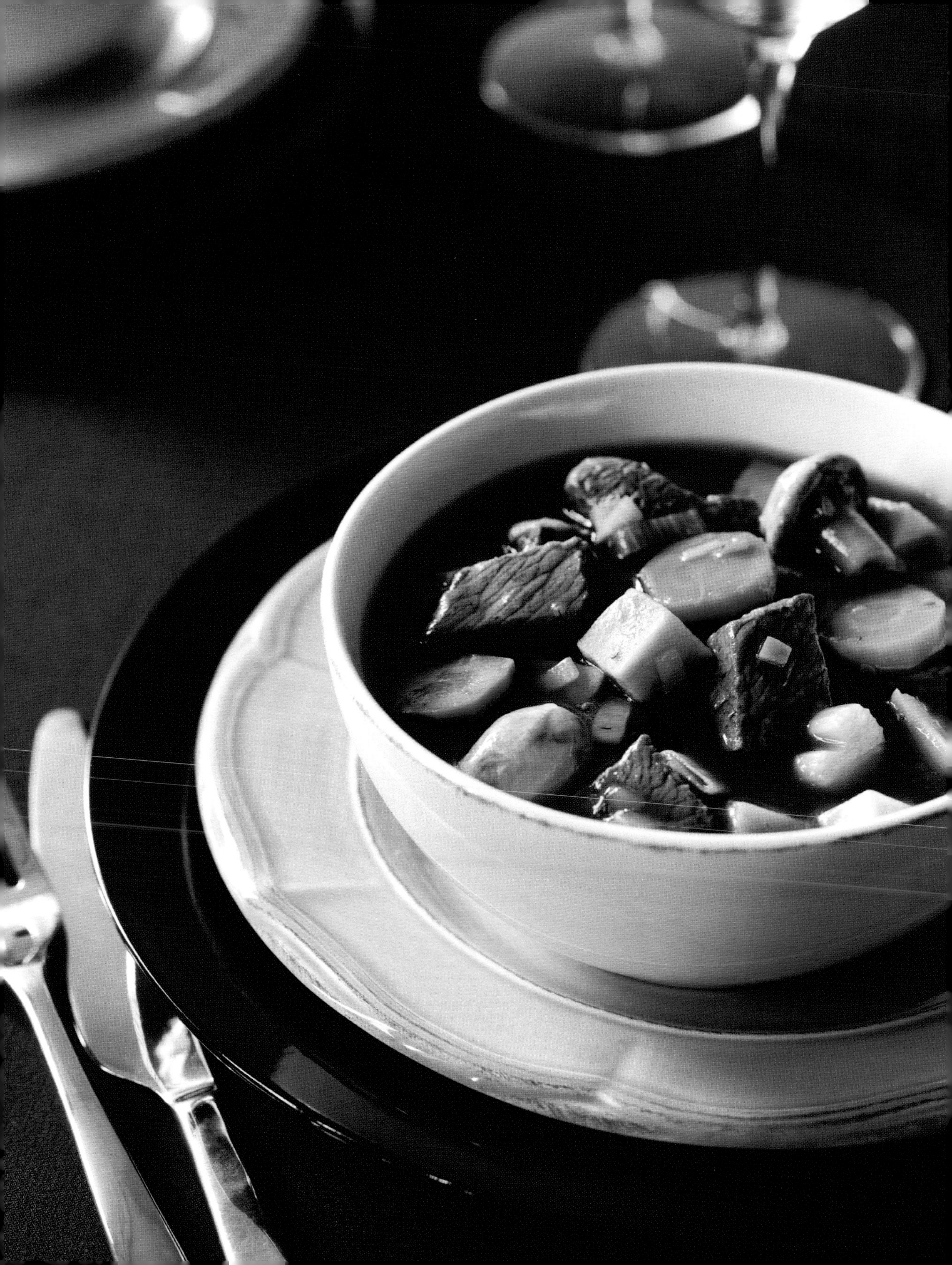

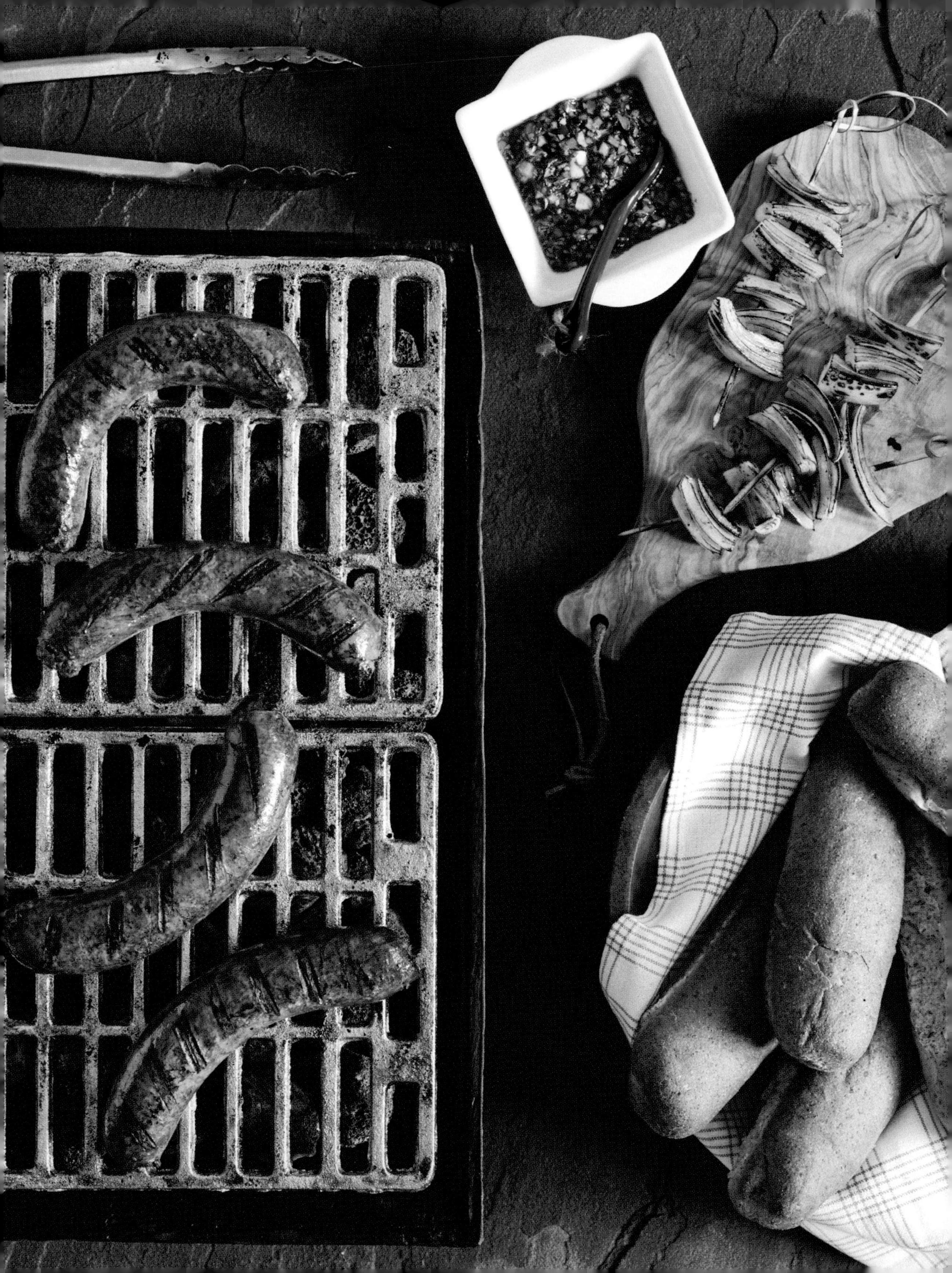

# SIZZLE YOUR SAUSAGE
## WITH SPICY CHILI PEPPER SAUCE

We thought that title would get your attention! This recipe brings sausage on a bun to a whole new level – for taste and for health. Just be sure you put the sauce away rather than leaving it on the table, or you'll be reaching for more buns to sop it up with!

### WHAT YOU'LL NEED»

4 bison, elk or venison sausages

1 Vidalia or other sweet onion, cut in large chunks

4 Ezekiel, spelt, kamut or other whole-grain buns

½ cup / 120 ml Cilantro Chili Pepper Sauce

### HOW TO MAKE IT»

1. Begin by preparing your chili pepper sauce – see recipe below.
2. Grill the sausage over indirect medium heat until browned (18 to 25 minutes). Turn the meat occasionally, until the juices run clear. While the meat is cooking, place the onion wedges onto skewers and grill until they turn translucent.
3. Lightly toast the buns on the grill – put them on about 5 minutes before the meat is done, and watch carefully!
4. Spread the toasted bun on both sides with cilantro chili pepper sauce, assemble the sausage and onions on top and enjoy served with sliced raw vegetables – carrot, celery or cucumber.

**NUTRITIONAL VALUE FOR ONE SAUSAGE ON A BUN WITH TWO TBSP OF SAUCE:**

Calories: 311 | Calories from Fat: 116 | Total Fat: 13 g | Saturated Fat: 6 g | Total Carbs: 24 g | Fiber: 3.7 g | Protein: 27 g | Sodium: 627 mg | Cholesterol: 0 mg

**Preparation time:** 10 minutes
**Cooking time:** 18– 25 minutes
**Yield:** 4 servings

## CILANTRO CHILI PEPPER SAUCE

### WHAT YOU'LL NEED»

3 fresh **chili peppers**, seeded and minced

1 Tbsp / 15 ml **sesame oil**

3 **garlic cloves**, pressed or minced

1 pinch **sea salt**

½ cup / 120 ml **malt vinegar**

2 Tbsp / 30 ml **fish sauce**

2 Tbsp / 30 ml **honey**

3 Tbsp / 45 ml **low-sodium soy sauce**

1 tsp / 5 ml **fresh lime juice**

1 bunch **cilantro**, chopped finely

1 **cooking onion**, minced

### HOW TO MAKE IT»

**1.** Combine all ingredients in a bowl. Cover and refrigerate. Keeps for a few days.

**Preparation time:** 10 minutes
**Yield:** 1 ½ cups

# THEY SAY SHE'S FROM "CHILI"

Chili and football just go together, somehow. But chili doesn't have to be the artery-clogging dish it usually is. Here's a recipe to keep you satisfied and healthy. Before long you'll have so much energy from Eating Clean you'll be back on the field *playing* football in addition to watching it on Monday nights.

**WHAT YOU'LL NEED»**

2 lbs / 900 g lean ground bison
2 Tbsp / 30 ml best-quality olive oil
1 medium yellow onion, chopped
1 head of garlic, roasted (see page 292)
1 large carrot, peeled and grated
1½ cups / 360 ml chopped sweet red bell pepper
3 medium poblano chilies, seeded and chopped
3 medium jalapeño chilies, seeded and chopped
2 Tbsp / 30 ml cumin seeds
3 Tbsp / 45 ml chili powder (not chili pepper!)
¼ tsp / 1½ ml red pepper flakes
3 x 14 oz / 398 ml cans of diced tomatoes
1 cup / 240 ml canned red kidney beans, drained and rinsed
1 cup / 240 ml canned white kidney beans, drained and rinsed
1 cup / 240 ml canned great northern beans, drained and rinsed
1 cup / 240 ml canned corn kernels, drained and rinsed
4 squares dark chocolate, 75% cocoa (preferably Chilean)
2½ cups / 600 ml vegetable stock
2 Tbsp / 30 ml unsulfured blackstrap molasses
Juice of one fresh lime
Juice of one fresh lemon
½ cup / 120 ml beer
2 tsp / 10 ml basil
2 tsp / 10 ml oregano
Sea salt to taste
Freshly ground black pepper to taste

**HOW TO MAKE IT»**

1. In a large saucepan or Dutch oven, heat olive oil over medium heat. Add onion, grated carrot, garlic and bison. Cook until meat is lightly browned and onions are translucent.
2. Stir in peppers, chilies, chili powder, cumin seeds, red pepper flakes, sea salt and black pepper. Cover and cook over low heat for 10 minutes.
3. Stir in the remaining ingredients. Blend well. Cover and let simmer for 20 minutes. Remove from heat and serve immediately. This dish can be served over brown rice or baked sweet potato, or alongside a thick slice of sprouted-grain bread.

**NUTRITIONAL VALUE FOR ONE CUP:**
Calories: 338 | Calories from Fat: 48 | Total Fat: 5 g | Saturated Fat: 1 g | Total Carbs: 30 g | Fiber: 6.5 g | Protein: 20 g | Sodium: 880 | Cholesterol: 53 mg

**Preparation time:** 15 minutes
**Cooking time:** 45 minutes
**Yield:** 12 cups

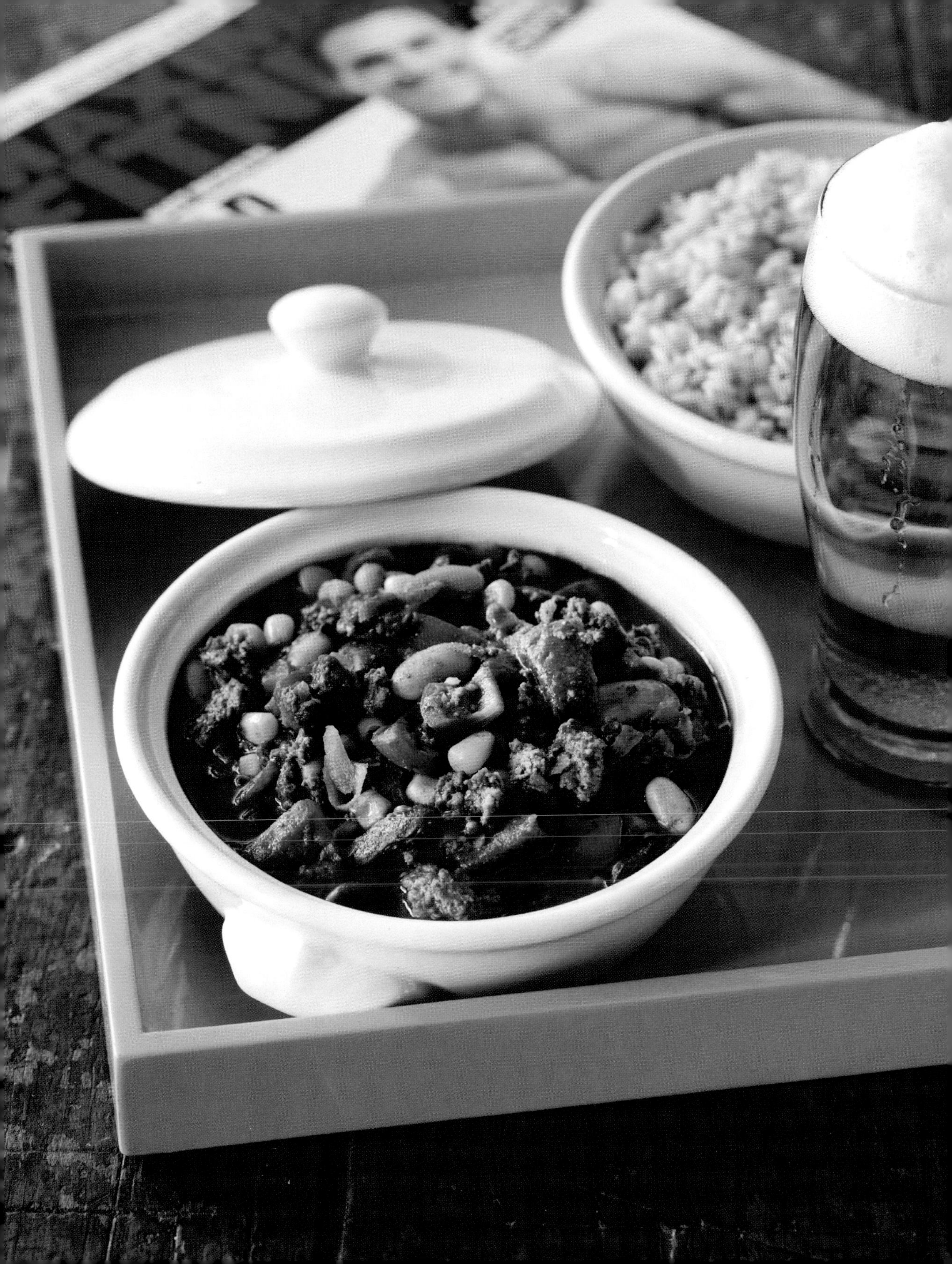

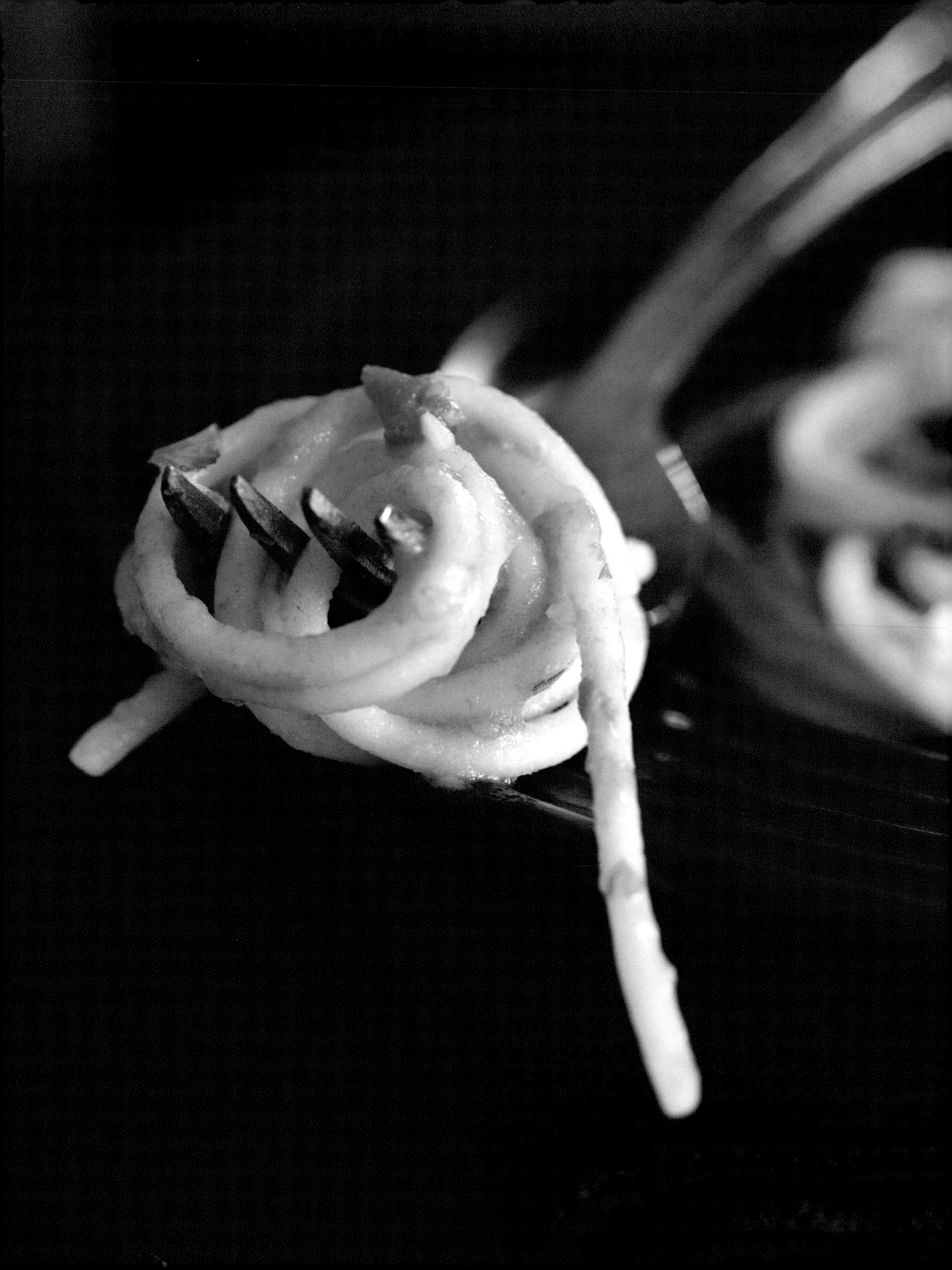

# PASTA LEGERRO

The perfect main course for a romantic vegetarian dinner. Impress her with your thoughtfulness, and give both of you some Clean energy for the night ahead. Pasta is, after all, considered the perfect food for an evening of passion.

### THE RED SAUCE»

3 cups / 720 ml cherry tomatoes, halved
2 cups / 480 ml roma tomatoes, sliced and halved
2 cups / 480 ml low-sodium vegetable stock
1 medium sweet potato, peeled and diced
4 Tbsp / 60 ml white wine, separated
2 Tbsp / 30 ml best-quality olive oil
½ cup / 120 ml rice milk
½ tsp / 2½ ml sea salt
½ tsp / 2½ ml freshly ground black pepper

### THE PASTA»

¼ lb / 115 g brown rice spaghetti noodles
2 Tbsp / 30 ml best-quality olive oil
2 garlic cloves, pressed or minced
¼ cup / 60 ml parsley

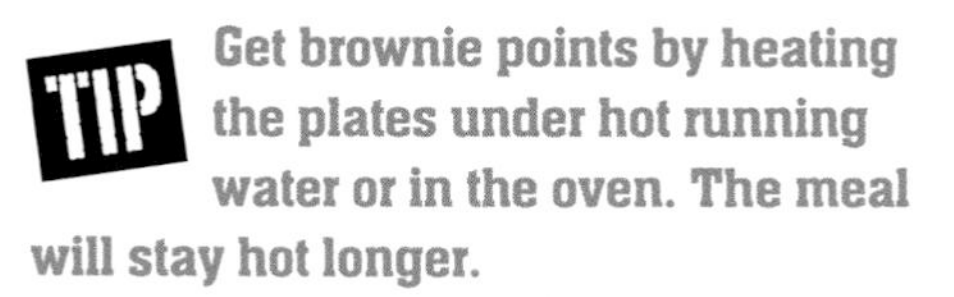

**TIP** Get brownie points by heating the plates under hot running water or in the oven. The meal will stay hot longer.

**NUTRITIONAL VALUE FOR ONE CUP OF PASTA WITH HALF CUP OF SAUCE:**
Calories: 280 | Calories from Fat: 43 | Total Fat: 5 g | Saturated Fat: 1.5 g | Total Carbs: 48 g | Fiber: 5.5 g | Protein: 6 g | Sodium: 122 mg | Cholesterol: 0 mg

### METHOD FOR SAUCE»

1. Sauté tomatoes in 2 Tbsp / 30 ml of olive oil over medium heat for 5 minutes.
2. Add vegetable stock and 2 Tbsp / 30 ml white wine along with the sweet potato. Simmer for 25 minutes.
3. Purée this tomato mix in a food processor and then put puréed mixture back in the pan. Add the rice milk. Add the rest of the white wine along with salt and freshly ground black pepper to taste.
4. Simmer for 2 to 3 minutes and remove from heat.

### METHOD FOR PASTA»

1. Bring a pot of water to boil and cook pasta.
2. Prepare garlic and parsley, and mix with olive oil.
3. When pasta is finished, strain it and put it in a large bowl. Toss with olive oil, garlic and parsley mixture until well distributed.
4. Divide the pasta in two bowls and ladle sauce over top. Sprinkle with salt and pepper to taste.

**Preparation time:** 30 minutes
**Cooking time:** 45 minutes
**Yield:** 2 servings

# SLEEPING ON THE COUCH TONIGHT **FIVE-BEAN STEW**

Don't let the title scare you. Sure, the after-effects of beans are well known, but they do pack a nutritional wallop, and done this way they taste amazingly good. Don't want to be relegated to the couch? Make sure your lovely lady eats some too, and you can make, ahem, beautiful music together!

### WHAT YOU'LL NEED»

1 Tbsp / 15 ml best-quality olive oil
1 large red onion, chopped
4 cloves garlic, pressed or minced
3 large carrots, grated
1 large leek, rinsed and chopped – discard tough dark green ends
1 Tbsp / 15 ml fresh thyme
1 tsp / 5 ml sea salt
1 tsp / 5 ml freshly ground black pepper
½ cup / 120 ml chopped fresh cilantro
1 x 15 oz / 445 ml can lima beans
1 x 15 oz / 445 ml can kidney beans
1 x 15 oz / 445 ml can pinto beans
1 x 15 oz / 445 ml can black beans
1 x 15 oz / 445 ml can cannellini beans, drained and rinsed
2 cups / 480 ml water
2 Tbsp / 30 ml rice vinegar
1 Tbsp / 15 ml honey
1 Tbsp / 15 ml Dijon mustard
4 Tbsp / 60 ml chopped fresh parsley, divided
Juice of one fresh lime

### HOW TO MAKE IT»

1. Sauté onion in olive oil in a large pot over medium-heat for about 5 minutes. Add garlic and sauté for about 5 minutes more. Add carrots and leek, and cook until softened. Add thyme, sea salt and black pepper and cook for a minute or so.
2. Add the beans – drain and rinse only the cannellini beans. Add vinegar, honey, mustard, water, cilantro and half of the parsley. Bring to a boil and reduce to a simmer over low heat. Cook, loosely covered so steam can escape, for 2 hours. Stir every so often.
3. Remove from the heat. Add lime juice and the rest of the parsley. Serve hot.

**Preparation time:** 20 minutes
**Cooking time:** 2½ hours
**Yield:** 10 cups

**NUTRITIONAL VALUE FOR ONE CUP:**
Calories: 216 | Calories from Fat: 23 | Total Fat: 2.6 g | Saturated Fat: 0.66 mg | Total Carbs: 38 g | Fiber: 10.5 g | Protein: 11 g | Sodium: 866 mg | Cholesterol: 0 mg

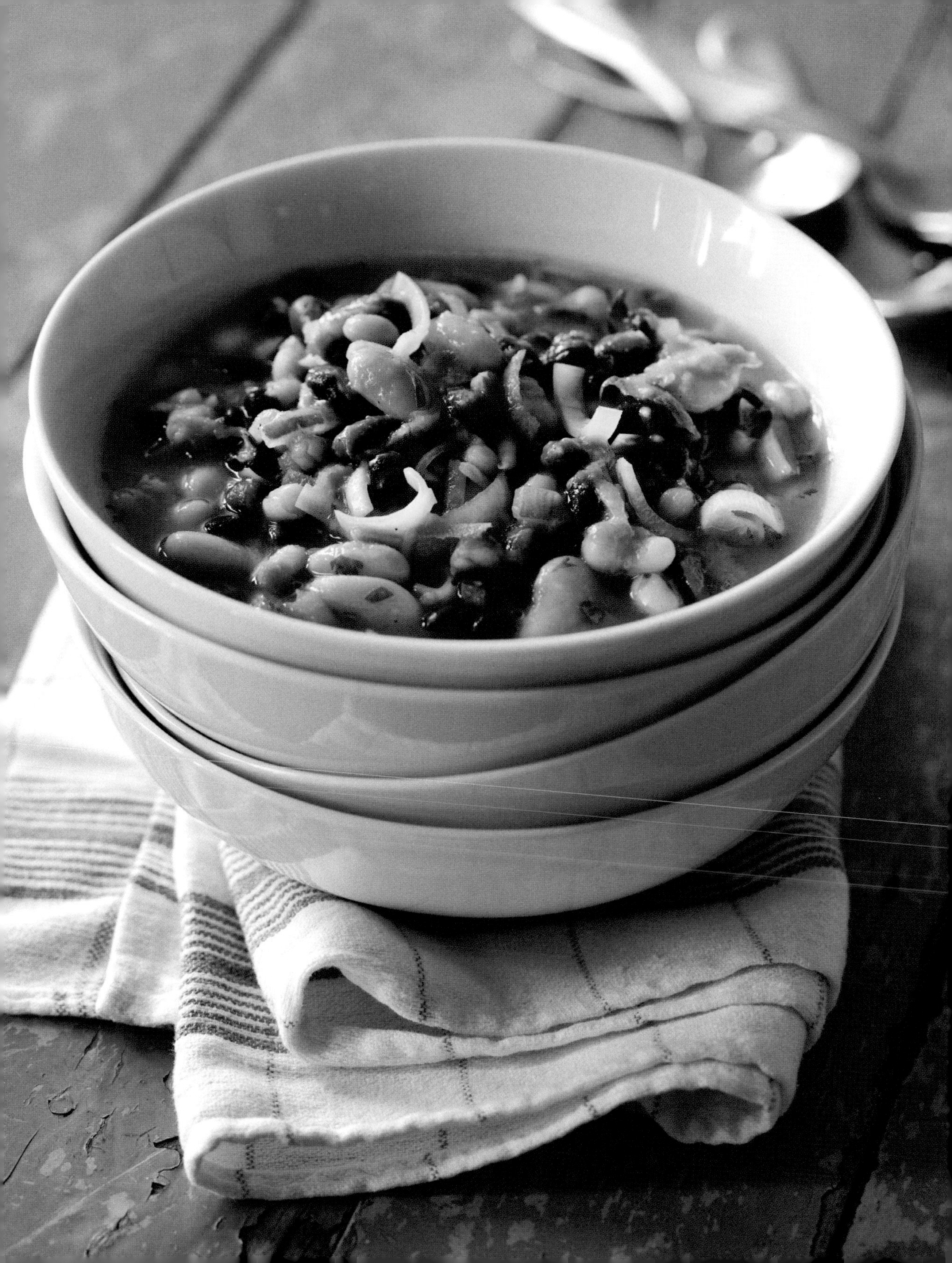

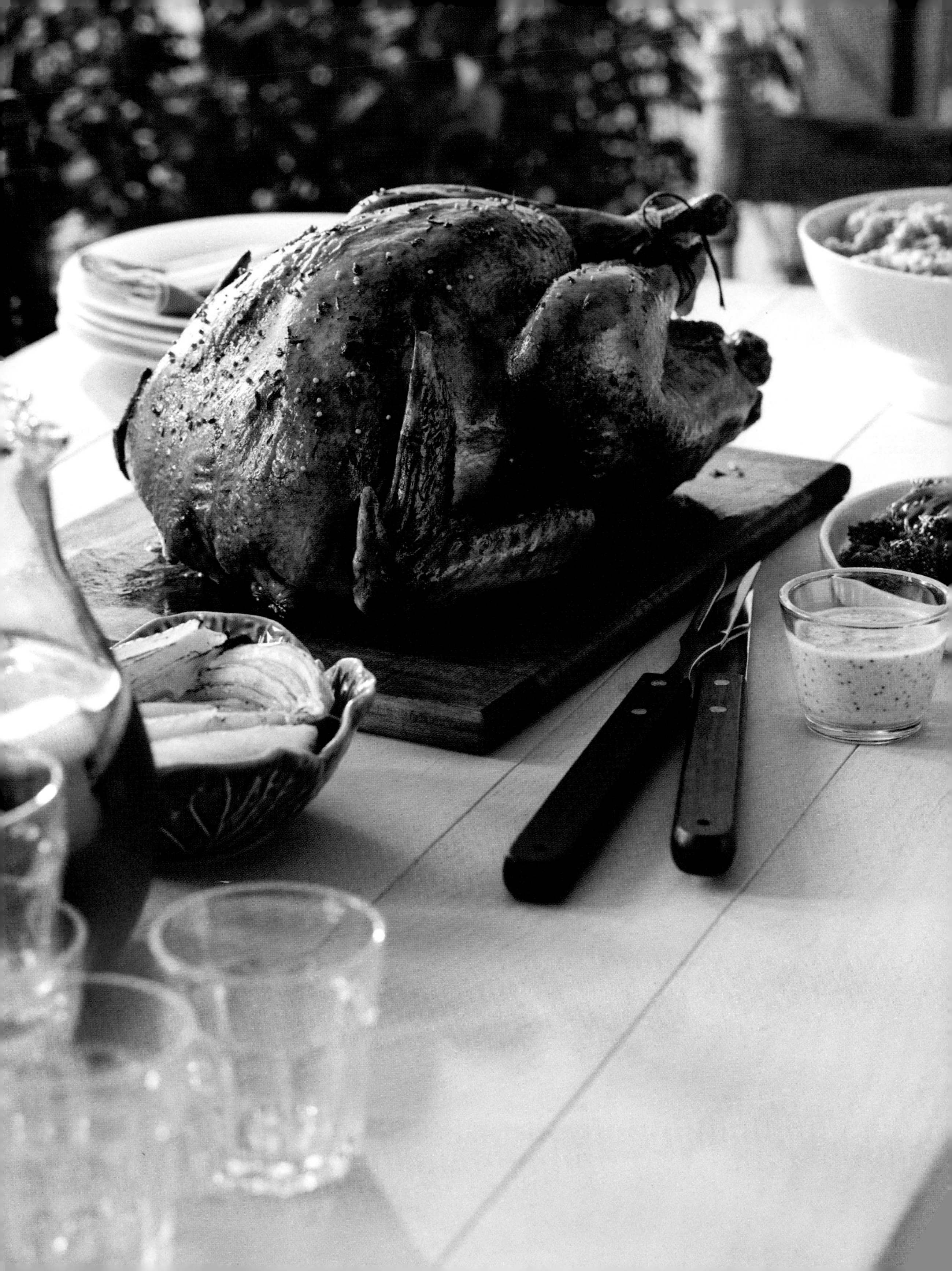

# BBQ ROASTED TURKEY

I have made turkey this way with my foodie brothers. They love the gutsy taste grilling adds to the bird. I like it because I don't have to clean up a dirty oven! Surprise your wife when you tell her you're cooking the turkey next Thanksgiving.

### WHAT YOU'LL NEED »

1 x 14 lb / 6.3 kg turkey
⅓ cup / 80 ml balsamic or white-wine vinegar
⅓ cup / 80 ml best-quality olive oil
2 Tbsp / 30 ml fresh rosemary
2 Tbsp / 30 ml fresh thyme
1 tsp / 5 ml Homemade Dijon mustard (recipe pg 226)

### HOW TO MAKE IT »

1. Remove neck and giblets. Rinse the entire turkey, inside and out. Pat dry. Skewer neck skin to back with metal skewers. Using kitchen string, tie the legs together and tie the wings to the body.
2. In a bowl, whisk together vinegar, oil, rosemary and mustard. Set aside.
3. Place foil drip pan under the barbeque grate. Heat one burner of a two-burner barbeque, or two outside burners of a three-burner barbeque to medium. Place turkey on greased grill over heated burners.
4. Close lid. Cook, brushing every 45 minutes with vinegar mixture. Monitor heat and keep temperature between 250°F and 300°F / 121°C - 148°C for 3½ to 4 hours or until meat thermometer inserted in thigh registers to 180°F / 82°C.
5. Transfer to a cutting board. Make a tent with foil over the bird and let stand for 20 minutes before carving.

**NUTRITIONAL VALUE FOR FOUR-OUNCE BREAST, WHITE MEAT, NO SKIN:**
Calories: 191 | Calories from Fat: 43 | Total Fat: 4.8 g | Saturated Fat: 0.9 g | Total Carbs: 0 g | Fiber: 0 g | Protein: 34.1 g | Sodium: 94 mg | Cholesterol: 97 mg

**Preparation time:** 30 minutes
**Cooking time:** 2 hours

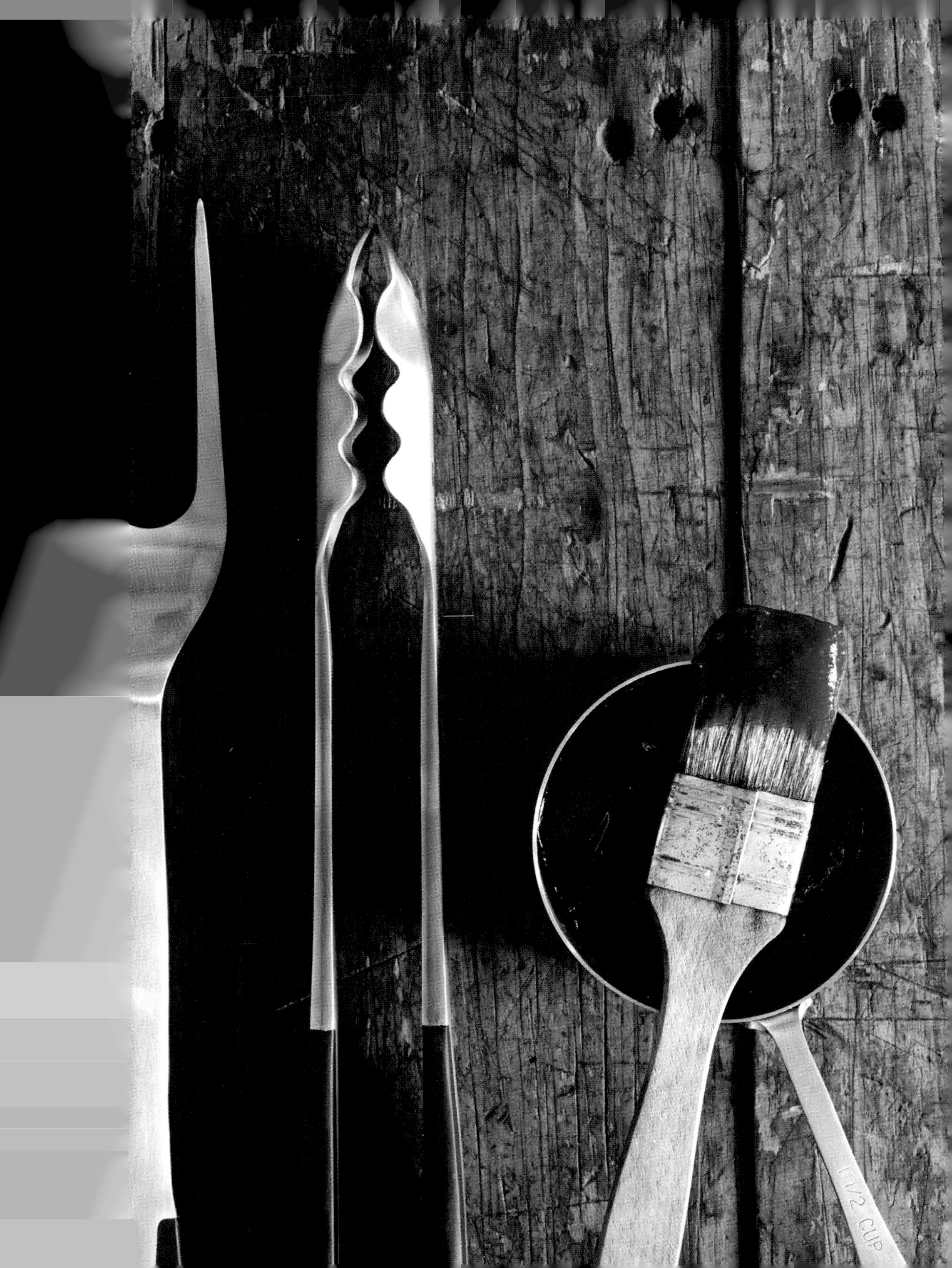
1 1/2 CUP

# GRILLING AND SNACKS

## The outdoor cooking experience

It's no secret that men love their grills. A man might not mind if a woman cooks at the stove, but if she gets near his barbecue, she'd better watch out! And while Eating Clean doesn't mean you have to give up your favorites, such as burgers and potato skins, there's no harm in testing your grilling skills with some cedar-plank salmon, either. Also in this section is some fare for men to share with their buddies during the game – wings and pizza, anyone?

# VEGETABLE GRILLING GUIDE

**Grilled veggies please even the staunchest vegetable hater. Here are some tips for perfect grilling.**

- Cut the veggies into pieces that will cook quickly and evenly. They should be of fairly equal thickness.
- Soak the veggies in water for 30 minutes to keep them from drying out. (Do not soak mushrooms.)
- Pat dry, and coat lightly with olive oil.

## WHEN GRILLING:

### ASPARAGUS

- Cut off ends.
- Turn every minute.
- Cooking time: 4 minutes.

### BELL PEPPERS

- Slice pepper in half down the middle of the pepper top to bottom, remove the stems and seeds and white bits.
- Flatten each half.
- Cooking time: 2-3 minutes.

### CHILI PEPPERS

- Grill whole chili.
- Cooking time: 2-3 minutes.

### CORN ON THE COB

- Gently pull back the husks, but don't remove them. Do remove the silk, and cut off the very tip.
- Fold husks back over after soaking and oiling, then twist the ends.
- Cooking time: 5-7 minutes.

### EGGPLANT

- Cut disks for large eggplants, in half for small eggplants.
- Cooking time: 2-3 minutes.

### GARLIC

- Take the whole bulb and cut off the root end.
- Cooking time: 10 minutes.
- Use as a paste to spread on bread or wraps.

### MUSHROOMS

- Rinse off dirt and pat dry. Use grill basket for small mushrooms.
- Cooking time: 6-8 minutes.

### ONIONS

- Remove the skin and cut horizontally about ½" thick.
- Cooking time: 3-4 minutes.

### TOMATOES

- Cut in half, top to bottom.
- Cooking time: 2-3 minutes.

### POTATOES

- Wash thoroughly and pat dry. Wrap in aluminum foil after brushing with oil. Grill for 35 minutes, turning occasionally.
- Cooking time: 20-25 minutes.

### ZUCCHINI AND SMALL SQUASH

- Slice ½" thickness. Brush with oil and grill.
- Cooking time: 2-3 minutes.

## GRILL PACKETS

**These tinfoil packets are easy to assemble and easy to clean up ...**

- Place meat of choice along with vegetables you are roasting (carrots, garlic, onions, anise root, leeks, baby potatoes, sweet potatoes, asparagus and broccoli are some good choices) on a large piece of tinfoil.
- Splash some olive oil and seasoning on top.
- Wrap up by pulling the length across the meat and rolling in the center – then fold outside edges in.
- Place on a medium-high preheated grill for 20 to 25 minutes or until the meat is cooked through.



**Why pay for unhealthy condiments when you can make tastier, healthier and cheaper versions yourself?**

## KAN'T KET-CHUP

**WHAT YOU'LL NEED»**

1 x 6 oz / 170 g can **tomato paste**
⅓ cup / 80 ml **water**
2 Tbsp / 30 ml **vinegar**
½ tsp / 2½ ml **dry mustard**
¼ tsp / 1¼ ml **sea salt**
¼ tsp / 1¼ ml **cinnamon**
1 pinch **cloves**
1 pinch **allspice**
1 pinch **cayenne pepper**
⅓ cup / 80 ml **Sucanat**

**HOW TO MAKE IT»**

**1.** Mix all ingredients together well and pour into a glass mason jar with a tight lid. Chill overnight.

## TICKLED PICKLED MAN-MADE RELISH

**WHAT YOU'LL NEED»**

1½ cups / 360 ml **apple cider vinegar**
1 tsp / 5 ml **mustard seeds**
1 tsp / 5 ml **coriander**
2 Tbsp / 30 ml **honey**
8 large **dill pickles**, chopped finely
1 **red pepper**, peeled, seeded, grilled and chopped
1 **yellow pepper**, peeled, seeded, grilled and chopped
1 **white onion**, finely chopped
Bunch **fresh dill**, minced

**HOW TO MAKE IT»**

**1.** Bring the vinegar, coriander and mustard seed to a boil in a medium saucepan. Cook until liquid is reduced by half and slightly syrupy.
**2.** Remove from heat, add remaining ingredients and gently toss to coat. Season with salt and pepper to taste. Cover and refrigerate.

# GOOD OL' BURGERS

No men's diet book could be complete without a burger recipe. We've included some recipes for ketchup and relish (on the previous page), but go crazy with healthy veggie toppings – try a sauté of onions and mushrooms.

**WHAT YOU'LL NEED»**

1 cup / 240 ml high-protein cereal flakes
½ cup / 120 ml soy milk
1 Tbsp / 15 ml low-sodium beef broth
3 Tbsp / 45 ml onion, minced
2 egg whites
1 lb / 454 g lean ground beef
Ezekiel whole-wheat buns

**NUTRITIONAL VALUE FOR ONE BURGER WITH BUN, KETCHUP AND RELISH:**
Calories: 464 | Calories from Fat: 82 | Total Fat: 9 g | Saturated Fat: 3 g | Total Carbs: 54 g | Fiber: 9.5 g | Protein: 42 g | Sodium: 665 mg | Cholesterol: 86 mg

**HOW TO MAKE IT»**

**1.** Combine the first five ingredients in a large bowl. Let the cereal flakes soak up the milk for 5 minutes. Add lean ground beef. Mix well with clean bare hands. Shape into patties and grill for 7-10 minutes on each side or until the burgers reach desired doneness.

**2.** Serve with grilled tomatoes and onions along with fresh lettuce leaves, homemade ketchup, relish and dijon mustard (see page 226).

**Preparation time:** 30 minutes
**Cooking time:** 14 – 20 minutes
**Yield:** 4 burgers

## T-SHIRT TANNED POTATO SKINS

**Potato skins are a famed greasy side dish at roadhouses everywhere. Enjoy this Clean version without the guilt!**

**WHAT YOU'LL NEED»**

3 lbs / 1.35 kg **baking potatoes**, scrubbed – use organic potatoes if possible, since you will be eating the skins.
2 heads **roasted garlic** (see recipe below)
1 Tbsp / 15 ml best-quality **olive oil**
1 tsp / 5 ml **sea salt**
½ tsp freshly ground **black pepper**
1 Tbsp / 15 ml **herbal seasoning** of your choice (I like Herbamare)

**ROASTED GARLIC**

Remove loose, papery skin from outer part of garlic heads. Slice off the top portion of the head of garlic, being careful not to break it apart. Place the heads of garlic in a shallow baking dish. Drizzle a half-tablespoon of olive oil over each head of garlic. Place in the oven with the potatoes.

**NUTRITIONAL VALUE FOR THREE POTATO SKINS:**
Calories: 119 | Calories from Fat: 14 | Total Fat: 1.5 g | Saturated Fat: 0.2 g | Total Carbs: 24 g | Fiber: 3 g | Protein: 3 g | Sodium: 48 mg | Cholesterol: 0 mg

**HOW TO MAKE IT»**

**1.** Preheat oven to 350°F / 177°C and prepare baking sheet with a layer of parchment paper.

**2.** Scrub each potato and then carefully pierce with a fork to allow for more even baking. Be careful not to pierce yourself!

**3.** Bake for 50 minutes, or until tender. Roast the garlic at the same time. Remove from oven. Let cool for 15 minutes.

**4.** Once cool, quarter each of the baked potatoes along the length. Be gentle with the skins, as these will be baked again. Scoop most of the baked flesh out, leaving about a quarter-inch of potato flesh on the skin. Set aside this flesh for use in another dish – potato makes a great soup thickener, or you can use it for a quick mashed-potato dish.

**5.** Increase the heat in the oven to 425°F / 220°C.

**6.** Squeeze the roasted garlic into a small bowl. Add salt, herb seasoning and pepper and mash together with a fork. Spread garlic mixture onto each potato skin. Place the potatoes on the prepared baking sheet and bake for 20 minutes in the hot oven.

**Preparation time:** 15 minutes
**Cooking time:** 50 + 20 minutes
**Yield:** 10 servings

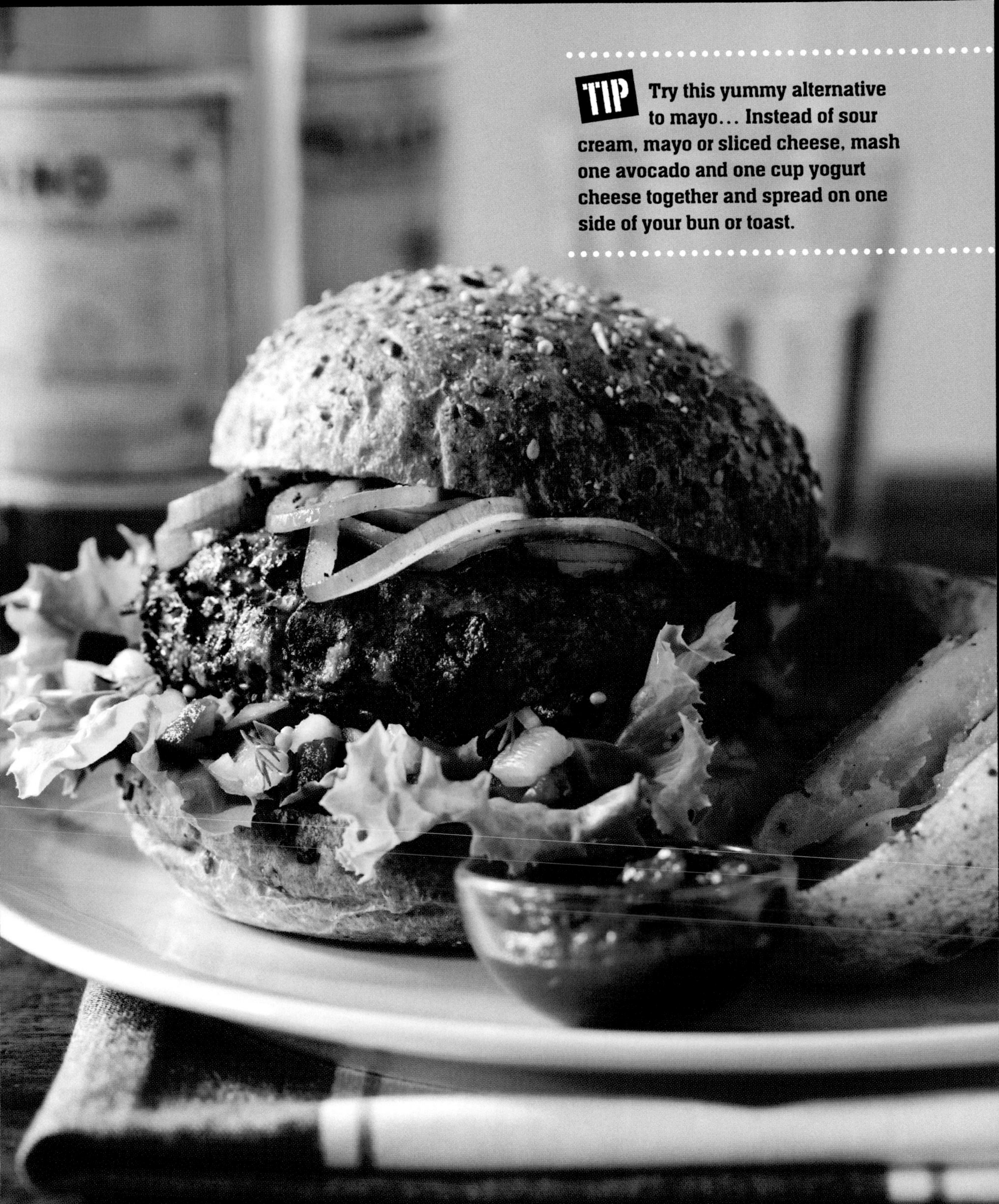

**TIP** Try this yummy alternative to mayo… Instead of sour cream, mayo or sliced cheese, mash one avocado and one cup yogurt cheese together and spread on one side of your bun or toast.

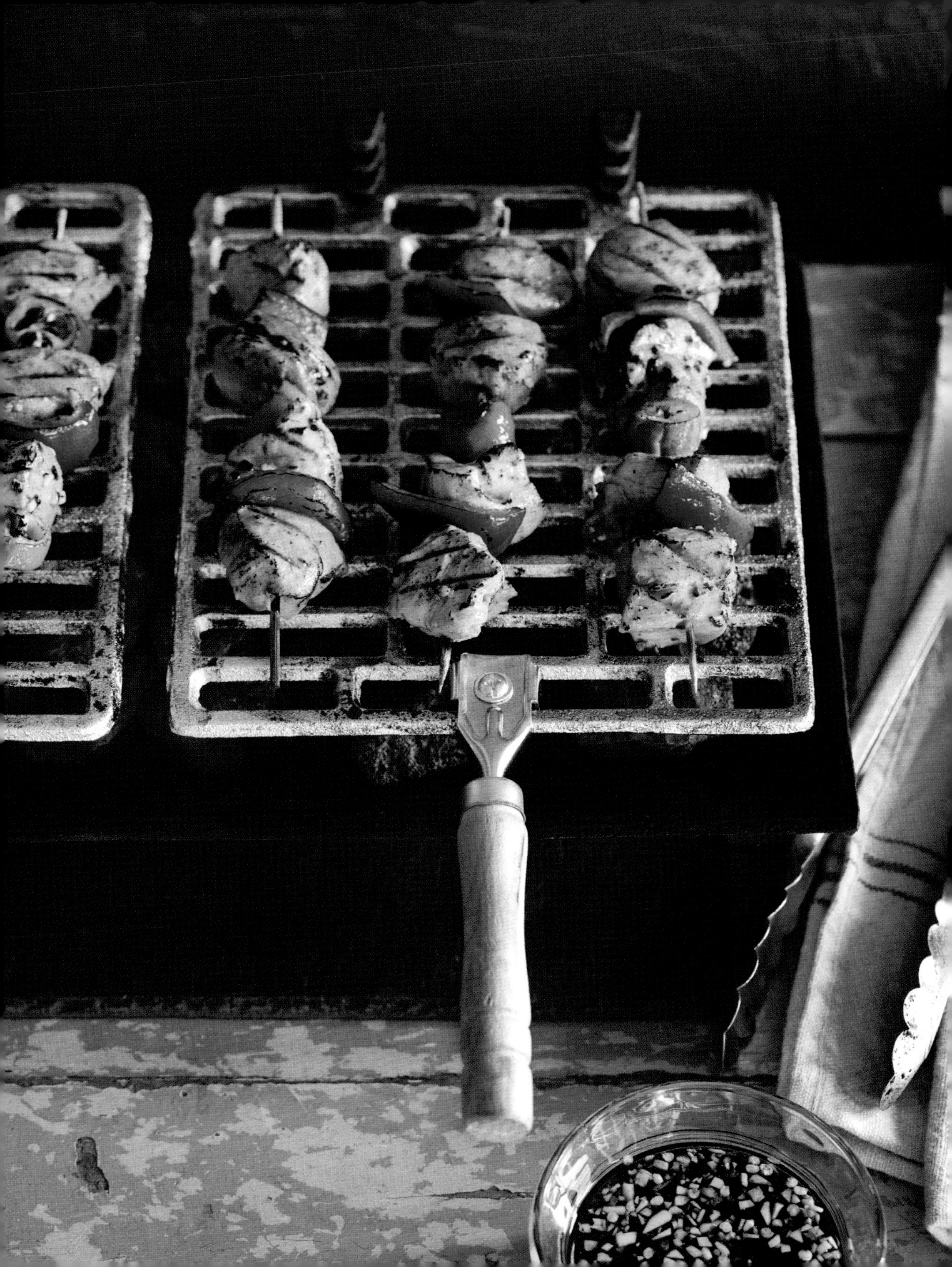

# GETTIN' A LITTLE HOT AND SPICY ... PORK SATAY

In Asian food balance is very important, and the most common combination of flavors to create that balance is sweet, hot and sour. This recipe does not disappoint, as it offers the sweetness of honey, the sour from vinegar and the heat from jalapeño. Now you can tell everyone how well balanced you are!

### WHAT YOU'LL NEED »

2 Tbsp / 30 ml light teriyaki sauce
1 Tbsp / 15 ml red-wine vinegar
1 Tbsp / 15 ml best-quality olive oil
2 garlic cloves, pressed or minced
1 Tbsp / 30 ml honey
½ tsp / 2½ ml red-pepper flakes
¾ lb / 340 g pork tenderloin, cut into 1-inch / 2½-cm cubes
1 red pepper, seeded and cut into wedges
1 jalapeño pepper, seeded and thickly sliced

### HOW TO MAKE IT »

**1.** In a medium bowl, mix the teriyaki sauce, red-wine vinegar, garlic, olive oil, honey and red pepper flakes.

**2.** Preheat the outdoor grill to high and lightly oil the grate.

**3.** Place the pork on the skewers, alternating with red pepper wedges and thick jalapeno slices.

**4.** Cook on the prepared grill, turning frequently and brushing with the teriyaki mixture. Cook for 10 to 12 minutes, or until done to your liking.

**5.** Serve with baked brown rice or rice noodles.

**NUTRITIONAL VALUE FOR ONE SKEWER:**
Calories: 167 | Calories from Fat: 57 | Total Fat: 6 g | Saturated Fat: 1.5 g | Total Carbs: 8.5 g | Fiber: 2.2 g | Protein: 11 g | Sodium: 480 m | Cholesterol: 0 mg

**Preparation time:** 15 minutes
**Cooking time:** 10 – 15 minutes
**Yield:** 4 skewers

# NICE B-ASS

We hear it again and again – fish is one of the best sources of protein going. Along with protein, sea bass offers the extraordinary health benefits of fish oil, including improved cardiovascular health, weight loss and a boosted immune system, and it acts as a natural anti-inflammatory. Best of all, this dish tastes fantastic with its smoky cedar flavor – and it looks impressive on the plate!

**WHAT YOU'LL NEED»**

1 bunch small green onions
4 x 10-inch / 25½ cm squares of cedar paper
4 x 3 oz / 85 g square fillets sea bass
2 tsp / 10 ml avocado oil, divided
2 tsp / 10 ml sea salt, divided
2 tsp / 10 ml freshly ground black pepper, divided
1 lemon, sliced
4 stems fresh basil, for garnish
Cooking string

**Preparation time:** 20 minutes
**Cooking time:** 10 – 12 minutes
**Yield:** 4 servings

**NUTRITIONAL VALUE FOR ONE SERVING:**
Calories: 146 | Calories from Fat: 41 | Total Fat: 4.5 g | Saturated Fat: 1 g | Total Carbs: 3.5 g | Fiber: 1.5 g | Protein: 21.5 g | Sodium: 800 mg | Cholesterol: 46 mg

**HOW TO MAKE IT»**

**1.** Moisten the cedar paper and string by immersing in cold water for 10 minutes.

**2.** Meanwhile, chop the green onion into slices. Discard the stringy, dark green ends. Look for nice, fresh light green strips.

**3.** Remove cedar from water and lay flat. Place a piece of sea bass in the center of each paper.

**4.** Drizzle ½ tsp / 2½ ml of the avocado oil over each piece of sea bass and season with salt and pepper. Place a small handful of onions and slice of lemon with each filet.

**5.** Fold the cedar paper around the bass to form a tube, overlapping the edges and tying it closed with cooking string.

**6.** Set the sea bass packets over the grill and cook for 5 to 6 minutes, turning occasionally. The cedar paper will char and may smolder slightly, but it should not burn.

**7.** Remove the tubes from the grill with tongs and transfer to plates, giving two parcels per plate. Open the cedar but leave the fish inside. Lay a sprig of fresh basil atop the fillets.

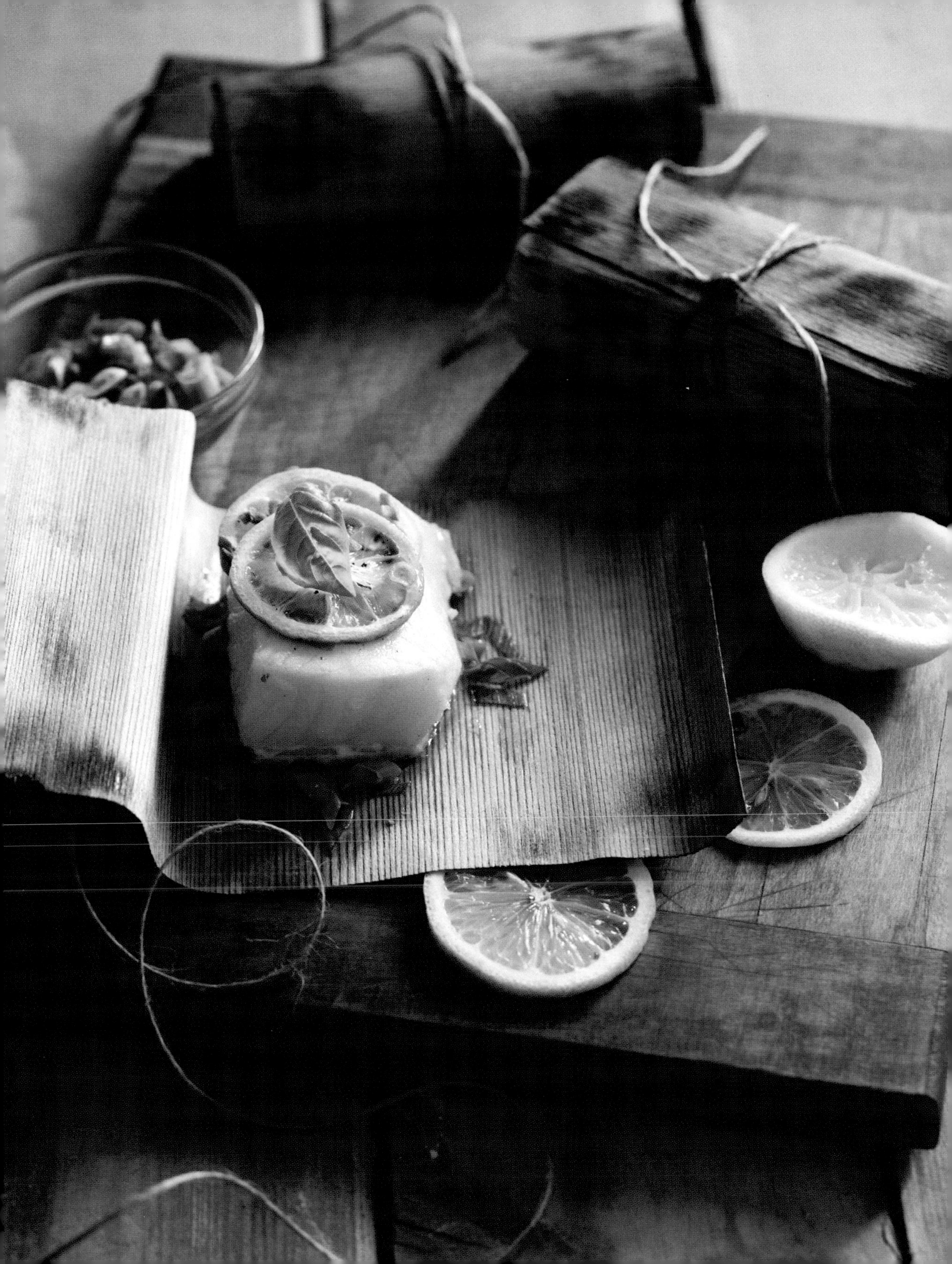

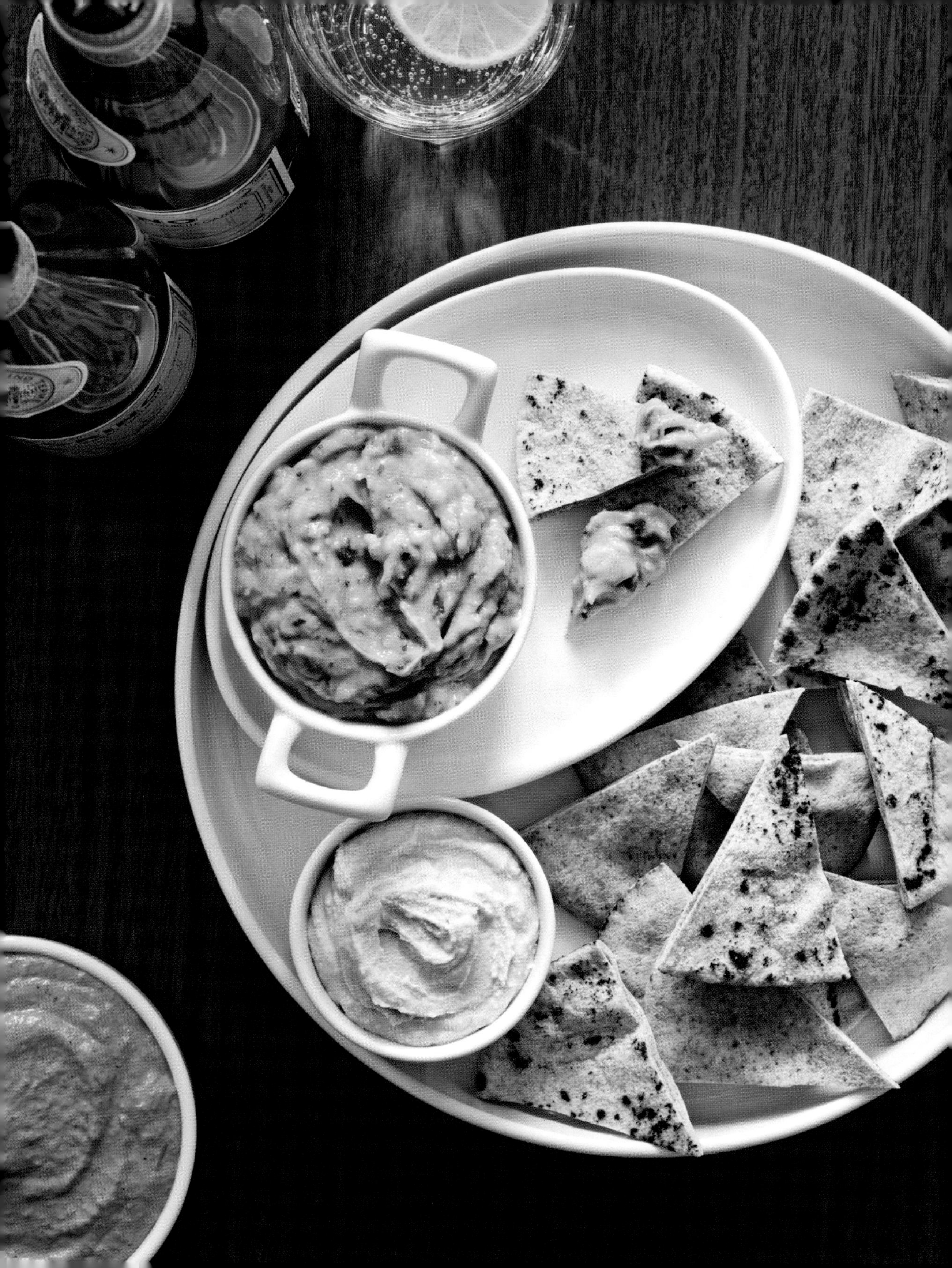

# PITA CHIPS & DIP

When we have company over we need to have something to nibble on. Toasted pita chips are the perfect answer, served with one dip, or an array.

## TOASTED PITA **Prep time:** 2 min. • **Cook time:** 6 min.

Preheat oven to 400°F / 205°C. Brush whole-wheat pitas very lightly with olive oil. Cut into eighths. Lay on baking sheet and place in preheated oven. Turn after 4 minutes, and bake for another 2 minutes.

## ROASTED RED PEPPER DIP

**WHAT YOU'LL NEED»**

4 **sweet potatoes**, baked and cooled
2 **cloves garlic**
2 Tbsp / 30 ml best-quality **olive oil**
2 Tbsp / 30 ml **red wine vinegar**
½ cup / 120 ml bottled **roasted red peppers**
¼ cup / 60 ml **fresh cilantro**, chopped
1 fresh **chili pepper**
1 large **ripe fresh tomato**, peeled, seeded and chopped
1 small **sweet onion**, chopped

**HOW TO MAKE IT»**

Blend together in a food processor till smooth.

**NUTRITIONAL VALUE FOR TWO TBSP:**
Calories: 64 | Calories from Fat: 21 | Total Fat: 2.5 g | Saturated Fat: 0.3 g | Total Carbs: 10.3 g | Fiber: 1.6 g | Protein: 1 g | Sodium: 28 mg | Cholesterol: 0 mg

**Prep time:** 10 min.

## EAT-CLEAN GUACAMOLE

**WHAT YOU'LL NEED»**

3 ripe **avocados**
Juice of ½ **fresh lime**
1 Tbsp / 15 ml chopped **cilantro**
½ **red** or **purple onion**, minced well
1 **clove garlic**, passed through a garlic press
**Sea salt** and freshly ground **black pepper** to taste
1 small **sweet onion**, chopped

**HOW TO MAKE IT»**

Peel avocados. Place all ingredients in medium bowl and mix until just combined. Don't over mix.

**NUTRITIONAL VALUE FOR TWO TBSP:**
Calories: 130 | Calories from Fat: 89 | Total Fat:2.5 g | Saturated Fat: 0.9 g | Total Carbs: 10 g | Fiber: 6 g | Protein: 2 g | Sodium: 25 mg | Sugar: 2 g

**Prep time:** 12 min.

## INDIAN HUMMUS

**WHAT YOU'LL NEED»**

3 Tbsp / 45 ml best-quality **olive oil**, divided
1 inch / 2.5 cm piece of **ginger**, peeled and thinly sliced
¼ cup / 60 ml **cashews**
1 tsp / 5 ml each **salt, ground cumin** and **ground coriander**
¼ tsp / 1¼ ml each **chili pepper, turmeric** and **cinnamon**
2 **garlic cloves**, smashed
1 x 19 oz / 540 ml can **chickpeas**, rinsed
Juice of 2 **limes**
2 Tbsp / 30 ml each chopped fresh **cilantro** and **mint**. Freshly ground **black pepper** to taste

**NUTRITIONAL VALUE FOR TWO TBSP:**
Calories: 130 | Calories from Fat: 43 | Total Fat: 5 g | Saturated Fat: 0.7 g | Total Carbs: 9 g | Fiber: 2 g | Protein: 3 g | Sodium: 101 mg | Cholesterol: 0 mg

**HOW TO MAKE IT»**

**1.** Heat two tablespoons of oil in a pan on medium-low heat. Turn heat to low and add the ginger to the pan, letting it simmer for 10 minutes. Do not burn or brown! Set aside to cool.
**2.** Meanwhile, heat one tablespoon oil in a thick-bottomed pan. Cook the cashews, stirring, for 10 minutes. Squeeze the limes overtop cashews. Add salt, cumin, coriander, chili pepper, turmeric and cinnamon. Cook for another two minutes, stirring to coat the cashews in the spices. Set aside to cool.
**3.** Once cooled, add all the cooked and uncooked ingredients to a food processor. Use a spatula to get all of the spicy oils from your pans into the mixture. Blend to a purée and add salt, pepper or chili pepper to taste.

**Prep time:** 10 min. • **Cook time:** 15 min.

# Y'ARGH PIRATE PLANKED SALMON

**WHAT YOU'LL NEED»**

Wild salmon filet (skin on) 1"/ 2.5 cm thick, large enough to feed your party
½ cup / 120 ml best-quality olive oil
Juice of one fresh lemon
1 lemon, cut into quarters
2 Tbsp / 30 ml fresh chopped dill
1 bunch green onions, trimmed
1 purple sweet onion, sliced into rings
2 sweet bell peppers
1 cedar plank to fit the fillet

**HOW TO MAKE IT»**

**1. Pre-Soaking the Plank**

- The plank must be pre-soaked prior to placing on the grill. The plank must soak for at least 2 hours and as long as 24 hours. The most common method is to place the planks in the kitchen sink and place enough weight on top of them to keep them completely immersed under water.
- Warm water helps to open the pores of the cedar plank.
- Beer, vinegar or spices added to your soaking water will seep into the planks and thus your food, so give these ideas a try to add zesty flavor.

**NUTRITIONAL VALUE FOR FOUR OUNCES OF SALMON WITH VEGGIES:**

Calories: 315 | Calories from Fat: 211 | Total Fat: 23.5 g | Saturated Fat: 4 g | Total Carbs:7.5 g | Fiber: 2 g | Protein: 19 g | Sodium: 59 mg | Cholesterol: 53 mg

**2. Preparing the Planks**

- Remove planks from their water bath. Dry with a clean kitchen towel. Lightly coat the top surface with olive oil.
- Preheat the grill on high for 10 minutes with the lid closed.
- Turn heat down to medium high and place plank on grill for 5 minutes.

**3. Preparing the Salmon**

- Wash the salmon with fresh water and pat it dry with a paper towel before placing it on the plank.
- Place the salmon skin side down on the plank and add rosemary, lemon juice, olive oil, lemon wedges, peppers and onions.

**4. Planking the Salmon**

- Close the lid and cook at a medium heat for about 15-25 minutes. Do not turn the salmon over on the plank.
- Check every 5 minutes for flare-ups (keep a spray bottle on hand to keep those flames tame).
- The difference between rare, medium and well-done ranges from 15 - 25 minutes on the grill.

**5. Serving the salmon**

- Remove the plank from heat source using tongs or oven mitts (the plank will be hot) and carefully transfer the salmon to a serving dish using a turner or lifter. Serve immediately.

**Soaking time:** 2 – 24 hours
**Preparation time:** 30 minutes
**Cooking time:** 15 – 25 minutes

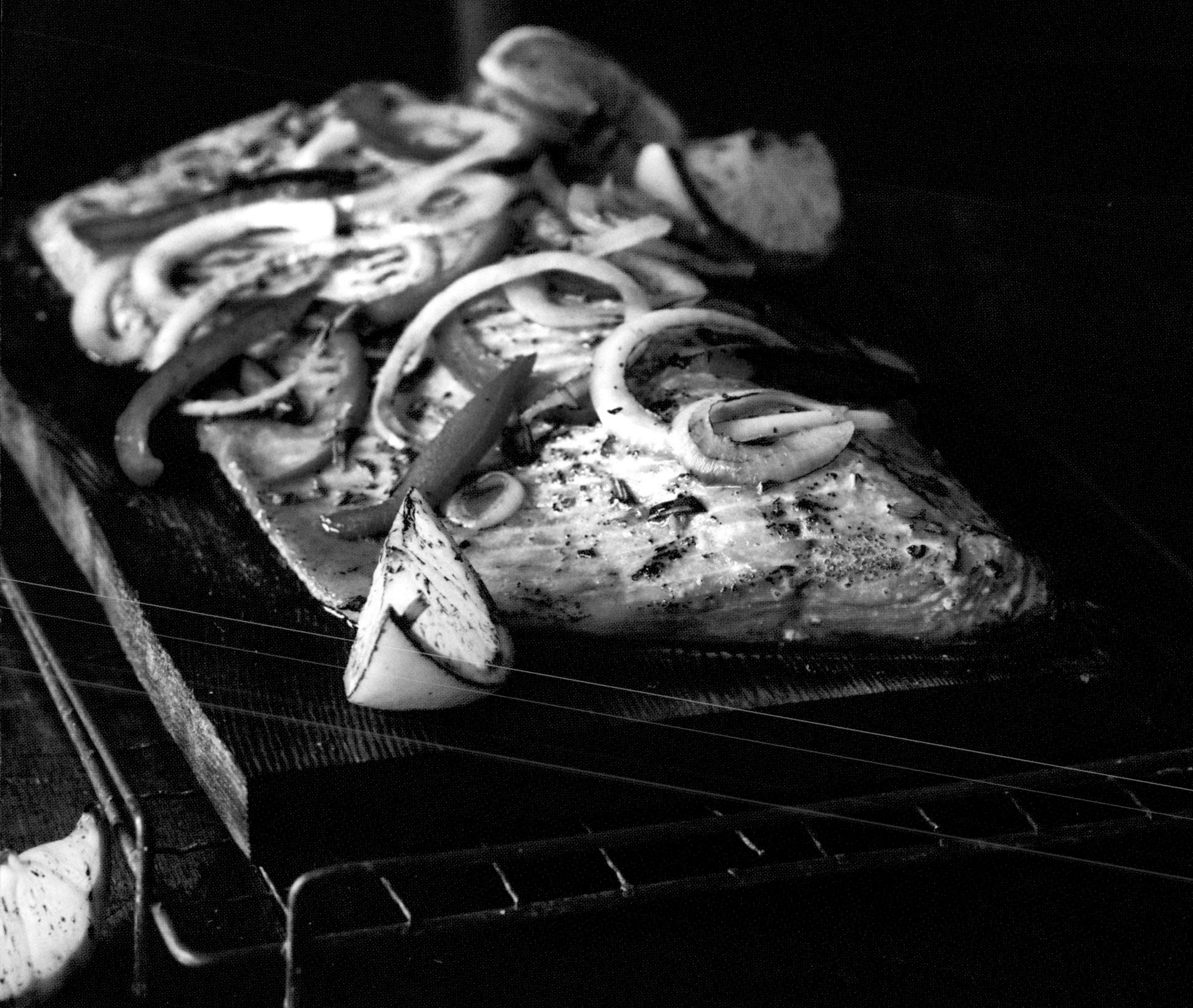

**TIP** Using cedar planks is one way to smoke fish or meat; another method is cedar papers. These papers now come in a variety of flavors including cedar, pine and hickory. Wood papers are flexible enough to hold a single-portion fillet of salmon, a hunk of fresh mozzarella or half of a ripe summer peach. The papers, first soaked in water, cook directly on the grill. The sheets can be rolled in tubes around shrimp, cinched with a strip of scallion green and grilled. The papers provide intense flavor, so they are best used with subtle foods. Try fish, tofu or summer fruit.

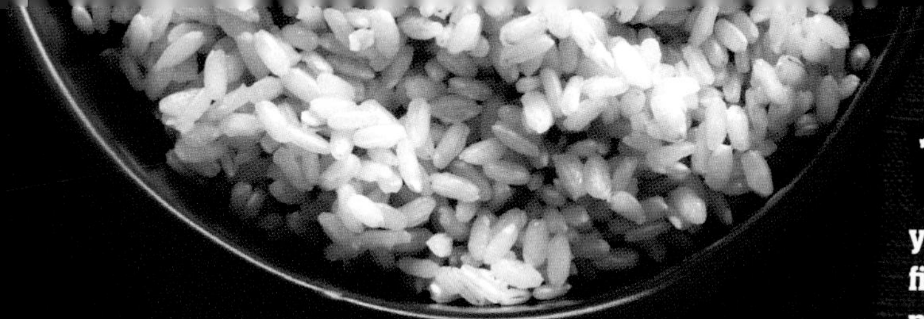

**TIP** Kabobs, satays or skewers – no matter what you call them you can transform meat, vegetables, fish or fruit into a tantalizing taste experience simply by skewering them, grilling, and serving at your next do.

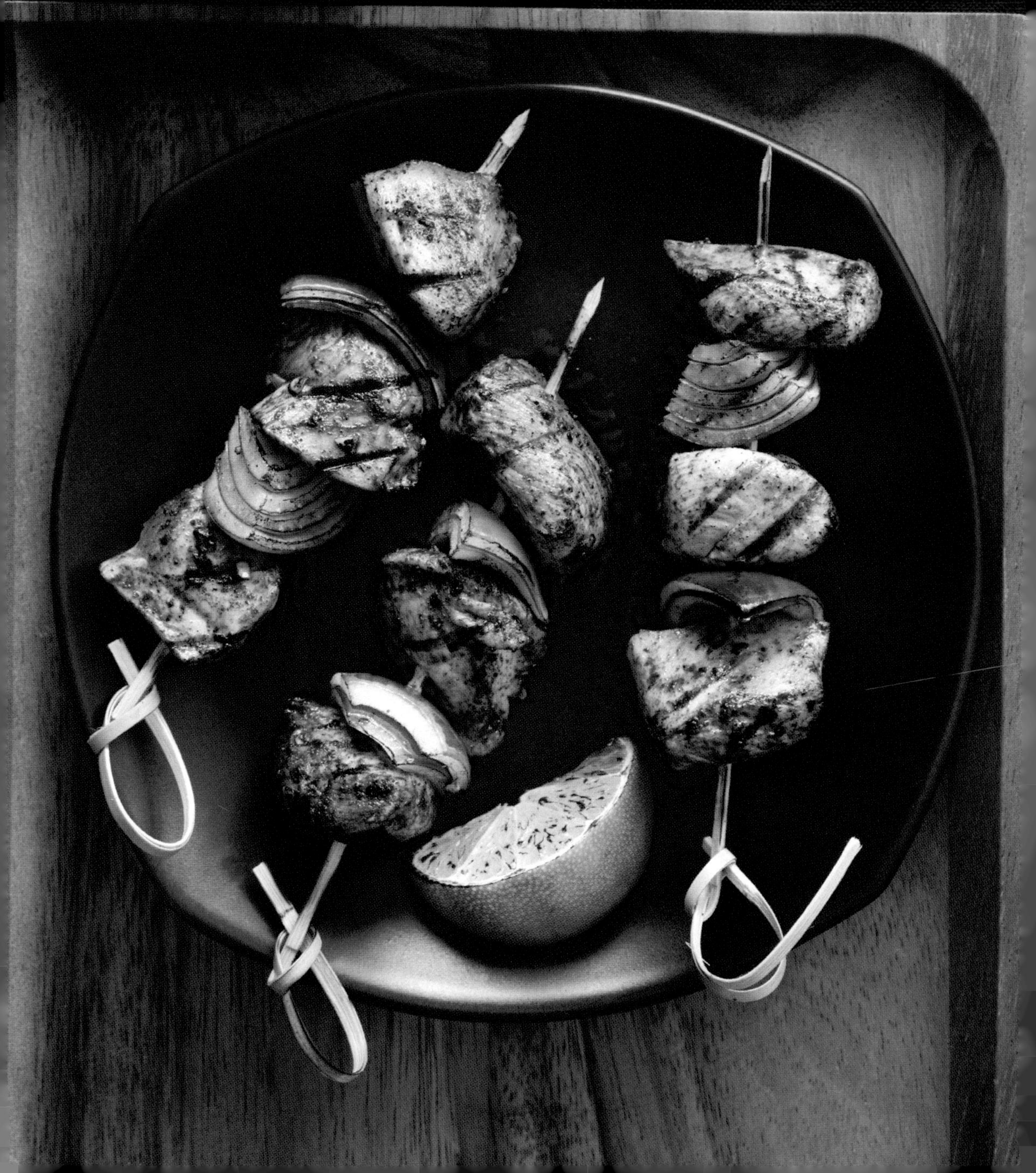

# CHILI CHICKEN KABOBS

## THE TRINIDADIAN MEN SAY: "LIME DOWN"

### WHAT YOU'LL NEED»

3 Tbsp / 45 ml best-quality olive oil

1½ Tbsp / 22 ml balsamic vinegar

Juice of one fresh lime

1 tsp / 5 ml chili powder

½ tsp / 2½ ml paprika

1 large onion, chopped into thick pieces

2 garlic cloves, pressed or minced

1 tsp / 5 ml cayenne pepper

Sea salt, to taste

Freshly ground black pepper, to taste

1 lb / 454 g boneless skinless chicken breast, cut into 1½-inch / 4-cm pieces

**NOTE:** Use pork, beef or bison tenderloin or turkey as alternative kabob meats. A sturdy, meaty fish such as salmon works well here too.

### HOW TO MAKE IT»

**1.** In a small bowl whisk together the olive oil, vinegar and lime juice. Season with chili powder, paprika, cayenne pepper, salt, pepper and pressed garlic.

**2.** Place the chicken in a shallow baking dish with the sauce and stir to coat.

**3.** Preheat the grill to medium high. Thread the chicken onto the skewers, alternating with chopped onion pieces. Discard the marinade.

**4.** Lightly oil the grill grate. Grill the skewers for 10 to 15 minutes or until the chicken juices run clear.

### REMEMBER TO...

- Cut meats, veggies or fruit to a uniform size: 1½ inches / 4 cm works well.
- Group foods with similar cooking times. Tomatoes are generally not the best for grilling – they turn to mush and can fall of the skewer and down into the grill before the other food is finished cooking.

**NUTRITIONAL VALUE FOR ONE KABOB:**
Calories: 186 | Calories from Fat: 75 | Total Fat: 8.5 g | Saturated Fat: 1 6 | Total Carbs: 6 g | Fiber: 1 g | Protein: 25 g | Sodium: 334 mg | Cholesterol: 61 mg

**Preparation time:** 15 minutes
**Cooking time:** 10 – 15 minutes
**Yield:** 4 kabobs

# PITA PIZZA

No fancy skills or time needed for this recipe. Just chop up some veggies, spread sauce on a pita, sprinkle some cheese and throw it all in the oven. Done!

**WHAT YOU'LL NEED »**

1 x 7-inch / 18 cm Ezekiel or brown-rice wrap for each pizza

Toppings (see right for ideas)

**HOW TO MAKE IT »**

**1.** Preheat oven to 350°F / 175 °C.

**2.** Place your pita on the baking sheet sprayed with Eat-Clean Cooking Spray (see page 262). Dress pita with your desired toppings and place in the oven.

**3.** Bake until the toppings become warm and the cheese melts (about 7 to 10 minutes).

**Preparation time:** 5 minutes
**Cooking time:** 7-10 minutes

**NUTRITIONAL VALUE FOR ONE PIZZA WITH TOMATO SAUCE, CHICKEN, FETA CHEESE, ONION AND BROCCOLI:**
Calories: 319 | Calories from Fat: 62 | Total Fat: 6.9 g | Saturated Fat: 3.5 g | Total Carbs: 36 g | Fiber: 8 g | Protein: 33 g | Sodium: 1000 mg | Cholesterol: 52 mg

**VEGETABLES**

- Eggplant
- Zucchini
- Mushrooms
- Bell peppers
- Sweet onions
- Black olives
- Sundried tomatoes
- Artichokes
- Spinach
- Broccoli florets
- Fresh tomatoes
- Fresh basil

**CLEAN SAUCES**

- Tomato Hot and Spicy Sauce (see page 233)
- Basil Pesto (see page 242)

**PROTEINS**

- Grilled chicken breast, cut into strips
- Grilled turkey breast, cut into strips
- Marinated grilled tofu, cut into strips

**BETTER CHEESE CHOICES**

- Low-fat mozzarella
- Low-fat feta cheese
- Goat cheese
- Hard parmesan

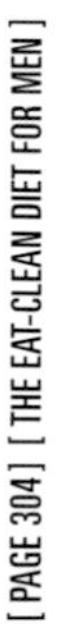

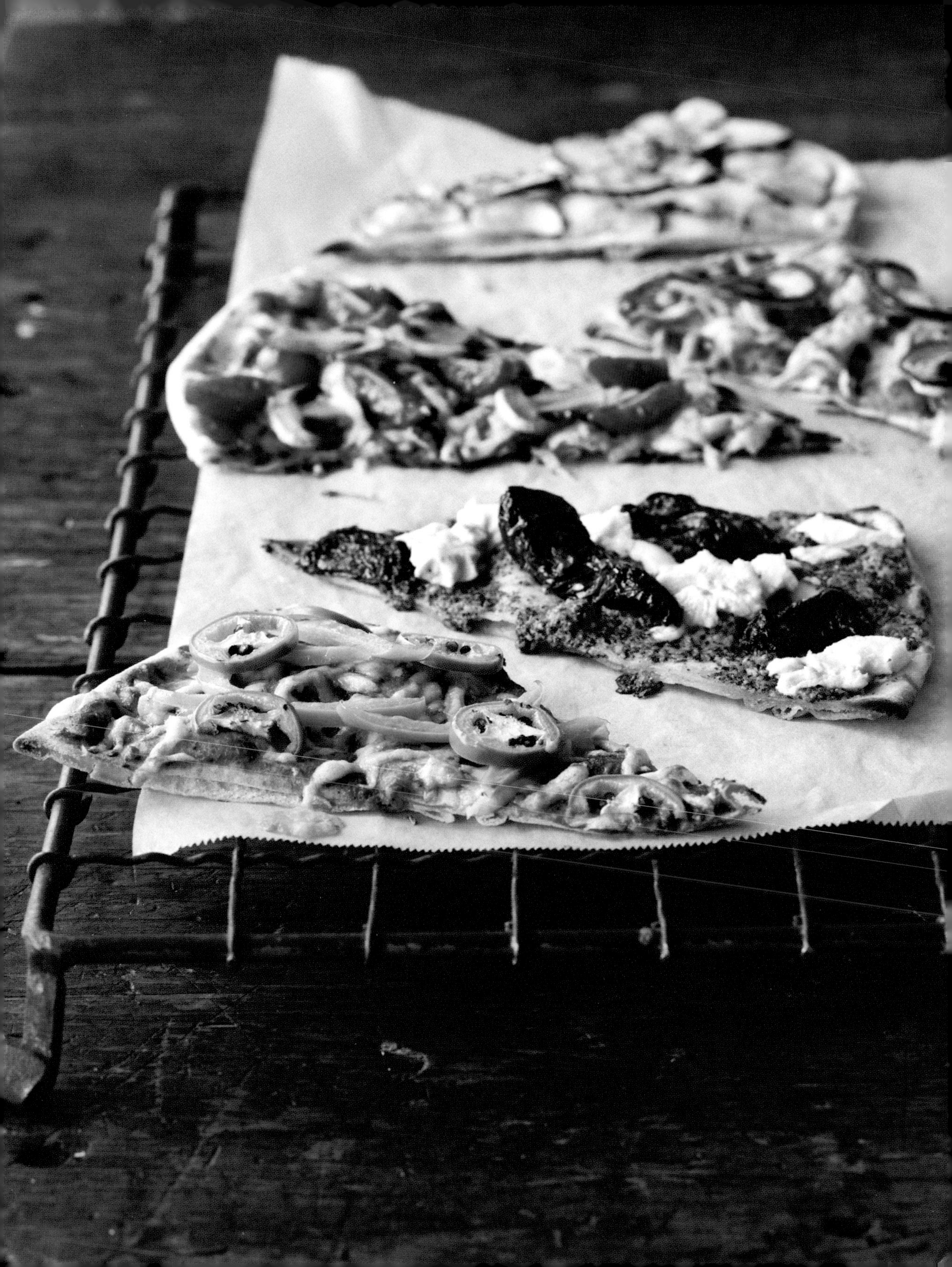

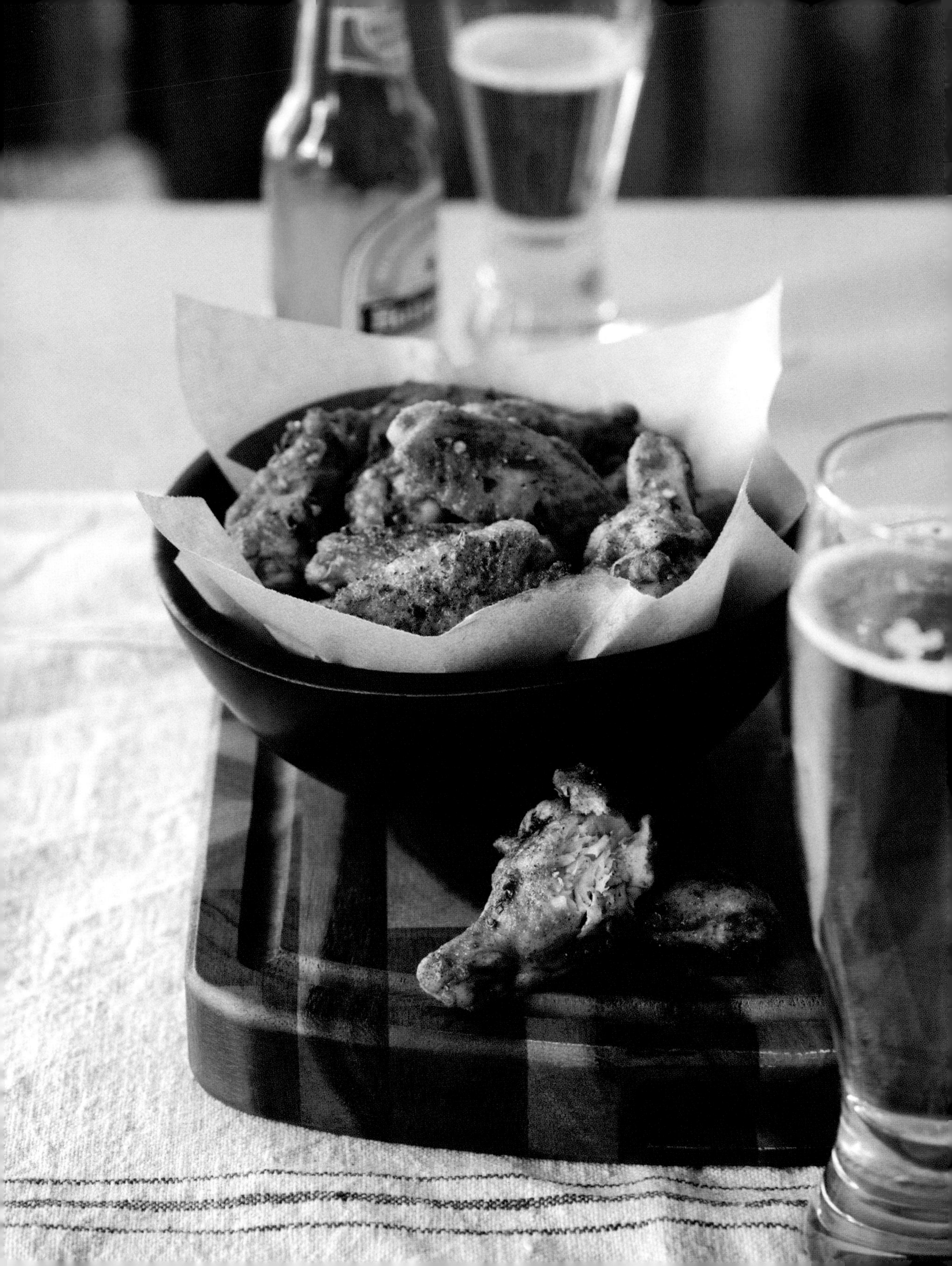

# CHICKEN WINGS

Chicken wings almost always spell party time, especially when must-see sporting events hit the big screen. Make this version of spicy wings – high in flavor but low in fat. Delicious, too!

### WHAT YOU'LL NEED»

2 dozen chicken wings
¾ cup / 180 ml spelt, kamut or other whole-grain flour
2 Tbsp / 30 ml paprika
1 tsp / 5 ml garlic powder
Sea salt and freshly ground black pepper to taste
¼ cup / 60 ml best-quality olive oil
Pinch red pepper flakes
Bay leaf
2 lemons, halved
10 roasted garlic cloves
¼ cup / 60 ml chopped fresh oregano
¼ cup / 60 ml light beer
2 cups / 480 ml low-sodium chicken broth

**TIP The wings will be spicy enough on their own thanks to the seasonings, but if you want a dipping sauce use homemade ketchup (see recipe page 291), which you can spice up the way you like.**

**NUTRITIONAL VALUE FOR 6 WINGS:**
Calories: 445 | Calories from Fat: 89 | Total Fat: 10 g | Saturated Fat: 8 g | Total Carbs: 9 g | Fiber: 3 g | Protein: 30 g | Sodium: 1000 mg | Cholesterol: 120 mg

### HOW TO MAKE IT»

1. Rinse the chicken wings in cold water and pat dry with paper towels.
2. Place flour in a shallow platter and season it by adding paprika, garlic powder, salt and pepper. Mix well.
3. Dredge the wings in the flour – that means roll the wings around in the flour to coat every bit of them. You can also place the flour and spices in a large sealable plastic bag and shake to coat.
4. Heat oil in a skillet and brown the chicken wings on all sides.
5. Remove the chicken from the pan and set aside on a platter.
6. Add pepper flakes, bay leaf, lemons, garlic, oregano, beer and chicken broth to the pan. Cook for 2 minutes to evaporate the alcohol.
7. Return the chicken wings to the pan.
8. Cover the pan and simmer for 15 minutes, or braise in a preheated 375°F / 190°C oven for 20 minutes.

**Preparation time:** 10 minutes
**Cooking time:** 35 minutes
**Yield:** 4 servings

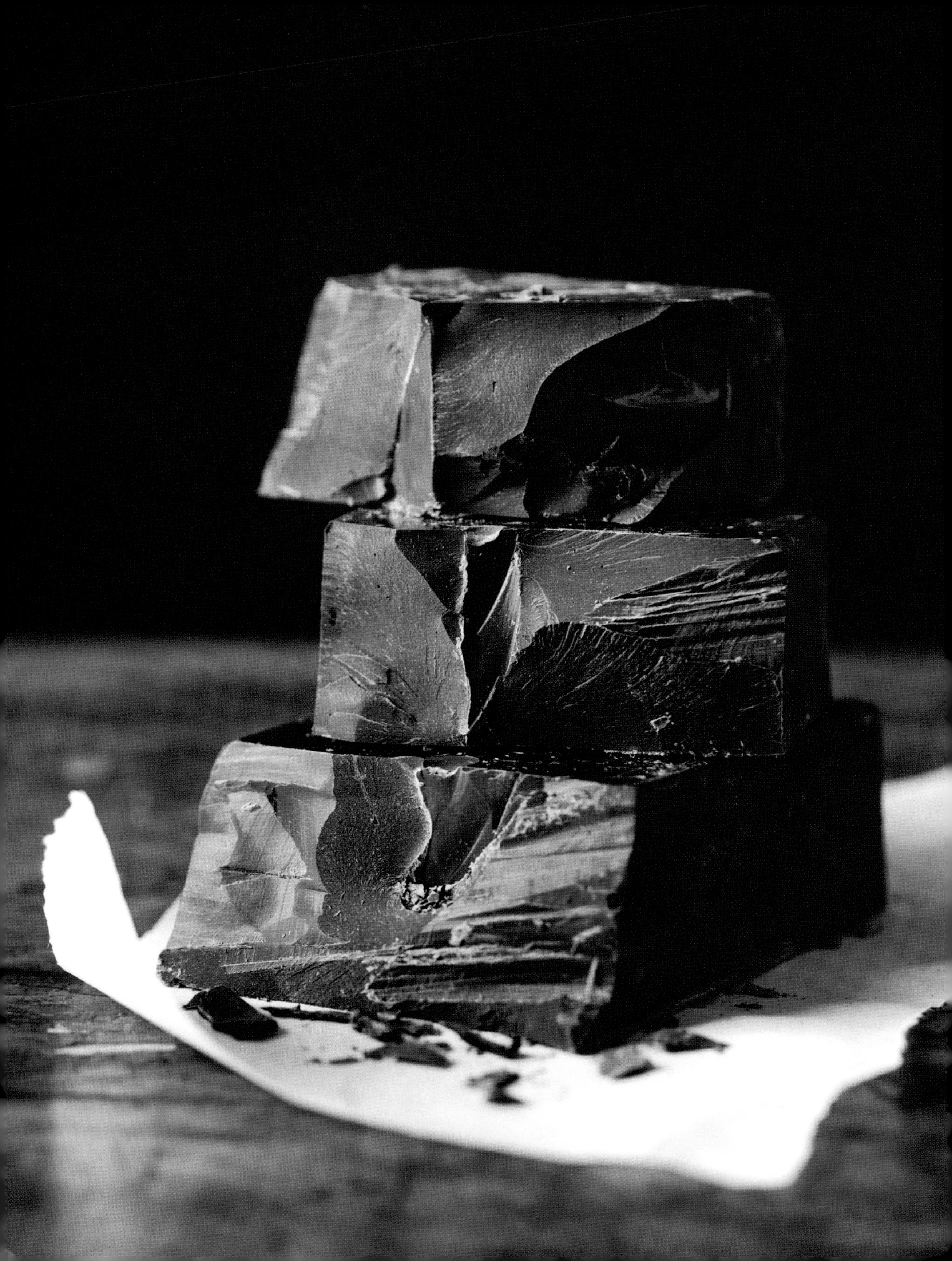

# DESSERTS

Eating Clean is a way of life, and that means you have to live it! No life would be complete without an occasional treat, but those treats do not have to destroy your body with artery-clogging, chemically charged ingredients. The best treats are those that taste great and don't leave you feeling like you have a hangover. We use all-natural ingredients without excessive sugars and fats, and they taste better than anything you'll pull ready-made from a box. Dig in!

# BROWNIES WITH A TWIST

Everyone loves brownies and their rich chocolaty goodness. A cup of coffee gives these brownies a little extra bite.

### WHAT YOU'LL NEED »

1 cup / 240 ml very strong coffee or espresso

½ cup / 120 ml olive oil-based margarine or Do-It-Yourself Olive Butter (see below for recipe)

1½ cups / 360 ml Sucanat or raw sugar

¾ cup / 180 ml best-quality cocoa powder

2 eggs, beaten

1 cup / 240 ml whole-wheat pastry flour

1 cup / 240 ml dark chocolate chips

½ cup / 120 ml chopped walnuts (optional)

Eat-Clean Cooking Spray (see page 262)

**NUTRITIONAL VALUE FOR ONE BROWNIE:**
Calories: 225 | Calories from Fat: 138 | Total Fat: 15 g | Saturated Fat: 4 g | Total Carbs: 28 g | Fiber: 2.5 g | Protein: 3.3 g | Sodium: 57 mg | Cholesterol: 23 mg

**Preparation time:** 30 minutes
**Cooking time:** 25 – 35 minutes
**Yield:** 16 brownies

### HOW TO MAKE IT »

1. Preheat oven to 350°F / 177°C. Spray 9x9-inch / 23x23-cm baking pan with cooking spray.
2. Melt margarine in saucepan over low heat.
3. Add cocoa powder to coffee and mix until the cocoa is dissolved. Add to the melted margarine.
4. Slowly stir the sugar into the coffee and margarine mixture, stirring until the sugar dissolves.
5. Add eggs and mix until just combined.
6. Remove the mixture from heat. Fold flour into the mixture until just combined. Do not overmix.
7. Fold in chocolate chips and walnuts. Again, do not overmix.
8. Spread batter into the prepared pan and bake for 25 to 35 minutes, or until the top is no longer shiny.
9. Let brownies cool before cutting them.

## DO-IT-YOURSELF OLIVE BUTTER SPREAD

### WHAT YOU'LL NEED »

½ cup / 120 ml **low-salt butter** at room temperature

½ cup / 120 ml best-quality **olive oil**

### HOW TO MAKE IT »

Place both ingredients in a food processor. Process until well combined. The mixture should resemble thick yogurt. Transfer into a serving bowl, preferably ceramic, glass or porcelain. Cover with plastic wrap and refrigerate.

**Preparation time:** 5 minutes
**Yield:** 16 one-tbsp servings

**NUTRITIONAL VALUE PER ONE-TBSP SERVING:**
Calories: 110 | Calories from Fat: 110 | Total Fat: 15 g | Saturated Fat: 12 g | Total Carbs: 0 g | Fiber: 0 g | Protein: 0 g | Sodium: 40 mg | Sugar: 0 g

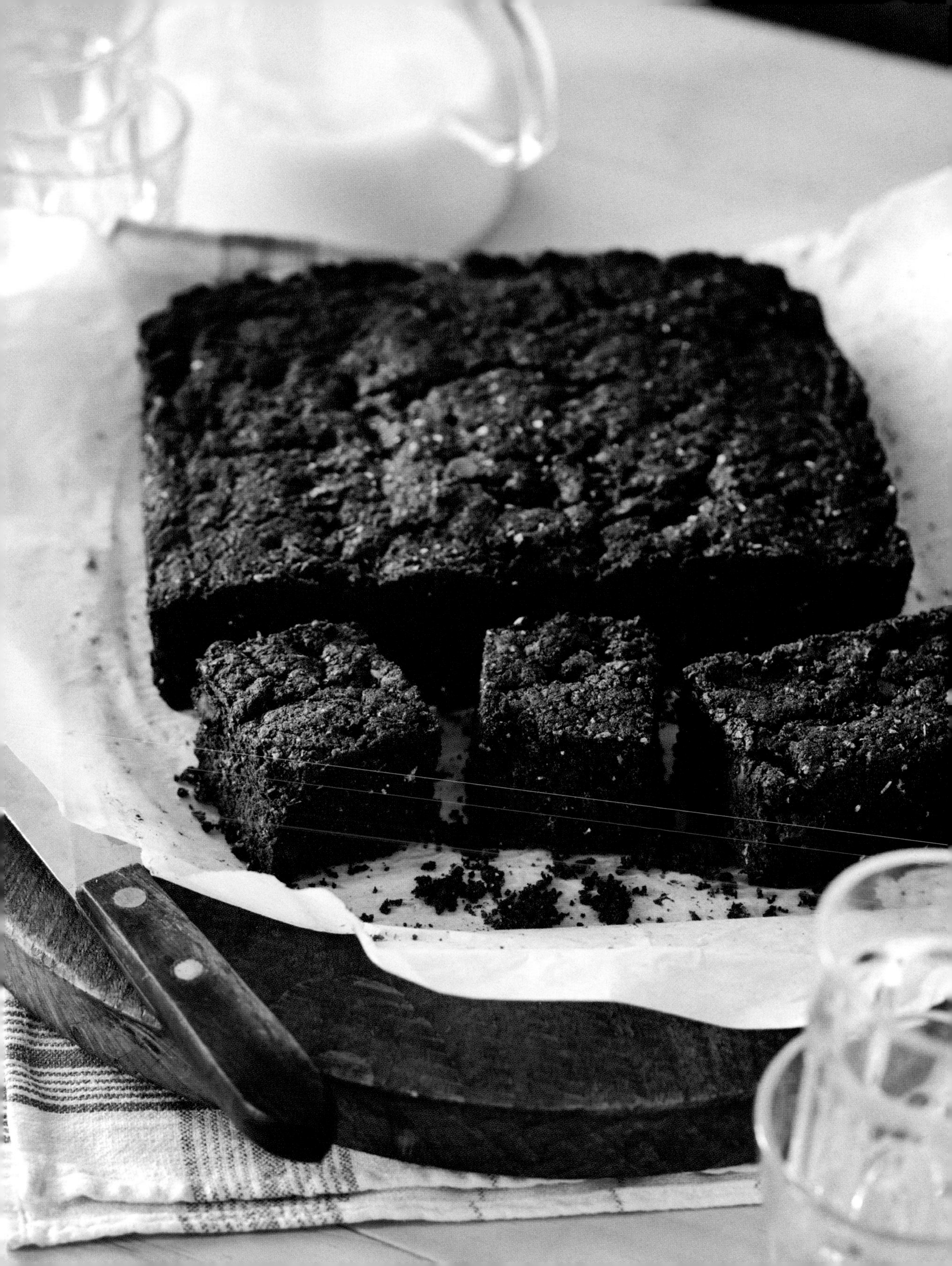

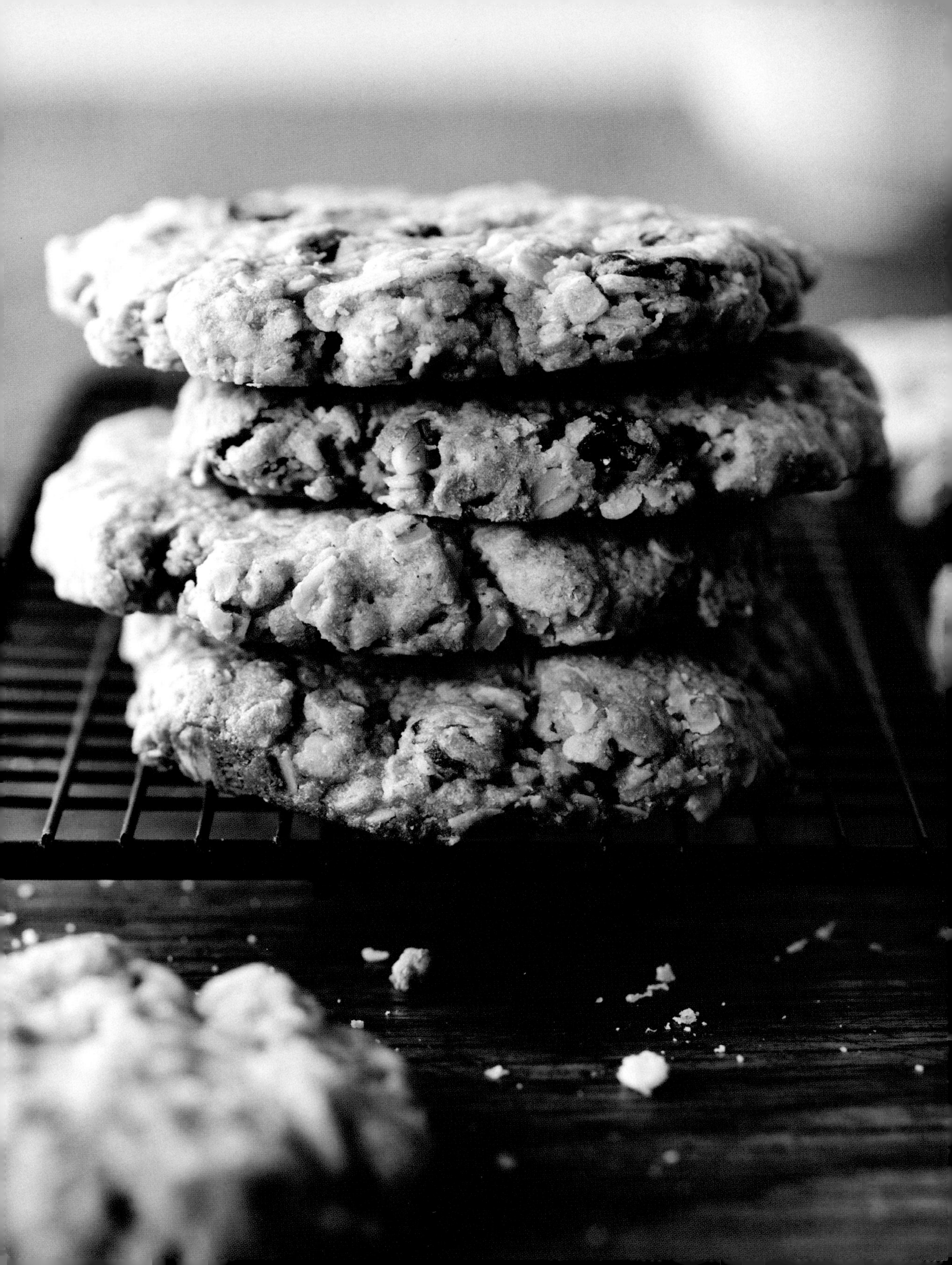

# OATMEAL PEANUT BUTTER COOKIES

Oatmeal and peanut butter – a delicious and nutritious combination. Kids and adults alike will be reaching for these.

### WHAT YOU'LL NEED»

1⅔ cups / 400 ml all-natural peanut butter

1 cup / 240 ml olive oil-based margarine or Do-It-Yourself Olive Butter (see page 310)

2 cups / 480 ml Sucanat or raw sugar

2 large omega-3 eggs

1 egg white

3 Tbsp / 45 ml honey

1 Tbsp / 15 ml best-quality vanilla

1½ tsp / 7½ ml sea salt

3 cups / 960 ml old-fashioned rolled oats

1 cups / 480 ml whole-wheat pastry flour

1 cup / 240 ml dark raisins (optional)

1 cup / 240 ml walnuts, coarsely chopped (optional)

### HOW TO MAKE IT»

1. Preheat the oven to 350°F / 177°C. Line baking sheets with parchment paper or Silpat sheets.
2. Cream the peanut butter, margarine, sugar and eggs together in a large bowl until smooth. Beat in the honey, vanilla and sea salt.
3. Use a large wooden spatula or your clean hands to work in the flour and oats until well combined. Add raisins and walnuts if desired. Mix well.
4. Shape the dough into large balls and press into flat cookies. Place them on the baking sheets and bake for 12-15 minutes.
5. Cool on wire racks.

**NUTRITIONAL VALUE FOR ONE COOKIE WITHOUT RAISINS OR WALNUTS:**

Calories: 305 | Calories from Fat: 156 | Total Fat: 17 g | Saturated Fat: 4 g | Total Carbs: 27.5 g | Fiber: 3 g | Protein: 7 g | Sodium: 136 mg | Cholesterol: 23 mg

**Preparation time:** 30 minutes
**Cooking time:** 15 minutes
**Yield:** 24 cookies

# CARROT CAKE
## WITH CRYSTALLIZED GINGER

Carrot cake is a perennial favorite for dessert or snack. The crystallized ginger makes this version a standout!

### WHAT YOU'LL NEED »

2 whole omega-3 eggs

2 omega-3 egg whites (discard yolks)

2 cups / 480 ml Sucanat or raw sugar

1/3 cup / 80 ml olive oil

2½ cups / 600 ml whole-wheat flour

1 tsp / 5 ml sea salt

1 tsp / 5 ml baking powder

2 tsp / 10 ml baking soda

2 tsp / 10 ml cinnamon

½ cup / 120 ml crystallized ginger, chopped

4 cups / 960 ml carrots, grated

Zest of one whole lemon

### YOGURT CHEESE ICING

#### WHAT YOU'LL NEED »

¼ cup / 60 ml **honey**

2 Tbsp / 20 ml **icing sugar**

1 packet of **unflavored gelatin**

1 cup / 240 ml **yogurt cheese** (see page 222)

2 Tbsp / 30 ml best-quality **vanilla**

#### HOW TO MAKE IT »

Blend together in a bowl with a hand blender until thoroughly mixed, smooth and spreadable.

**NUTRITIONAL VALUE FOR ONE SLICE OF CAKE WITH TWO-TBSP ICING:**

Calories: 237 | Calories from Fat: 60 | Total Fat: 7 g | Saturated Fat: 1 g | Total Carbs: 42 g | Fiber: 3.5 g | Protein: 6 g | Sodium: 317 mg | Cholesterol: 24 mg

### HOW TO MAKE IT »

1. Preheat oven to 350°F / 177°C.
2. Prepare pan. Cover bottom of 9-inch / 22-cm springform pan with parchment paper. Grease the sides with a light coating of olive oil and dust with flour.
3. In a large bowl beat together eggs and sugar until fluffy. Beat in oil.
4. In a separate bowl combine dry ingredients: flour, salt, baking powder, cinnamon and baking soda. Combine with egg mixture in a large bowl.
5. Stir in ginger, carrots and lemon zest. Combine until just blended.
6. Pour into prepared springform pan.
7. Bake for one hour or until golden on top and toothpick inserted into cake comes out clean.
8. Remove outer ring of springform pan. Let cake cool.
9. Spread with yogurt-cheese icing if desired.

**TIP** **This recipe makes a great lunch-pail treat, too. Bake in two smaller loaf pans and cut into slices to pack into your lunch!**

**Preparation time:** 30 minutes
**Cooking time:** 1 hour
**Yield:** 16 servings

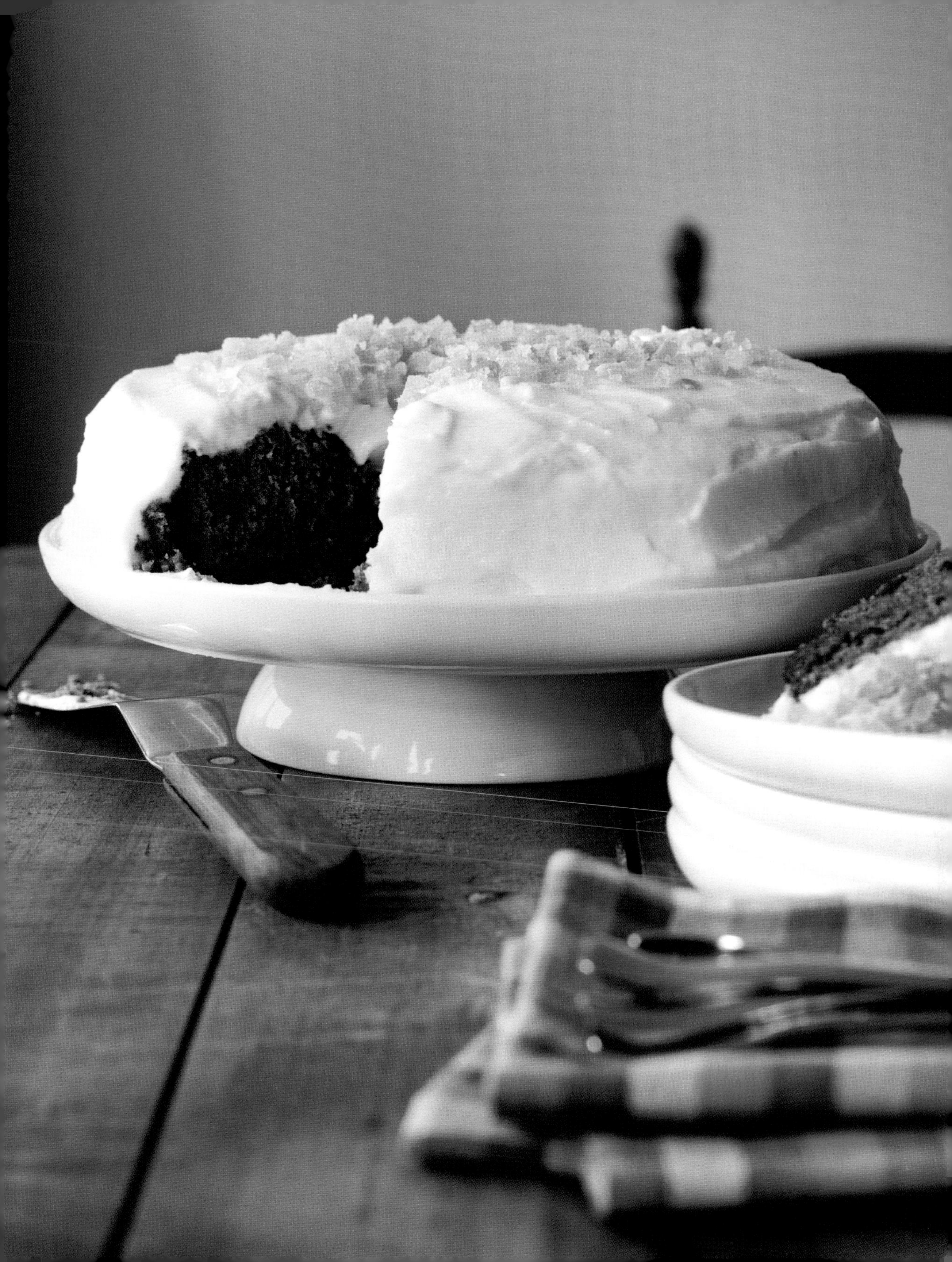

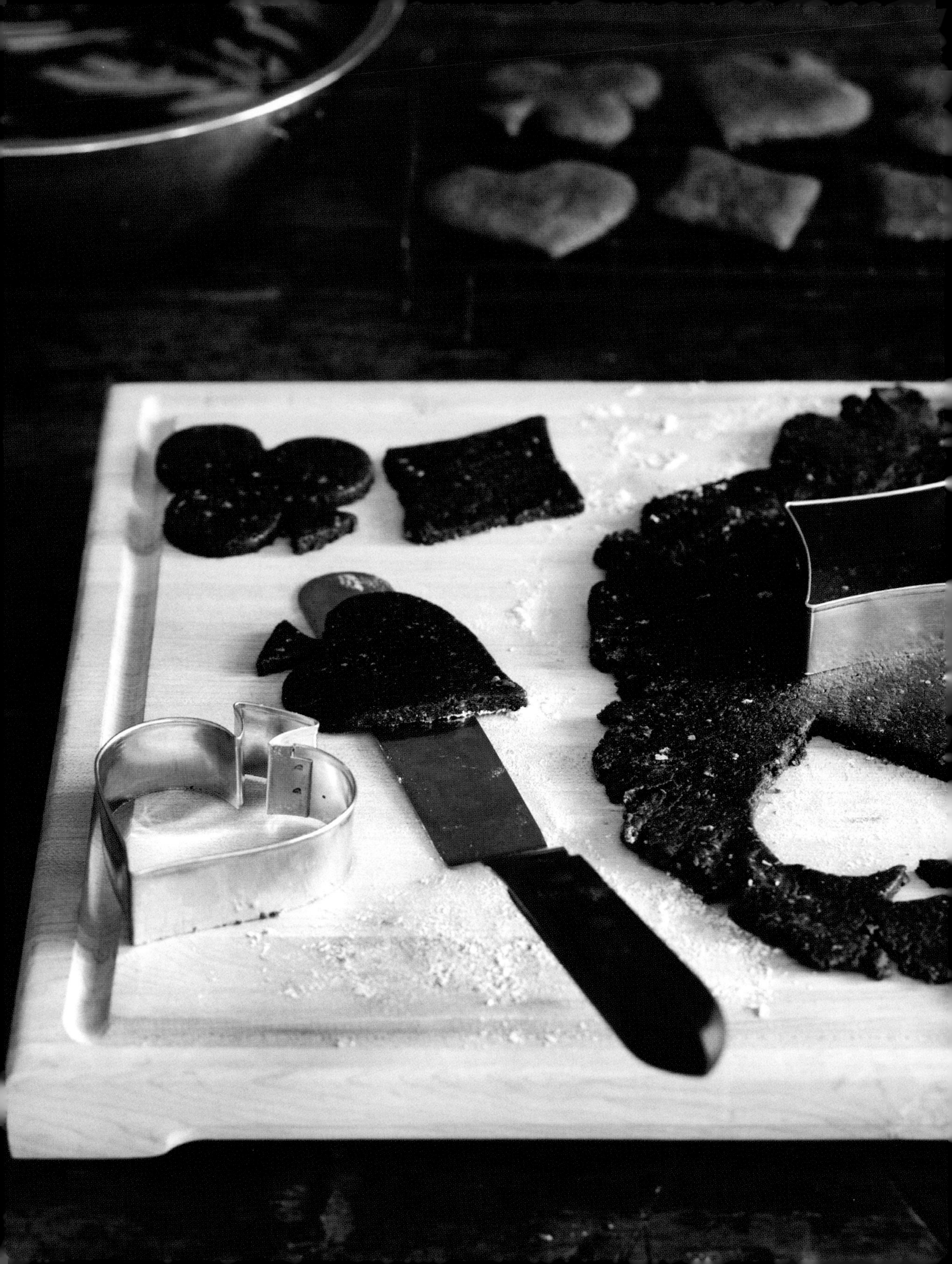

# CRUNCHY GINGERBREAD COOKIES

Even a big man will enjoy the homey flavor of a gingerbread cookie. Make a batch with your son, nephew or just for the boys. They are easy and delicious even for the least-skilled kitchen staff.

### WHAT YOU'LL NEED»

½ cup / 120 ml olive-oil based margarine or Do-It-Yourself Olive Butter (see page 310)

½ cup / 120 ml Sucanat or raw sugar

1 omega-3 egg

½ cup / 120 ml plus 2 Tbsp / 30 ml unsulfured Blackstrap molasses

3 cups / 720 ml spelt flour

1 tsp / 5 ml ginger

½ tsp / 2.5 ml each baking soda, sea salt, cloves and cinnamon

**Thanks to Cynthia Lee and Joe Caruso for this recipe, and thanks for the story on your Eat-Clean success!**

**Preparation time:** 40 minutes
**Cooking time:** 12 – 15 minutes
**Yield:** 60 medium sized cookies

**NUTRITIOINAL VALUE FOR ONE COOKIE:**
Calories: 44 | Calories from Fat: 15 | Total Fat: 1.6 g | Saturated Fat: 0.5 g | Total Carbs: 7 g | Fiber: 1 g | Protein: 1 g | Sodium: 37 mg | Cholesterol: 0 mg

### HOW TO MAKE IT»

1. Preheat oven to 325°F/ 163°C.
2. Place margarine and Sucanat in a large bowl and let sit for 15 minutes. Add egg and molasses to the bowl, and beat the mixture until it becomes somewhat fluffy and the sugar begins to dissolve.
3. In a separate mixing bowl mix flour, ginger, baking soda, salt, cloves and cinnamon.
4. Combine wet and dry ingredients. You may have to use your clean hands when the dough becomes too stiff. When dough is smooth and all ingredients are evenly combined divide into two. Wrap each half in plastic wrap and refrigerate. Refrigerate for one hour.
5. Between sheets of wax or parchment paper, roll out half of the dough to about ⅓"/ 1 cm thickness. Remove top sheet of wax or parchment paper. Use a cookie cutter to cut out shapes, re-rolling scraps.
6. Transfer cookies to a baking sheet lined with Silpat or parchment paper. Freeze the cookies for about 12 minutes.
7. Bake in 325°F / 163°C oven for 12-15 minutes or until the cookies are golden and firm to the touch.

# MOIST GINGERBREAD

We love the smells of gingerbread at any time of the year. Pungent ginger, cloves and cinnamon challenge the nostrils and tempt the tongue. Gentlemen, you can indulge your exotic spice desires with this delicious moist bread that is more like a cake. Cut it into squares and tuck it into your lunch. Better than a store-bought muffin any day.

**WHAT YOU'LL NEED»**

1 cup / 240 ml Sucanat or raw sugar

2 omega-3 eggs

1 cup / 240 ml pumpkin purée, baked squash or sweet potato

½ cup / 60 ml coconut oil

¼ cup / 60 ml of olive oil based margarine or Do-It-Yourself-Olive Butter (see page 310)

½ cup / 60 ml buttermilk or milk soured with 1 Tbsp / 15 ml lemon juice

1¾ cups / 420 ml spelt, kamut or other unrefined flour

1 tsp / 5 ml each ginger and baking soda

½ tsp / 2.5 ml each sea salt, cinnamon, nutmeg, ground cloves and allspice

¼ tsp / 1.25 ml baking powder

**Optional:** Use yogurt cheese icing to frost (see page 314)

**NUTRITIONAL VALUE FOR ONE SQUARE WITHOUT FROSTING:**

Calories: 325 | Calories from Fat: 175 | Total Fat: 20 g | Saturated Fat: 12.25 g | Total Carbs: 35 g | Fiber: 4 g | Protein: 5 g | Sodium: 267 mg | Cholesterol: 50 mg

**HOW TO MAKE IT»**

1. Preheat oven to 350°F / 177°C.
2. In a large mixing bowl beat sugar, eggs, pumpkin or alternative, oil and buttermilk. Beat until smooth.
3. In a separate mixing bowl combine flour, baking soda, spices, salt and baking powder.
4. Combine wet and dry ingredients and stir until blended. Do not overblend.
5. Pour into a prepared 9"/ 22 cm square pan. Bake in 350°F oven for 35 minutes. Remove and let cool.
6. Frost when completely cool, if desired.

**Preparation time:** 40 minutes
**Cooking time:** 35 minutes
**Yield:** 9 squares

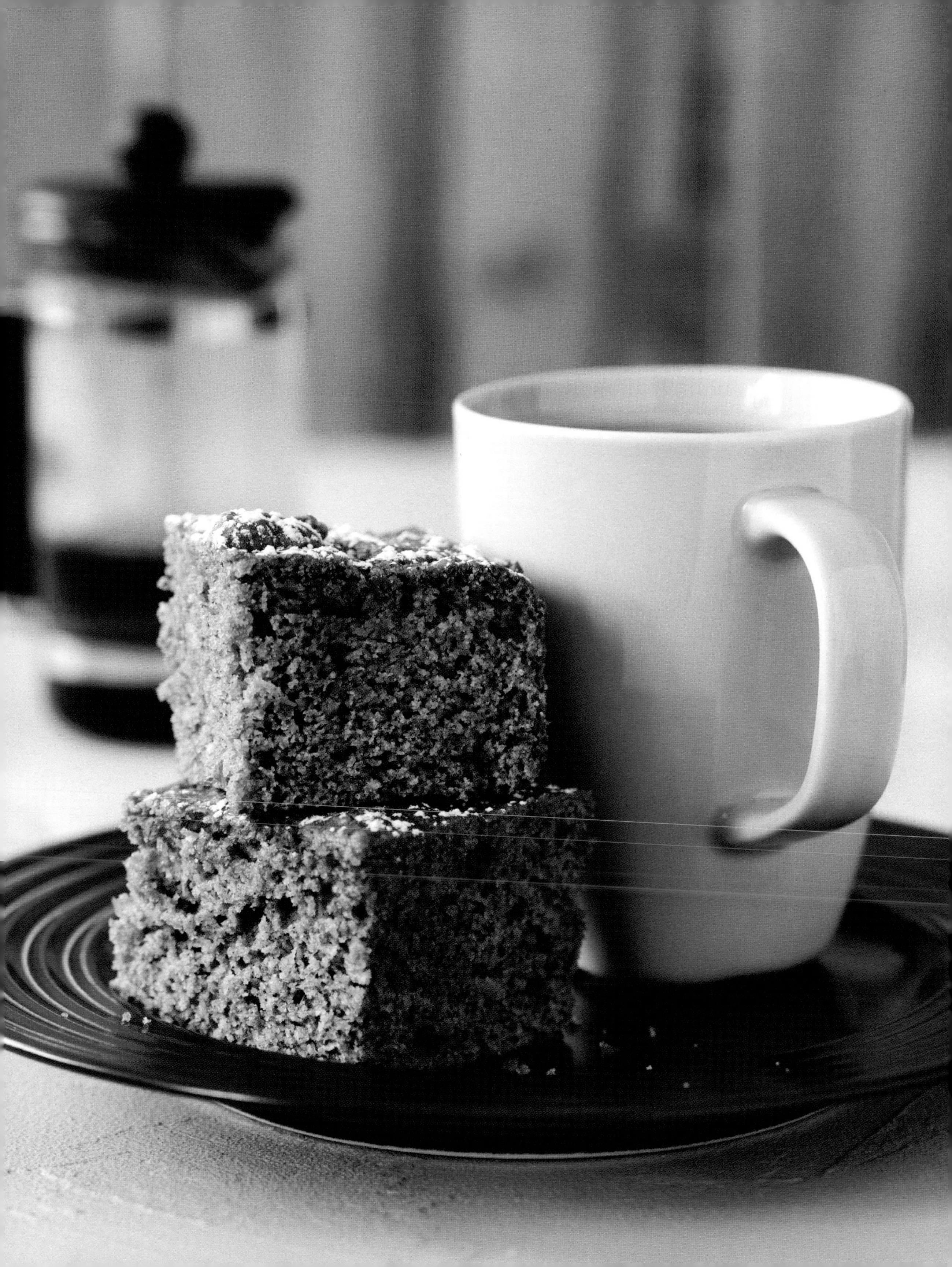

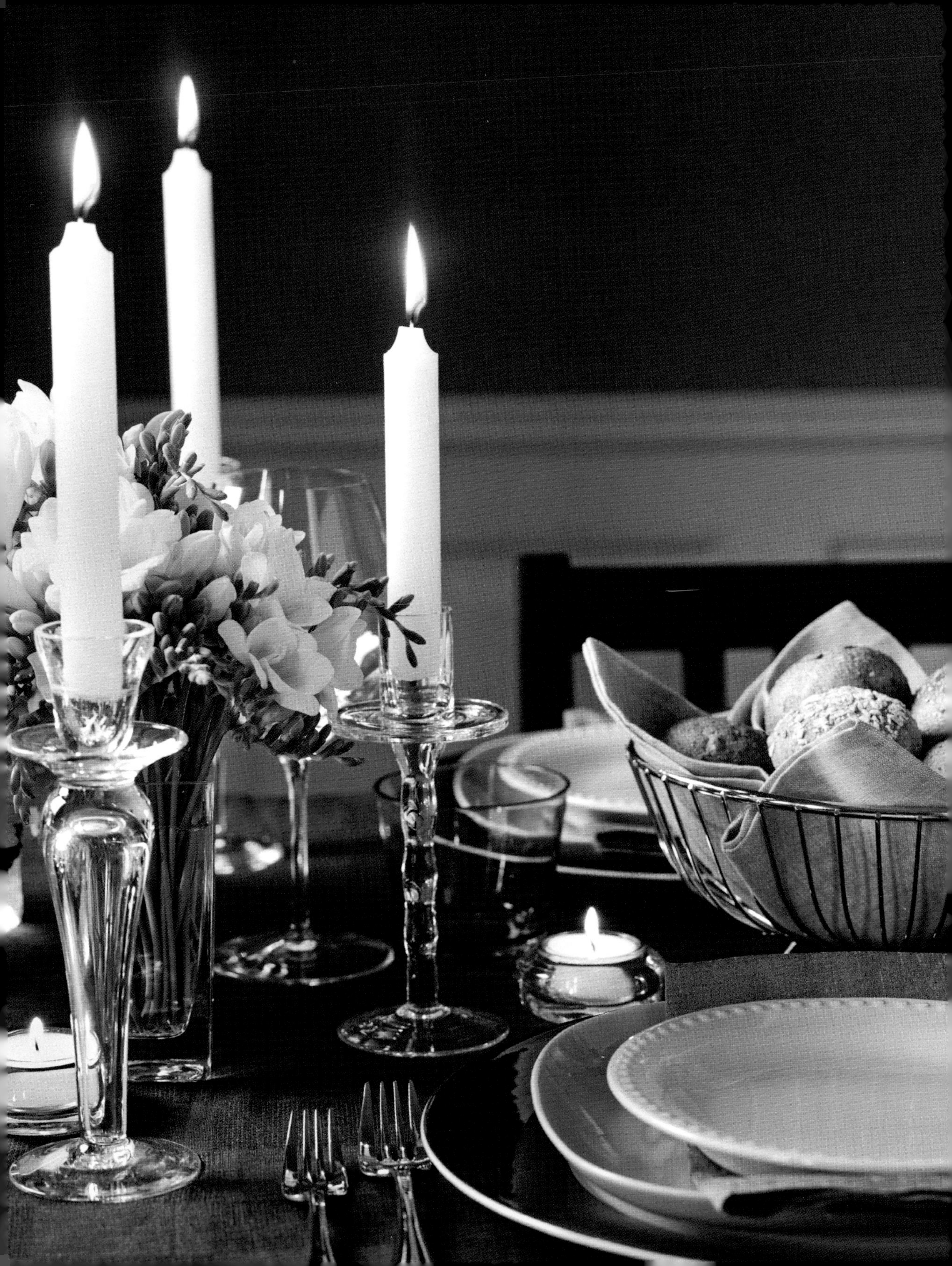

# ROMANTIC FOUR COURSE MEAL

Light the candles, get the places set just so, dim the lights and put some sensual music on the stereo. Forget the fancy restaurants – nothing will impress your special someone more than a romantic dinner à deux that's been cooked with your own loving hands. And because this is a Clean dinner, you won't feel overstuffed, bloated or lethargic when you're done. In fact, you should have plenty of energy for ... whatever comes later.

# ROMANTIC FOUR-COURSE MEAL

Hey there Mr. Romance – are you trying to win your lady's attention? Show off your culinary side by cooking your shining star a meal she'll never forget ...

# COOKING AN APHRODISIAC MEAL

If you are hoping to enhance your sexual power during this date you may want to use aphrodisiac foods – these recipes will be based on specific ingredients to increase sexual drive.

**Keep these tips in mind as you prepare your meal:**

❶ Ask your date if she has any dietary restrictions, dislikes, intolerance or allergies – cooking up some steak is all well and good until your date tells you she is a vegetarian.

❷ Have a selection of fine wines on hand – white and red. Buy your date a bouquet of roses or fresh mixed flowers and have them sitting on the table.

❸ Keep it simple and light. Four courses: salad, starter, main and dessert, should impress anyone and won't leave you flustered in the kitchen.

❹ Have a basket of fresh bread on the table – especially breads of interest like sprouted grains, naan, lavash or flatbreads. Have a small dish with olive oil and balsamic vinegar mixed together to dip the bread into.

❺ At the end of the meal, make sure to have freshly brewed coffee or tea prepared, along with a selection of dark chocolate and freshly washed strawberries.

❻ Serve the meal by candlelight. Keep the room lit dimly. Stay away from scented candles – your guest could be allergic to perfume and the scent may clash with the smells wafting from the kitchen. Invest in a variety of candle sizes – thick, thin, short and tall. Place them on the table and throughout the room.

❼ Make sure to leave yourself some time to get cleaned up – about an hour or so before your guest is to arrive. Clean up your kitchen as well. She will want to join you and admire your cooking skills.

❽ Let your date help you. Leave the salad until the end and have the vegetables handy for chopping.

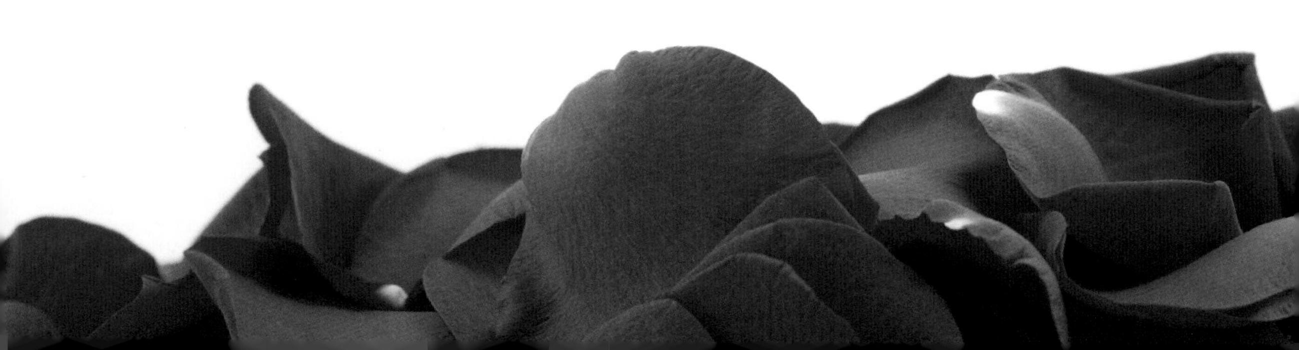

## ROMANTIC FOUR-COURSE MENU

**Salad**

*Bocconcini Salad*

❖

**Appetizer**

*Barbecued Prawns*

❖

**Main Course**

*Grilled Venison*

*with Steamed Asparagus and*

*Mashed Sweet Potatoes*

❖

**Dessert**

*White Chocolate Tofu Mousse*

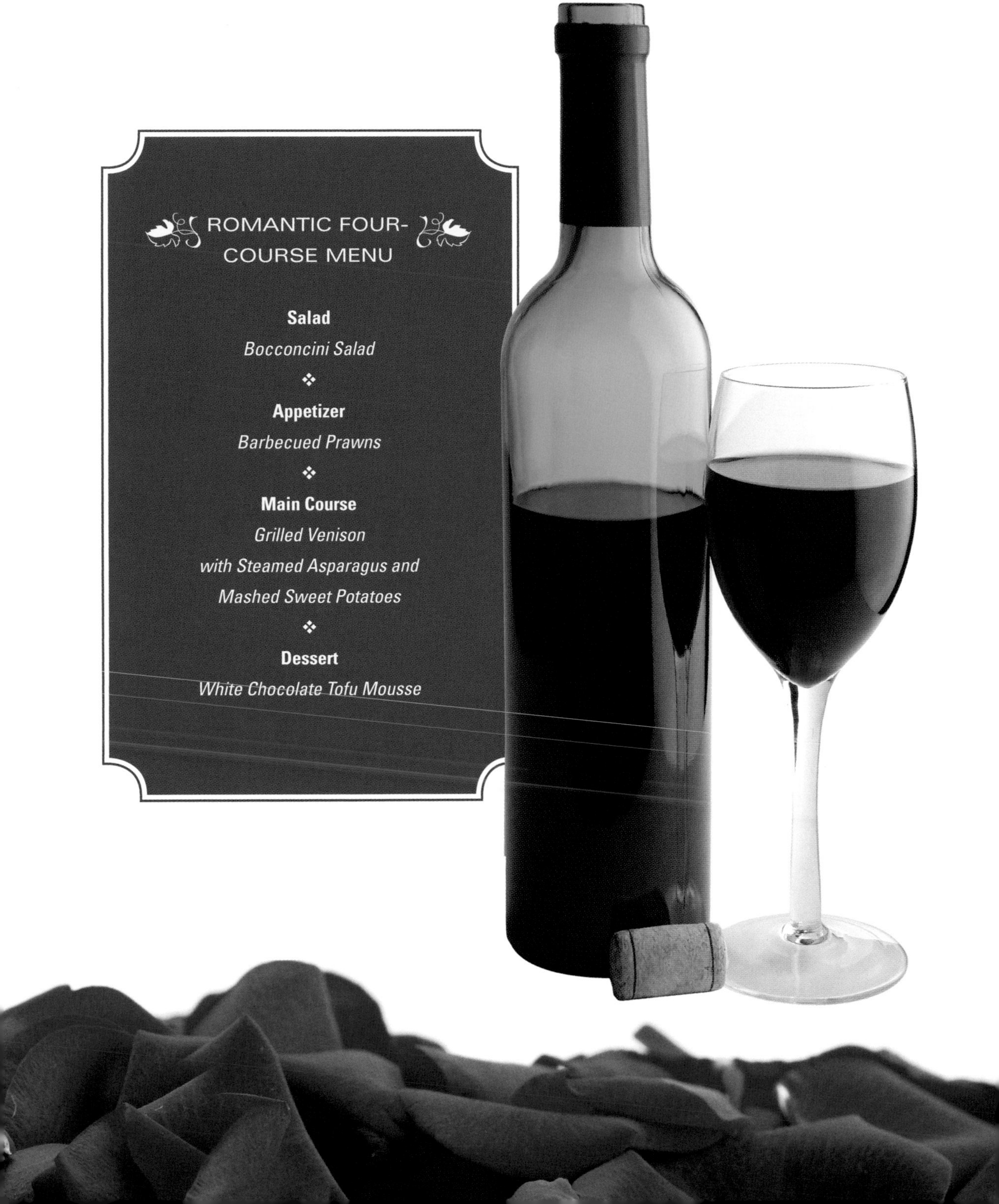

# BOCCONCINI SALAD

**WHAT YOU'LL NEED»**

2 cups / 480 ml cherry tomatoes, sliced in half

½ lb / 227 g cocktail-sized bocconcini cheese, cut into 1-inch / 2.5 cm cubes

2 garlic cloves, minced or pressed

¼ cup / 60 ml best-quality olive oil

1 Tbsp / 15 ml fresh basil, chopped

Sea salt, to taste

Freshly ground black pepper, to taste

**HOW TO MAKE IT»**

**1.** Slice the cherry tomatoes in half and place in a bowl with the bocconcini cubes, herbs, garlic, oil, salt and pepper. Mix gently to distribute the oil and flavors.

**2.** Divide between the two bowls and serve.

**NUTRITIONAL VALUE FOR ONE SERVING:**
Calories: 400 | Calories from Fat: 340 | Total Fat: 38 g | Saturated Fat: 10 g | Total Carbs: 7 g | Fiber: 2 g | Protein: 21.5 | Sodium: 284 mg | Cholesterol: 40 mg

**Preparation time:** 15 minutes
**Cooking time:** 0 minutes
**Yield:** 2 servings

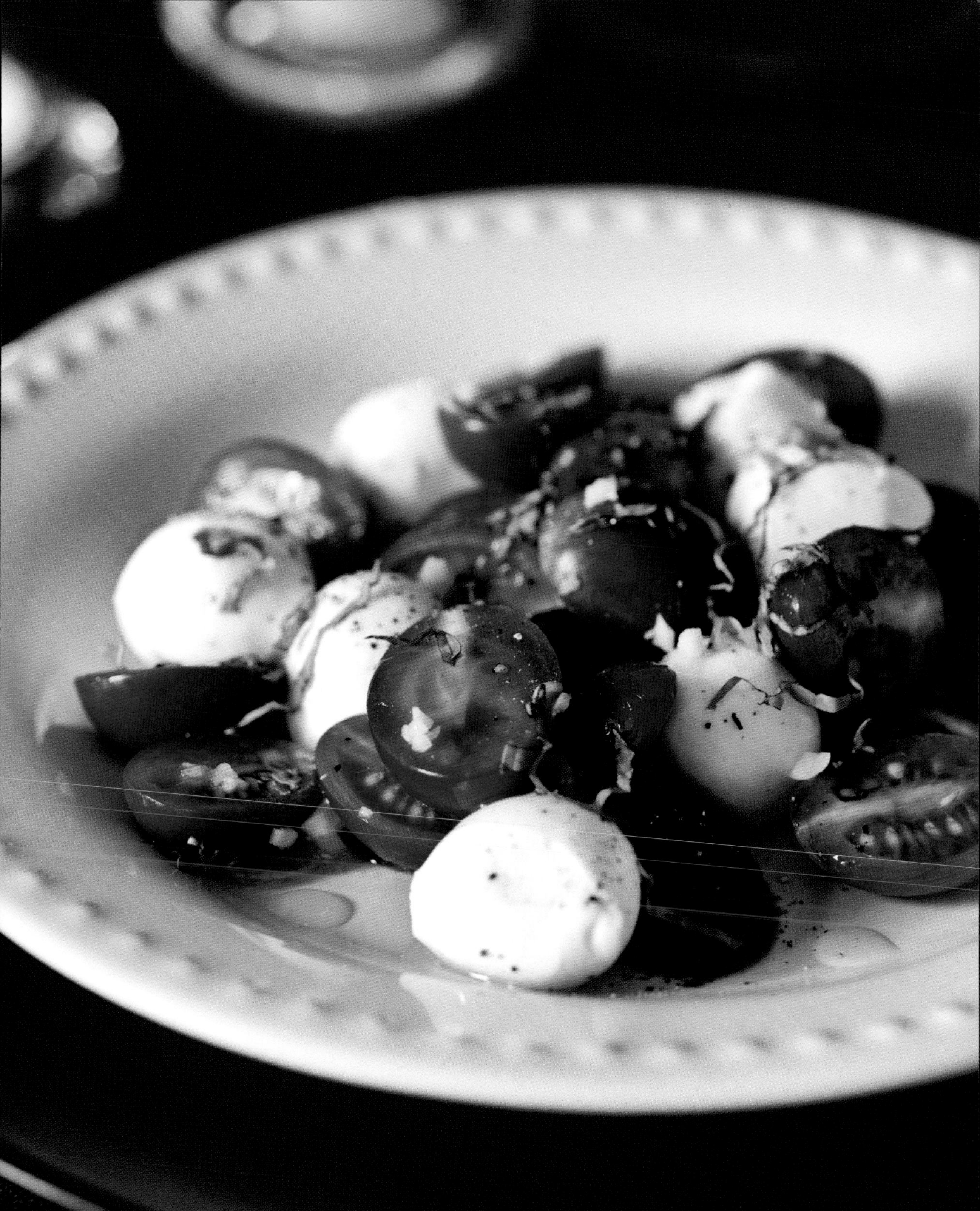

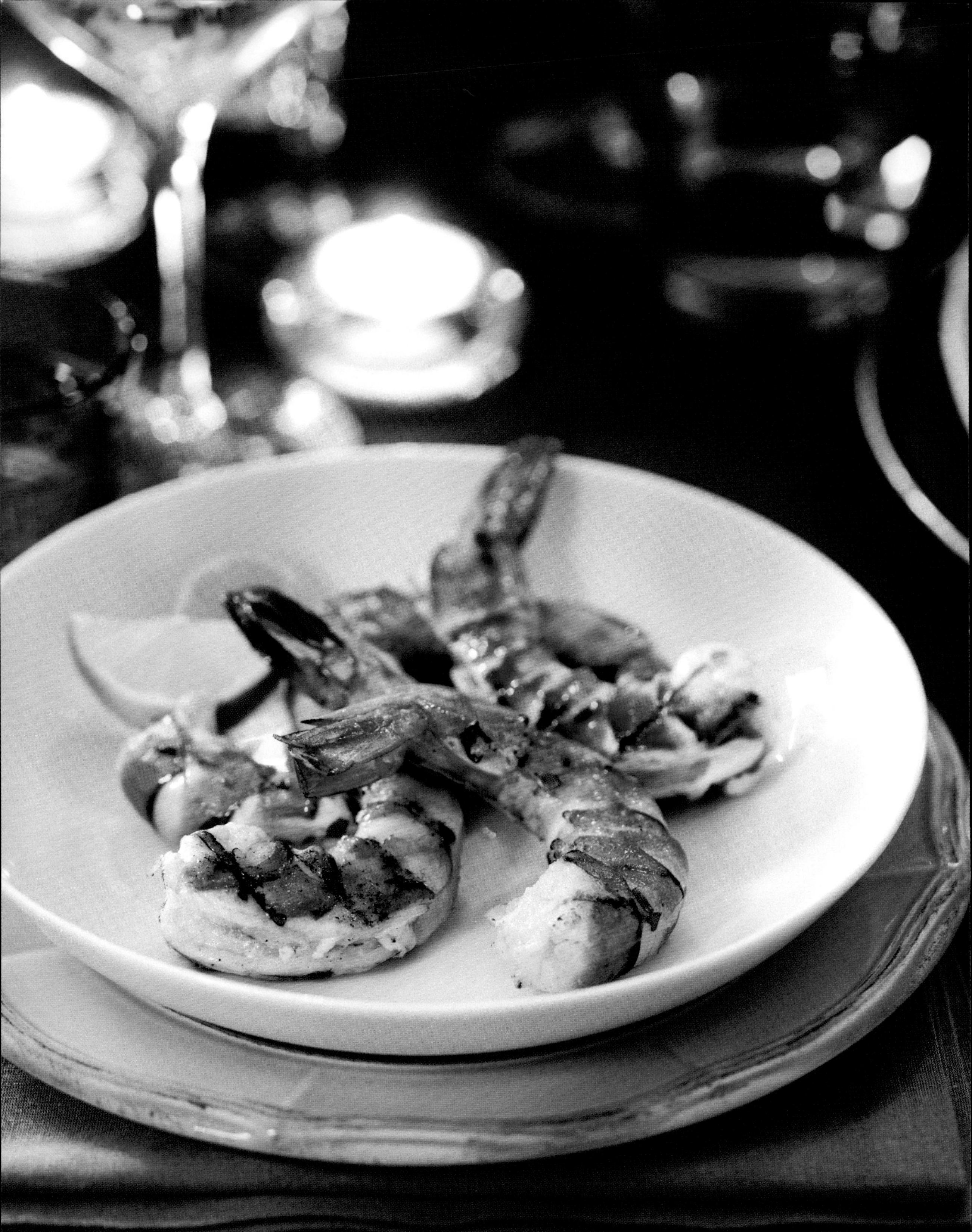

# BARBECUED PRAWNS

Keep this evening refreshing and exciting – wake up those taste buds and stimulate the atmosphere and conversation.

### WHAT YOU'LL NEED »

10 jumbo shrimp or prawns

1 cup / 240 ml lemon juice (preferably fresh)

¼ cup / 60 ml best-quality olive oil

2 Tbsp / 30 ml chopped fresh basil

2 tsp / 10 ml peeled and grated ginger

### HOW TO MAKE IT »

**1.** Mix oil, lemon juice, ginger and basil in a medium-sized glass bowl. Add prawns and toss to coat. Marinate in the fridge for one to two hours. I like to place a plate on top of the bowl to keep flavors in the bowl and not in the fridge.

**2.** Preheat the barbecue on medium heat and cook the prawns for 3 to 4 minutes on each side, brushing frequently with leftover marinade. Cook until opaque and done all the way through. You will have nice grill marks on your prawns when the cooking is finished.

**3.** Divide equally on a plate for you and your date.

**NUTRITIONAL INFORMATION FOR FIVE PRAWNS:**
Calories: 183 | Calories from Fat: 78 | Total Fat: 8.6 g | Saturated Fat: 1.3 g | Total Carbs: 1.5 g | Fiber: 0 g | Protein: 23 g | Sodium: 168 mg | Cholesterol: 172 mg

**Preparation time:** 5 minutes
**Cooking time:** 6–8 minutes
**Marination time:** 1–2 hours
**Yield:** 2 servings

# GRILLED VENISON
## WITH STEAMED ASPARAGUS AND MASHED SWEET POTATOES

Venison is rich tasting, satisfying and impressive, along with being nutritious and low in fat. Add fresh asparagus for that special touch. See recipes for asparagus and mashed sweet potatoes on following page.

### WHAT YOU'LL NEED »

2 x 8-ounce / 227 g venison steaks
¼ cup / 60 ml best-quality olive oil
1 pinch allspice
1 pinch ginger
½ tsp / 2½ ml garlic powder

### HOW TO MAKE IT »

**1.** Bring steaks to room temperature. Brush lightly with oil and dust with seasonings.
**2.** Follow tips for grilling steak at right.

**NUTRITIONAL VALUE FOR ONE VENISON STEAK:**
Calories: 240 | Calories from Fat: 133 | Total Fat: 14 g | Saturated Fat: 5 g | Total Carbs: 0.5 g | Fiber: 0.5 g | Protein: 25 g | Sodium: 85 mg | Cholesterol: 91 mg

### PROPER GRILLING FORM

- Trim excess fat from meat – the less fat the fewer flare-ups and the easier the clean-up.
- Keep the lid tightly closed on your grill. Keeping the lid closed allows the heat to circulate for even cooking and fewer flare-ups.
- A few key tools: a thermometer and timer will help you keep track of internal temperatures and cooking time. Long-handled tools will help prevent burns. Tongs are best for turning and forks are excellent for lifting.

**Preparation time:** 5 minutes
**Cooking time:** See chart below
**Yield:** 2 servings

### COOKING TIME FOR VENISON »

| THICKNESS | RARE | MEDIUM | WELL | HEAT |
|---|---|---|---|---|
| 1" | 8-10 min | 12-14 min | 16-20 min | High |
| 1½" | 10-14 min | 16-20 min | 22-26 min | High |
| 2 | 12-16 min | 18-22 min | 24-28 min | Medium |

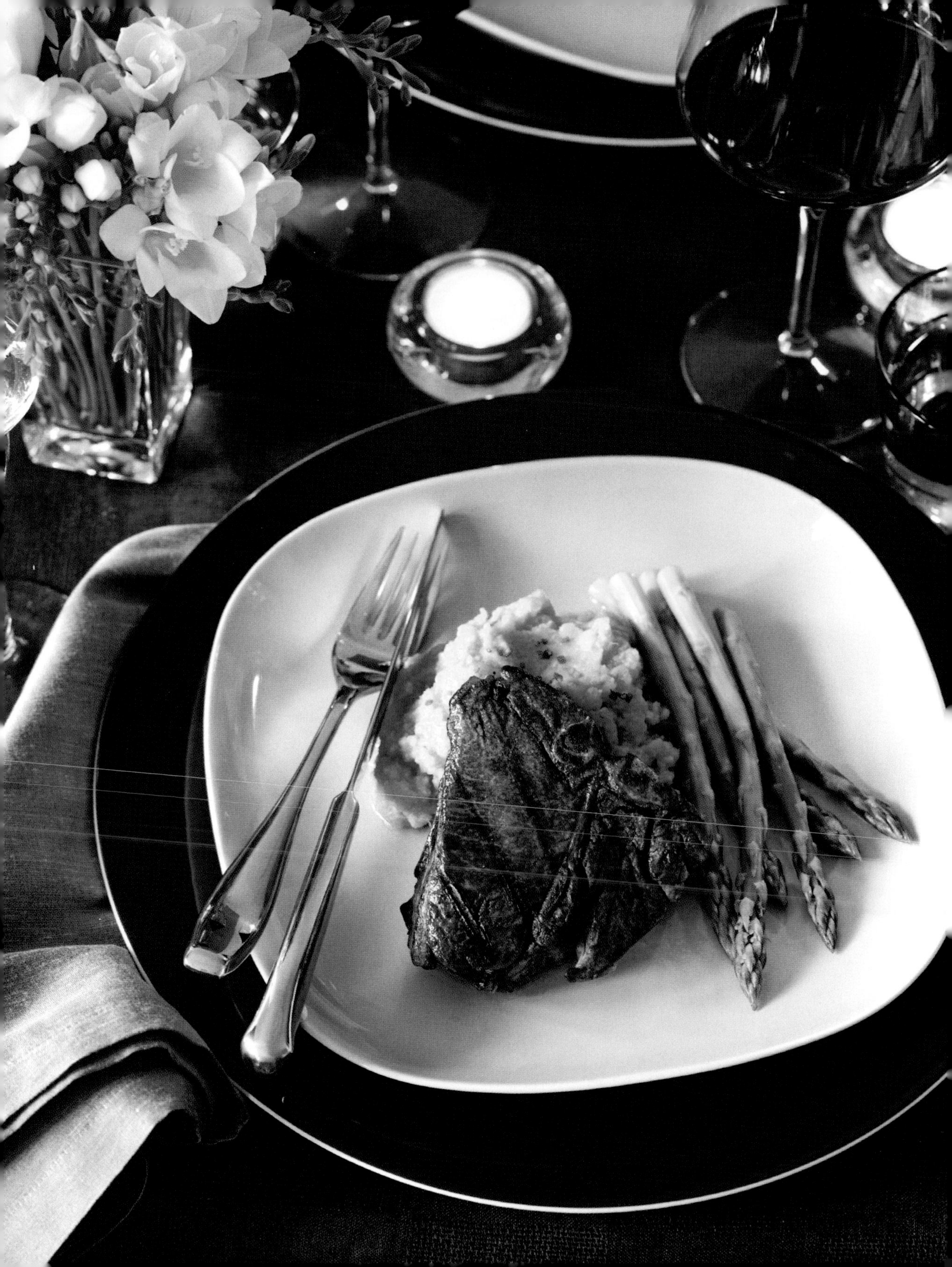

# STEAMED ASPARAGUS

**WHAT YOU'LL NEED»**

14 stalks asparagus

Boiling water

Fresh lemon juice

Sea salt

**HOW TO MAKE IT»**

**1.** Snap asparagus at the end. Discard tough, chewy end.

**2.** Place tips in a steamer basket over a pot of boiling water.

**3.** When the asparagus changes color to bright green, remove from the heat.

**4.** Serve with a splash of fresh lemon juice and a sprinkle of sea salt.

**TIP** If you like steamed asparagus, you'll love broiled asparagus. Turn the broiler in your oven to low, lay the washed asparagus on a broiling pan, brush with a light coating of olive oil and sprinkle with sea salt and freshly ground pepper. Place on an upper rack. Cook for a minute or two and then turn over and cook for a couple of minutes more.

**NUTRITIONAL VALUE FOR SEVEN STALKS OF STEAMED ASPARAGUS:**

Calories: 22 | Calories from Fat: 0 | Total Fat: 0 g | Saturated Fat: 0 g | Total Carbs: 4.4 g | Fiber: 2.4 g | Protein: 2.5 g | Sodium: 0 mg | Cholesterol: 0 mg

**Preparation time:** 2 minutes
**Cooking time:** 3–5
**Yield:** 2 servings

# MASHED SWEET POTATOES

### WHAT YOU'LL NEED »

¾ lb / 340 g sweet potatoes, scrubbed, peeled and cut into chunks
½ medium parsnip, peeled and cut into chunks
¼ tsp and 1 pinch / 3 ml sea salt
2 Tbsp / 30 ml low-sodium chicken stock or water
1½ Tbsp / 7½ ml pumpkinseed oil
Pinch / 0.3 ml ground nutmeg
Pinch / 0.3 ml ground cinnamon
White pepper, to taste

### HOW TO MAKE IT »

**1.** Place sweet potatoes and parsnip in a medium saucepan and cover with water. Add a pinch of salt and bring to a boil over high heat. Reduce heat and continue to cook for 15 to 20 minutes or until vegetables are tender. Remove from heat.

**2.** Drain, reserving cooking liquid.

**3.** Add chicken stock or water, pumpkinseed oil, sea salt, nutmeg, cinnamon and white pepper.

**4.** Mash potatoes and parsnips with a potato masher until smooth. Add a little reserved cooking liquid if the potato mixture is too stiff.

**5.** Transfer mashed vegetables to a casserole dish that has been coated lightly with Eat-Clean Cooking Spray (see page 262). Cover and keep warm in a low-temperature oven. Serve hot!

**NUTRITIONAL VALUE FOR HALF-CUP SERVING:**
Calories: 116 | Calories from Fat: 33 | Total Fat: 3.5 g | Saturated Fat: 0.5 g | Carbohydrates: 20 g | Fiber: 3.5 g | Protein: 1.5 g | Sodium: 244 mg | Cholesterol: 3.5 g

**Preparation time:** 10 minutes
**Cooking time:** 30 minutes
**Yield:** 2 servings

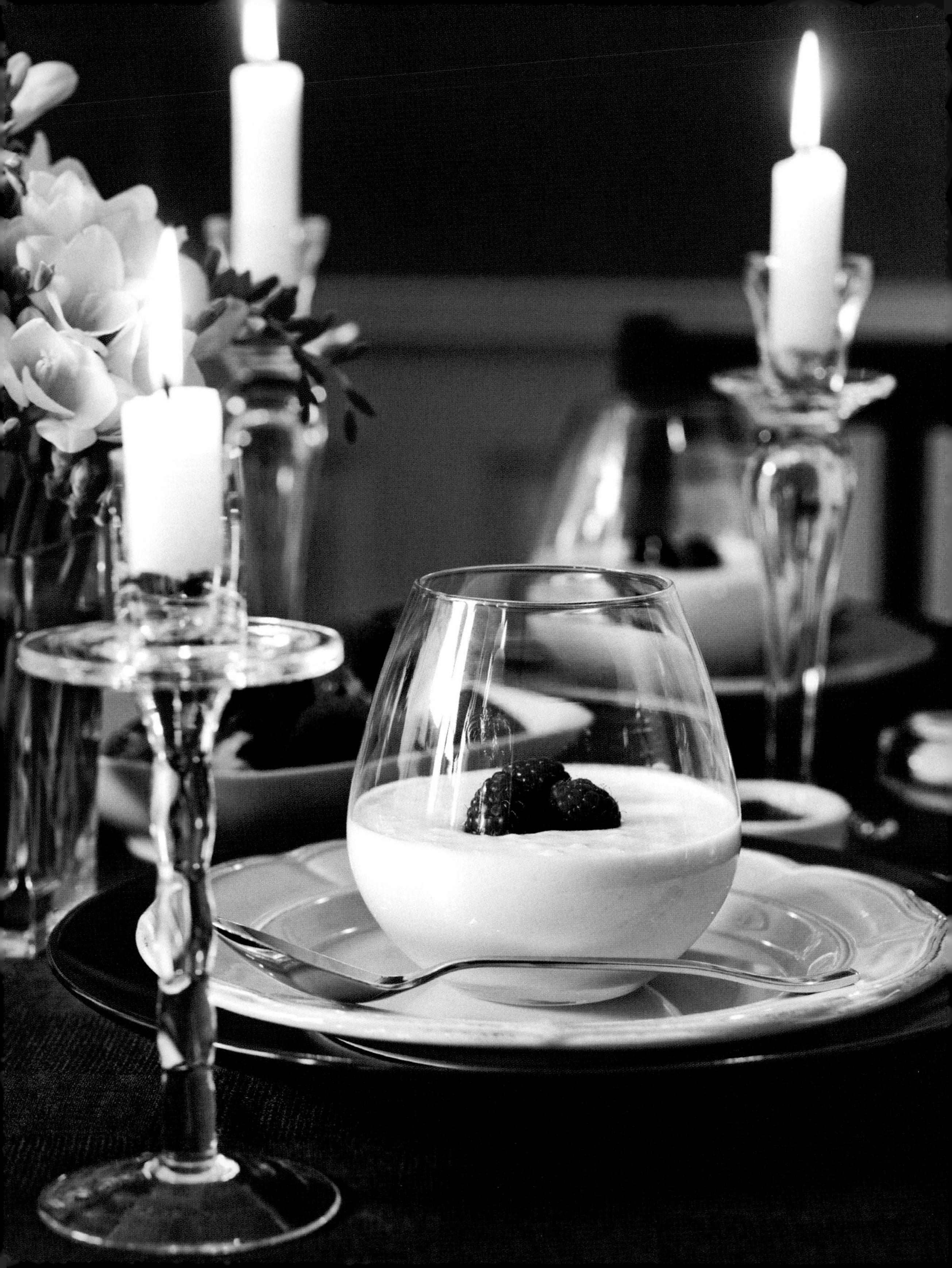

# WHITE-CHOCOLATE TOFU MOUSSE

Chocolate mousse is a woman's best friend. When you make it white chocolate with the added romantic touch of ripe red raspberries, she'll melt.

### WHAT YOU'LL NEED»

¾ cup / 180 ml white chocolate chips

12 oz / 360 ml unflavored silken tofu at room temperature, drained

½ cup / 120 ml warmed milk of choice (skim, almond, rice ...)

1 tsp / 5 ml best-quality vanilla

### HOW TO MAKE IT»

**1.** Melt white chocolate chips in a double boiler or in the microwave. Make sure to let the chocolate melt slowly. Stir until the chocolate is uniformly smooth.

**2.** In a food processor, combine the tofu, melted chocolate, warmed milk, and vanilla. Process until smooth.

**3.** Place the mixture into a fine-mesh strainer or sieve, pushing through with the back of a wooden spoon, into a medium decorative serving bowl.

**4.** Serve from the bowl or ladle into individual serving bowls.

**5.** Chill. Top with a few raspberries before serving.

**NUTRITIONAL VALUE FOR ONE SERVING:**

Calories: 286 | Calories from Fat: 125 | Total Fat: 14 g | Saturated Fat: 7 g | Total Carbs: 32 g | Fiber: 0 g | Protein: 8 g | Sodium: 58 mg | Cholesterol: 0.5 mg

**Preparation time:** 5 minutes
**Cooking time:** 5 minutes
**Yield:** 4 servings

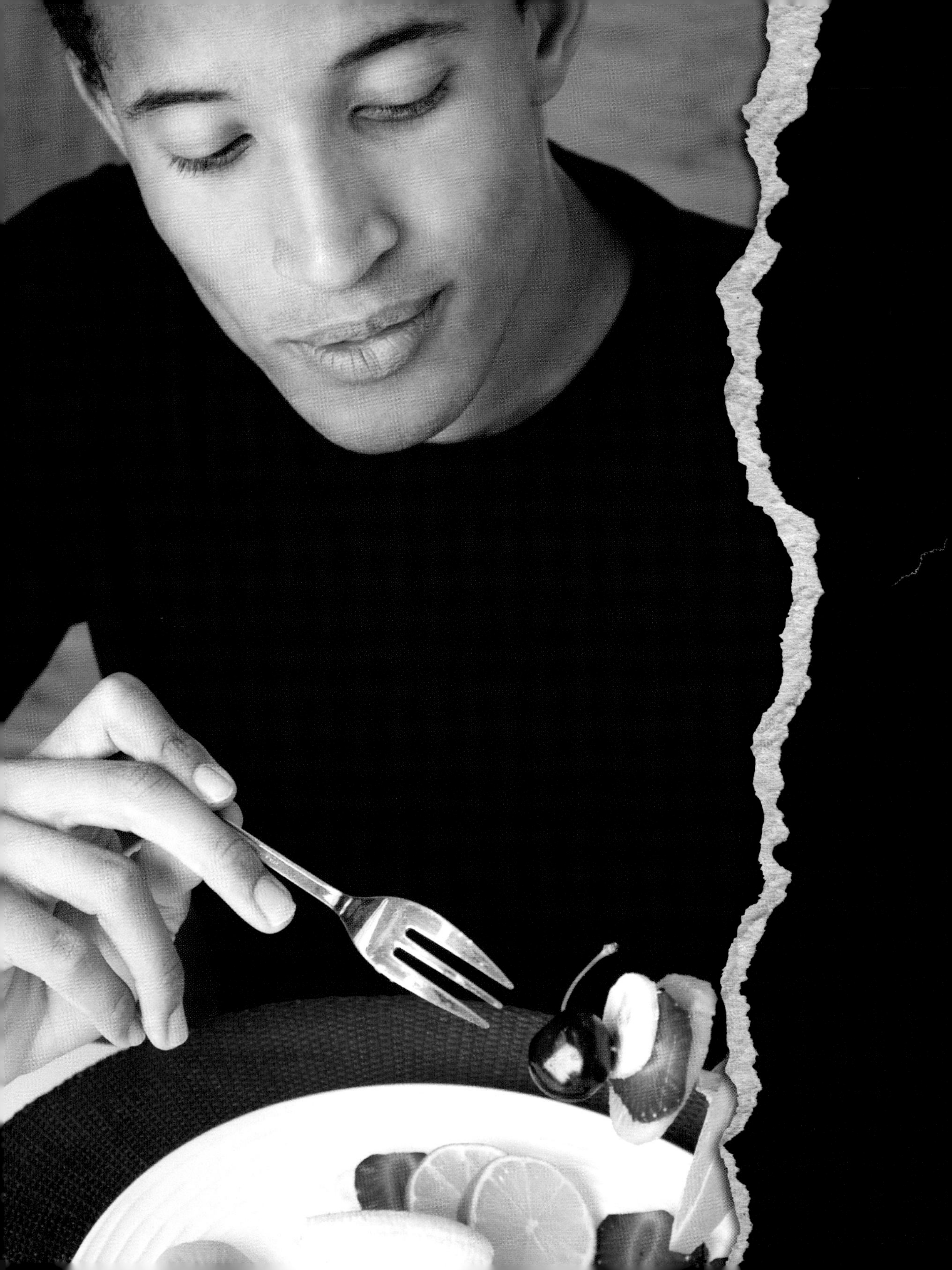

# [CHAPTER FOURTEEN]

## TWO-WEEK MENU AND SHOPPING LISTS

# MEAL PLAN: WEEK ONE

| | MORNING START | MIDMORNING BOOSTER | LUNCHTIME REFUEL |
|---|---|---|---|
| DAY 1 | Whole-grain Ezekiel toast spread with almond butter and sliced apples and sprinkled with flaxseed; water and black coffee. | Fat-free, sugar-free plain yogurt with mixed berries; water. | **Third-Base Turkey-Ball Sub**; sliced carrots and cucumbers; water. |
| DAY 2 | **NYC Bagel Breakfast**; sliced cantaloupe; black coffee and water. | Clean protein bar; orange; water. | **Pumpkin Soup**; grilled chicken; water. |
| DAY 3 | Oatmeal with sliced peaches, wheat germ, bee pollen, flaxseed; hard-boiled egg whites; water and black coffee. | Handful of walnuts with banana; water. | **She Grilled Me Salmon Sandwich**; water. |
| DAY 4 | Whole-wheat English muffin topped with nut butter, sprinkled with flaxseed and topped with sliced banana; water and black coffee. | **Banana Roll-Up**; water. | Leftover **Pasta Legerro** with grilled chicken; water. |
| DAY 5 | Cream of Wheat with flaxseed, wheat germ, bee pollen; scrambled egg whites; black coffee and water. | Nectarine with a handful of almonds. | **Bring Home the Bacon … Lettuce and Tomato**; kiwi; water. |
| DAY 6 | **Weekend Egg Sandwich**; green grapes; black coffee and water. | Celery stalks spread with nut butter and topped with raisins; water. | Whole-wheat pita stuffed with leftover bison tenderloin, mixed greens and balsamic vinaigrette; water. |
| DAY 7 | Whole-grain cereal with skim milk, flaxseed, wheat germ and bee pollen; sliced banana; hard-boiled egg whites; water and black coffee. | Sliced carrots, cucumbers, and tomatoes with hummus; water. | **Boys Don't Turn to Mush-Room Soup**; whole-grain toast; water. |

Here are some Eat-Clean menus and grocery lists to show you how you might choose to eat throughout the week. *They are simply suggested guidelines.* Just make sure to follow the Eat-Clean Principles and you'll be fine. Adjust portion sizes accordingly (refer to page 66).



| MIDAFTERNOON MUNCH | DINNER DELIGHT | BEFORE BED IF HUNGRY |
|---|---|---|
| **Banana Roll-Up**; water | Grilled chicken with roasted beets, cauliflower and parsnips and brown rice; water. | Scrambled egg whites with sliced tomato; water. |
| Sliced apple with nut butter; water. | **Y'argh Pirate Planked Salmon** served with brown rice and a variety of sliced heirloom tomatoes; water. | Fat-free, sugar-free plain yogurt with sliced strawberries; water. |
| Sliced, hard-boiled egg whites on whole-grain toast topped with salsa; water. | **Pasta Legerro** served with grilled chicken; water. | Smoothie made with rice milk, mixed berries and protein powder. |
| Trail mix with a combination of dried fruit and nuts; water. | **Black Beans and Rice** with scrambled egg whites; water. | Sliced apple with nut butter; water. |
| Smoothie made with protein powder, banana, strawberries and rice milk; water. | Bison tenderloin served with quinoa and green beans; water. | Scrambled egg whites with sliced oranges; water. |
| Nectarine with handful of cashews; water. | **Chicken Wings**; baked potato; sliced carrots and celery sticks; water. | Popcorn with a handful of almonds; water. |
| Whole-grain bread spread with nut butter and topped with sliced strawberries; water. | **Lazy Sunday Venison Stew** served over brown rice; water. | Fat-free cottage cheese with blueberries; water. |

# MEAL PLAN: WEEK TWO

| | MORNING START | MIDMORNING BOOSTER | LUNCHTIME REFUEL |
|---|---|---|---|
| DAY 1 | Fat-free yogurt with blueberries, flaxseed, bee pollen, wheat germ and a scoop of protein powder; Ezekiel toast; water and black coffee | Trail mix; water. | **Mr. Big's Fresh Fig and Pork Loin Sandwich**; sliced apple; water. |
| DAY 2 | Egg-white omelet made with tomatoes, spinach, onions and red pepper; hot oatmeal topped with flaxseed, wheat germ and bee pollen; black coffee and water. | Sliced cantaloupe with cottage cheese; water. | **Mega-Muscles Minestrone Soup**; toasted whole-wheat English muffin; water. |
| DAY 3 | **Power Breakfast**; black coffee and water. | Clean protein bar; handful of grapes; water. | Leftover roasted turkey on a whole-wheat wrap spread with hummus and topped with alfalfa sprouts, tomatoes and flaxseed; water. |
| DAY 4 | **Home Fries**; scrambled egg whites; ½ grapefruit; black coffee and water. | Yogurt with sunflower seeds and blueberries; water. | Sliced tofu atop mixed greens paired with chickpeas, black beans and corn and a squeeze of lemon juice; water. |
| DAY 5 | Whole-wheat toast topped with cashew butter and sprinkled with flaxseed; scrambled egg whites; chopped mango; black coffee and water. | **Tropical Smoothie**; water. | Canned tuna mixed with yogurt cheese spread on toasted whole-grain bread with lettuce and tomato; water. |
| DAY 6 | Whole-grain wrap spread with yogurt cheese and topped with chopped tomato, red bell peppers, alfalfa sprouts and sliced tofu; water and black coffee. | Fat-free cottage cheese with sliced strawberries; water. | **Big Fello Portobello Open-Faced Sandwich**; water. |
| DAY 7 | **Southern Sweet Potato Pancakes**; scrambled egg whites; sliced strawberries; black coffee and water. | Raw cauliflower, broccoli and tomatoes with hummus; water. | **Wrap You Up in Curried Chicken Love**; sliced cucumbers; water. |

Here are some Eat-Clean menus and grocery lists to show you how you might choose to eat throughout the week. *They are simply suggested guidelines*. Just make sure to follow the Eat-Clean Principles and you'll be fine. Adjust portion sizes accordingly (refer to page 66).



| MIDAFTERNOON MUNCH | DINNER DELIGHT | BEFORE BED IF HUNGRY |
|---|---|---|
| Cup unsweetened applesauce with handful of cashews; water. | **Bison and Broccoli**; rice noodles; water. | Oatmeal with flaxseed, protein powder and berries; water. |
| Hummus with green and red bell pepper slices; water. | Roasted turkey breast served with steamed asparagus and whole-wheat couscous; water. | Scrambled egg whites served with sliced tomato; water. |
| Scrambled egg whites with sliced green peppers, mushrooms, and tomatoes; water. | **Good Ol' Burgers** served with corn on the cob; water. | Leftover **Power Breakfast**; water. |
| Brown rice cake spread with nut butter and sprinkled with flaxseed; water. | Whole-grain pasta noodles with turkey meatballs and tomato sauce; green salad topped with balsamic vinegar and olive oil; water. | Smoothie made with fruit, fat-free milk and protein powder; water. |
| 1 clean protein bar with 1 peach; water. | **Italian Wedding Soup**; water. | Fat-free cottage cheese; 1 handful of raspberries; water. |
| 1 handful of almonds with 1 pear; water. | **Bhoona** served with brown rice; water. | Popcorn with 1 handful of walnuts; water. |
| Handful of raspberries with yogurt and sunflower seeds; water. | **Senegalese Mafé**; water. | Oatmeal with protein powder and applesauce; water. |

# GROCERY LIST FOR WEEK ONE

## PRODUCE

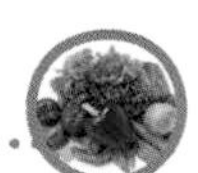

### Vegetables

- ❍ Bell pepper, red
- ❍ Carrots
- ❍ Cauliflower
- ❍ Celery
- ❍ Cucumbers
- ❍ Garlic
- ❍ Green beans
- ❍ Leeks
- ❍ Mixed greens
- ❍ Mushrooms, white button
- ❍ Onions:
  - Red
  - Purple
- ❍ Parsnips
- ❍ Pumpkin
- ❍ Romaine lettuce
- ❍ Sweet potatoes
- ❍ Tomatoes:
  - Cherry
  - Field
  - Heirloom
  - Plum
- ❍ Vidalia onions
- ❍ Yukon potatoes

### Fresh Herbs and Flavor Enhancers

- ❍ Fresh cilantro
- ❍ Fresh mint
- ❍ Fresh parsley
- ❍ Fresh oregano
- ❍ Ginger
- ❍ Jalapeno peppers
- ❍ Thai chili peppers

### Fruits

- ❍ Apples
- ❍ Avocados
- ❍ Bananas
- ❍ Blackberries
- ❍ Blueberries
- ❍ Cantaloupe
- ❍ Green grapes
- ❍ Kiwis
- ❍ Lemons
- ❍ Limes
- ❍ Nectarines
- ❍ Oranges
- ❍ Peaches
- ❍ Raspberries
- ❍ Strawberries

## BAKERY

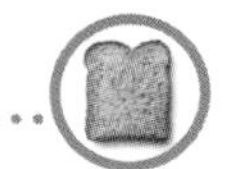

- ❍ Ezekiel bread
- ❍ Sprouted-grain submarine buns
- ❍ Sprouted-grain kamut bagels
- ❍ Whole-grain bagels
- ❍ Whole-grain bread
- ❍ Whole-grain pita
- ❍ Whole-grain wrap
- ❍ Whole-wheat English muffins

## MEAT, POULTRY & SEAFOOD

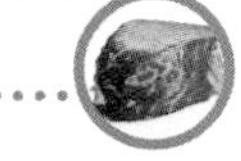

- ❍ Boneless, skinless chicken breast
- ❍ Chicken wings
- ❍ Lean, ground turkey breast
- ❍ Salmon filet
- ❍ Smoked salmon
- ❍ Turkey bacon
- ❍ Venison steaks

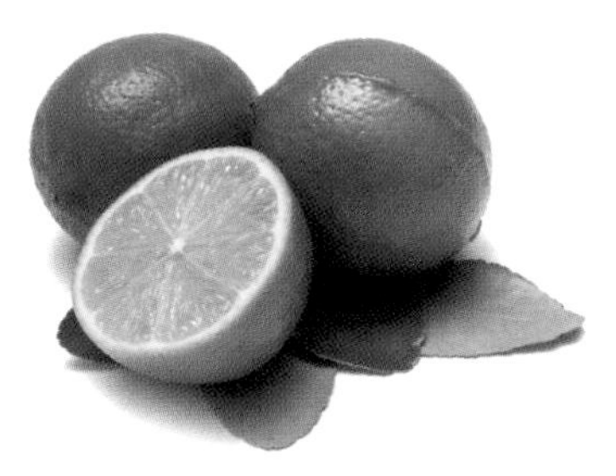

## DAIRY

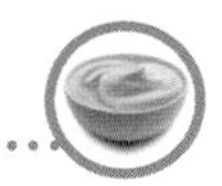

❍ Eggs
❍ Fat-free cottage cheese
❍ Plain fat-free yogurt
❍ Almond milk
❍ Rice milk
❍ Skim milk

## NUTS, SEEDS, OIL & SNACKS

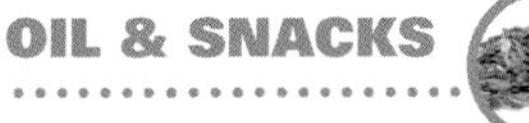

❍ Almonds
❍ Cashews
❍ Walnuts
❍ Olive oil
❍ Flaxseed
❍ Popcorn
❍ Protein bars
❍ Trail mix

## DRY GOODS, CEREALS

❍ Brown rice
❍ Brown-rice spaghetti noodles
❍ Cream of Wheat
❍ Oatmeal
❍ Protein powder
❍ Quinoa
❍ Raisins
❍ Spelt/kamut flour
❍ Wheat germ
❍ Whole-grain cereal

## DRIED HERBS & SPICES

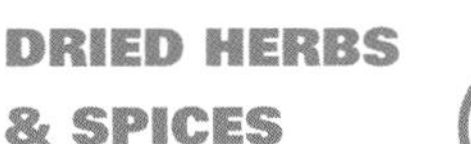

❍ Rosemary
❍ Paprika
❍ Basil
❍ Bay leaves
❍ Black pepper
❍ Chilis
❍ Chives
❍ Coriander
❍ Cumin
❍ Curry powder
❍ Garlic powder
❍ Mustard powder
❍ Parsley
❍ Red pepper flakes
❍ Sea salt
❍ Thyme
❍ Turmeric

## CANNED GOODS

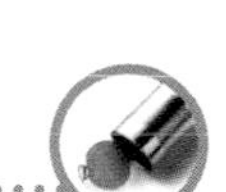

❍ Black beans
❍ Canned tomatoes
❍ Capers
❍ Corn
❍ Chickpeas
❍ Low-sodium chicken broth
❍ Low-sodium beef broth
❍ Low-sodium vegetable stock

## OTHER

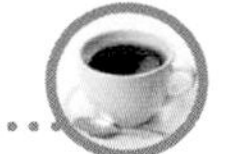

❍ Almond butter
❍ Balsamic vinaigrette
❍ Bee pollen
❍ Coffee
❍ Green tea
❍ Hot sauce
❍ Salsa

# GROCERY LIST FOR WEEK TWO

## PRODUCE

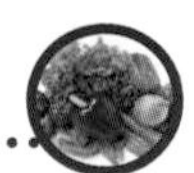

### *Vegetables*

- ❍ Alfalfa sprouts
- ❍ Asparagus
- ❍ Bell peppers, red and green
- ❍ Broccoli
- ❍ Cabbage
- ❍ Carrots
- ❍ Cauliflower
- ❍ Corn on the cob
- ❍ Cucumbers
- ❍ Garlic
- ❍ Leeks
- ❍ Mixed greens
- ❍ Mushrooms:
  - Button
  - Portobello
- ❍ Onions
- ❍ Potatoes
- ❍ Romaine lettuce
- ❍ Spinach
- ❍ Squash
- ❍ Sweet potatoes
- ❍ Tomatoes
- ❍ Zucchini

### *Fresh Herbs*

- ❍ Fresh basil

### *Fruits*

- ❍ Apples
- ❍ Bananas
- ❍ Blackberries
- ❍ Blueberries
- ❍ Cantaloupe
- ❍ Figs
- ❍ Grapefruit
- ❍ Grapes
- ❍ Lemons
- ❍ Mangos
- ❍ Oranges
- ❍ Peaches
- ❍ Pears
- ❍ Pineapple
- ❍ Raspberries
- ❍ Strawberries

### *Other Items From Produce Department*

- ❍ Tofu

## BAKERY

- ❍ Ezekiel bread
- ❍ Ezekiel buns
- ❍ Ezekiel wraps
- ❍ Rye baguette
- ❍ Sprouted-grain rye bread
- ❍ Whole-wheat English muffins
- ❍ Whole-wheat bread
- ❍ Whole-wheat wraps

## MEAT, POULTRY & SEAFOOD

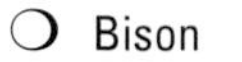

- ❍ Bison
- ❍ Bison sausages
- ❍ Boneless, skinless chicken breasts
- ❍ Lean, ground beef
- ❍ Lean, ground turkey
- ❍ Pork tenderloin
- ❍ Turkey breast

## DAIRY

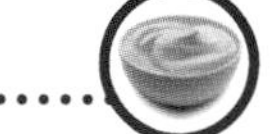

- ❍ Almond cheese
- ❍ Eggs
- ❍ Fat-free cottage cheese
- ❍ Plain, non-fat yogurt
- ❍ Skim milk
- ❍ Soy milk
- ❍ Parmesan cheese

## NUTS, SEEDS, OIL & SNACKS

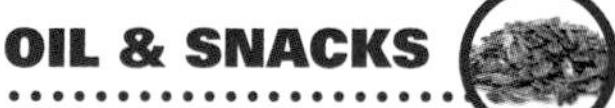

- ❍ Almonds
- ❍ Almond butter
- ❍ Cashews
- ❍ Cashew butter
- ❍ Peanut butter, natural
- ❍ Pecans
- ❍ Pumpkin seeds
- ❍ Sunflower seeds

- ❍ Walnuts
- ❍ Extra-virgin olive oil
- ❍ Peanut oil
- ❍ Flaxseed
- ❍ Brown rice cakes
- ❍ Popcorn
- ❍ Protein bars
- ❍ Trail mix

## CEREALS & DRY GOODS

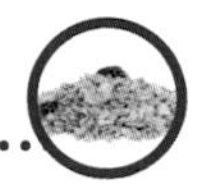

- ❍ High-protein cereal flakes
- ❍ Oat bran
- ❍ Whole-wheat flour
- ❍ Baking powder
- ❍ Brown rice
- ❍ Oatmeal
- ❍ Jasmine rice
- ❍ Rice noodles
- ❍ Shredded coconut
- ❍ Wheat germ
- ❍ Whole-wheat couscous
- ❍ Whole-wheat macaroni
- ❍ Whole-grain pasta

## DRIED HERBS & SPICES

- ❍ Basil
- ❍ Bay leaves
- ❍ Black and red peppercorns
- ❍ Cinnamon
- ❍ Coriander powder
- ❍ Curry powder
- ❍ Garam masala
- ❍ Hot chili pepper
- ❍ Mustard seeds
- ❍ Nutmeg
- ❍ Oregano
- ❍ Sea salt
- ❍ Thyme
- ❍ Turmeric

## CANNED GOODS

- ❍ Black beans
- ❍ Chickpeas
- ❍ Coconut milk, unsweetened
- ❍ Corn
- ❍ Italian tomatoes
- ❍ Low-sodium beef broth
- ❍ Low-sodium chicken broth
- ❍ Tomato paste
- ❍ Tomato sauce
- ❍ Tuna

## OTHER

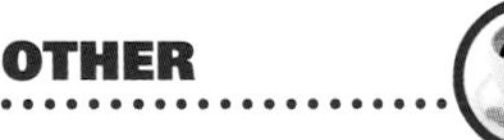

- ❍ Agave nectar
- ❍ Apple cider
- ❍ Applesauce
- ❍ Balsamic vinegar
- ❍ Bee pollen
- ❍ Coffee
- ❍ Hemp protein powder
- ❍ Lemon juice
- ❍ Protein powder
- ❍ Rice vinegar
- ❍ Salba
- ❍ Sundried tomatoes
- ❍ Vanilla extract
- ❍ White grape juice, frozen, concentrated

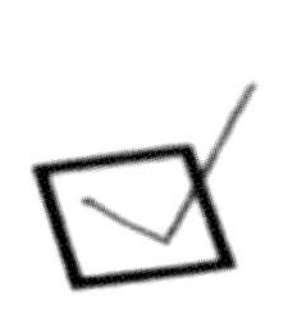

# [INDEX]

# [CREDITS]


## BACK COVER PHOTO CREDIT

**Paul Buceta (Hair & Makeup by Michelle Rosen)**

## INTERIOR PHOTO CREDITS

**Bigstockphoto.com:** Page 26 (caveman / modern man illustration), 48, 172.

**Cory Soreson:** Page 72 (model: Diego Sebastian), 151 (model: Diego Sebastian)

**Eric Jacobson:** Page 140.

**Jason Breeze:** Page 53 and 167 (model: Obi Kendol).

**Jean Héguy:** Page 132 (model: Zac Titus).

**PaulBuceta.com:** Page 2 (model: Tim Taylor), 6 (model: Tim Taylor), 11 (Robert Kennedy and Tosca Reno), 77 (model: Nathane Jackson), 55 (Tosca Reno after photo), 88 (model: Tim Taylor), 126 (Robert Kennedy and Tosca Reno).

**Ralph DeHaan:** Page 51 (model: Dexter Jackson).

**Robert Reiff:** Page 17 (model: Jeff Gum), 19 (model: Jeff Gum), 118 (model: Dan Gavin), 123 (model: Dan Gavin), 163 (model: Jesse Goddarz), 164 (model: Andrew Sinclair), 168 (model: Jeff Gum), 186 (model: Jeff Gum).

**Ted Hammond:** Page 160-162 (illustrations)

**Zeller & Butler:** Page 51 (model: Arnold Schwarzenegger).

All photos in the recipe section (Chapter 13) by **Donna Griffith.**
**(Food styling - Marianne Wren)**

**All other photos from istockphoto.com**

## PROP-STYLING CREDITS

**Gabriella Caruso Marques & Jessica Pensabene**

## ASSISTANT WRITING:

**Rachel Corradetti,** B.Sc. Honours Kinesiology

# [ACKNOWLEDGMENTS]

No book is written in solitude. We stand shoulder to shoulder with many who have inspired the creation of this latest addition to *The Eat-Clean Diet* series. Most important among these are the men who have demanded their own version of Eating Clean to satisfy their specific needs. Thanks to you we have learned plenty about what makes you tick and why this way of eating is of such significance in your own journey toward health. Women will naturally seek out answers to health and diet questions – it would seem the word "diet" is exclusively in the department of women. Not so! No man need pursue a "diet" in the "I can't eat that, I am on a diet," sense of the word. A man needs to eat and eat well. Thousands of you have contributed to the writing of this book. We are grateful for your patient counsel.

Dr. Lars Thompson, we want to thank you for your advice and guidance throughout the writing of this book and other work. We are grateful for your friendship and admire your achievements.

To the Eat-Clean Supreme Team, we are eternally grateful for your collective efforts. From pen and ink to blank pages and on to carefully selected images a book is born and delivered from your hands. Gabby Caruso, Wendy Morley, Vinita Persaud, Antonia McGuire, Rachel Corradetti and Jessica Pensabene you are our dream team! We also welcome the newest members of the book team, Brian Ross and Ellie Jeon, and Kim Dunlop, from *Oxygen*, who graciously lent us her time. We will go on to create many more books, I am sure.

Gabby, by the time this book is born your little one will also be born. We are excited to see you become a mother. We have no doubt you will be a caring new mom. You cannot fail to be. You have such a generous spirit. Congratulations Little Baby Caruso.

Trudy, thank you for your typing skills. Glad you are a pro at it! We know without you no one would be able to decipher Bob's words. And thank you for making sure the office runs smoothly.

Rachel, thank you for working hard to develop the menus and eating plans. It was no doubt difficult to carve out the time to do it since you are so busy with studies to become a Naturopathic Doctor. Nonetheless we are grateful for your help. You are the light in our eyes and heart.

We are continually amazed at how much our family supports us. Hugs and kisses to our children – Rachel, Kiersten, Braden, Chelsea and Kelsey-Lynn. You are our inspiration to do better every day! We love you all deeply and we are now a happy, crazy family on our own journey.

Thank you to all of those who read our books and columns and visit our websites. We honestly feel we have the biggest, happiest and healthiest extended family. What fun it is every day to wake up to correspondence from you. We read about your ups and downs, your celebrations and your faltering, and we know we still have our job to do – that is to be of service to all of you. Our desire to do this for you remains high. Please continue to write and contact us. Remember, we are always listening.

# OTHER TITLES IN THE EAT-CLEAN DIET SERIES BY TOSCA RENO

## The Eat-Clean Diet

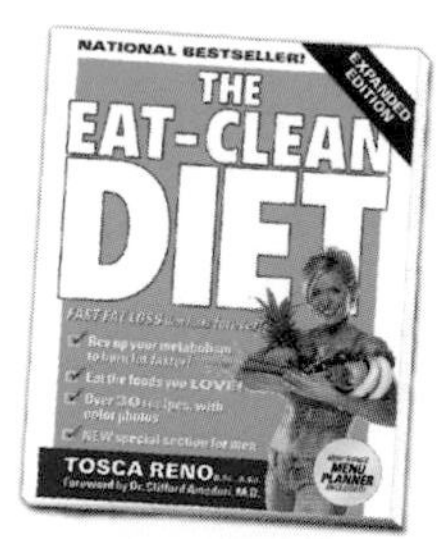


The first in *The Eat-Clean Diet* series, this book not only covers the basic principles of Clean Eating, it also includes two weeks of menu plans and over 30 recipes. Author Tosca Reno focuses on making Clean Eating work every day by packing a cooler and cooking planned leftovers. She gives you lots of tips for dealing with potential problems such as feeding your kids and eating out, to help you apply Clean Eating to your day-to-day life. You'll also learn how to use superfoods and supplements to fire up your metabolism. Let *The Eat-Clean Diet* transform you. You'll become a thinner, healthier version of yourself, with glowing skin, beautiful hair, strong nails and energy to spare. A best seller!

## The Eat-Clean Diet Cookbook

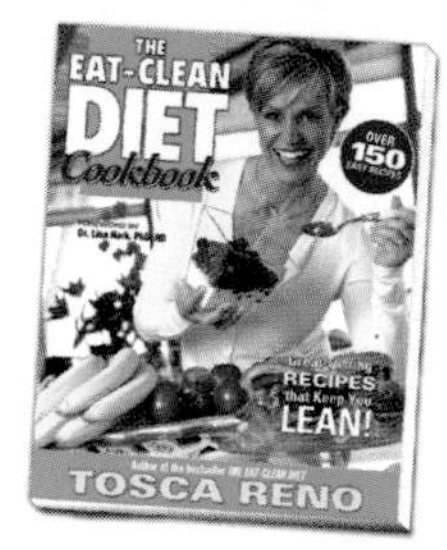


After the resounding success of *The Eat-Clean Diet*, the cookbook was a perfect follow-up. With over 150 recipes and gorgeous color photos filling the pages, this cookbook is bound to be your go-to guide for every Clean meal. From soups and sauces to main courses and desserts, Tosca touches on every food group and combines them into delicious meals – easy to prepare and definite crowd pleasers. Bonus info pages fill you in on the Eat-Clean Principles, protein facts, sugar substitutes and more. Grab your apron and heat up the oven because delicious, healthy food is on the menu tonight! A best seller!

## The Eat-Clean Diet Workout

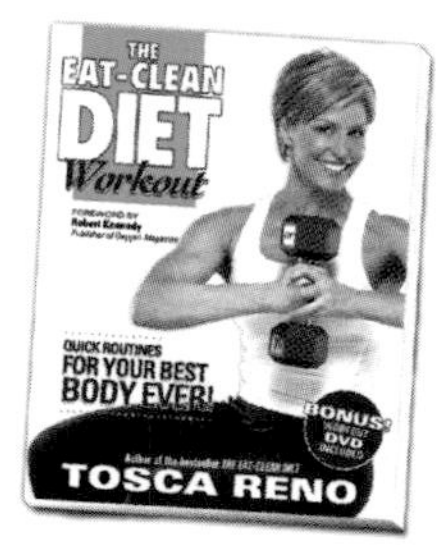


Eating Clean is a big part of the puzzle, but exercise is the missing piece. *The Eat-Clean Diet Workout* gives you the latest information on everything fitness related. As a seasoned competitor and fitness columnist, Tosca knows what she's talking about and she shares it all with you. There are chapters dedicated to each bodypart, as well as tried-and-true equipment, training plans and nutrition. Tosca even shares with you a sampling of her workout routines and secret tips from the best in the business. Whether you're a pro or a beginner, there is something for you in *The Eat-Clean Diet Workout*. Bonus 30-minute DVD!

## The Eat-Clean Diet Workout Journal

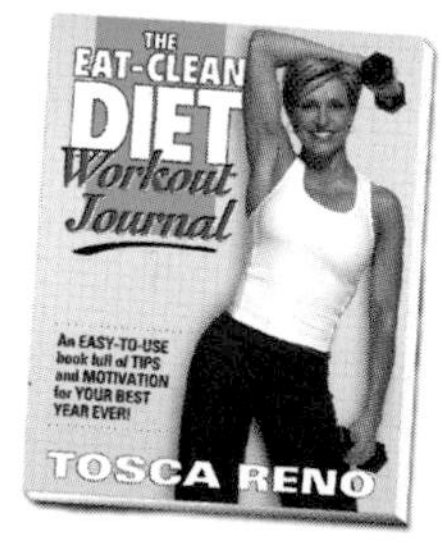


*The Eat-Clean Diet Workout Journal* is the perfect companion to your workout routine. This easy-to-use book is filled with daily journal pages, providing space for reps, sets, weights and exercises as well as cardio notes. Pair these pages with motivational tips, inspirational quotes, great photos and goal-setting sheets, and you're guaranteed to be in your best shape ever! Journaling increases success by as much as 50 percent.

## The Eat-Clean Diet for Family and Kids

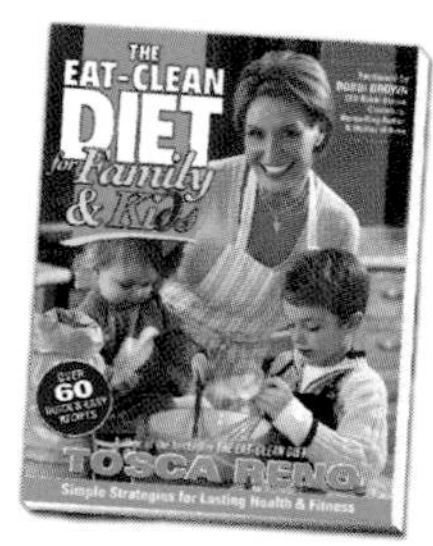


For the first time, children are not expected to live as long as their parents. How did we, as a society, end up this way? And more importantly, how can we bring about true health for our loved ones? Tosca Reno has changed the face of health, diet and fitness with her Clean-Eating revolution, and now she's delivering that message to the family. In her foreword, cosmetics icon, CEO and mother-of-three Bobbi Brown says, "Tosca Reno's newest book could not have come at a better time ... Healthy eating needs to start at home and it is our obligation as parents to set the right example for our kids." With tons of tips, tricks and advice in addition to 60 kid-friendly recipes, this book is sure to become your biggest resource.

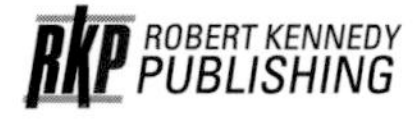